D0947538

Basic ICD-10-CM/PCS Coding Exercises

Fourth Edition

Lou Ann Schraffenberger, MBA, RHIA, CCS, CCS-P, FAHIMA

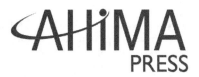

AHIMA
PRESS

This book includes the 2012 draft ICD-10-CM and ICD-10-PCS codes sets that are available online from the National Center for Health Statistics and the Centers for Medicare and Medicaid Services at http://www.cdc.gov/nchs/icd/icd10cm.htm and http://www.cms.gov/Medicare/Coding/ICD10/index.html.

The print version of the 2012 draft ICD-10-CM and ICD-10-PCS, published by Ingenix and OPTUMInsight™, was also used to code the exercises.

Copyright ©2012 by American Health Information Management Association. All rights reserved. No part of this publication may be reproduced, stored in a retrieval system, or transmitted, in any form or by any means, electronic, photocopying, recording, or otherwise, without the prior written permission of the publisher.

ISBN 978-1-58426-248-0

AHIMA Product No. AC210512

Jessica Block, MA, Assistant Editor
Claire Blondeau, MBA, Senior Editor
Katie Greenock, MS, Editorial and Production Coordinator
Karen Kostick, RHIT, CCS, CCS-P, Reviewer
Theresa Rihanek, MHA, RHIA, CCS, Reviewer
Ashley Sullivan, Project Editor

Limit of Liability/Disclaimer of Warranty: This book is sold, as is, without warranty of any kind, either express or implied. While every precaution has been taken in the preparation of this book, the publisher and author assume no responsibility for errors or omissions. Neither is any liability assumed for damages resulting from the use of the information or instructions contained herein. It is further stated that the publisher and author are not responsible for any damage or loss to your data or your equipment that results directly or indirectly from your use of this book.

The websites listed in this book were current and valid as of the date of publication. However, webpage addresses and the information on them may change at any time. The user is encouraged to perform his or her own general web searches to locate any site addresses listed here that are no longer valid.

All copyrights and trademarks mentioned in this book are the possession of their respective owners. AHIMA makes no claim of ownership by mentioning products that contain such marks.

For more information, including updates, about AHIMA Press publications, visit http://www.ahima.org/publications/updates.aspx.

American Health Information Management Association
233 North Michigan Avenue, 21st Floor
Chicago, Illinois 60601-5809

ahima.org

Contents

About the Author

Lou Ann Schraffenberger, MBA, RHIA, CCS, CCS-P, FAHIMA, is employed by Advocate Health Care as the manager of clinical data in their Center for Health Information Services. Advocate Health Care is an integrated healthcare delivery system of ten hospitals and other healthcare entities, based in Oak Brook, Illinois. Her position is dedicated to system-wide health information management (HIM) and clinical data projects, clinical coding education, and coding data quality issues. Prior to her current position, Lou Ann served as director of hospital health record departments, director of the Professional Practice Division of the American Health Information Management Association (AHIMA), and a faculty member at the University of Illinois at Chicago's health information management program. An experienced seminar leader, Lou Ann continues to serve as part-time faculty and a continuing education instructor in the health information technology and coding certificate program at Moraine Valley Community College. She has also contributed her knowledge and skills as a consultant for clinical coding projects with hospitals, ambulatory care facilities, physicians, and medical group practices. Lou Ann has been active in national, state, and local HIM associations. She is a current member of the Commission on Certification for Health Informatics and Information Management (CCHIIM), an AHIMA commission dedicated to ensuring the competency of professionals practicing health information management. She served as chair of the Society for Clinical Coding (2000). In 1997, Lou Ann was awarded the first AHIMA Volunteer Award. Lou Ann received the Legacy Award from the AHIMA Foundation in 2008 in recognition of her significant contribution to the HIM knowledge base through her authorship of coding books published by AHIMA.

About the Contributors

Three experienced clinical coding experts contributed to the 2012 version of this publication by reviewing the exercises and translating the ICD-9-CM answers to the revised ICD-10-CM/PCS answers from the draft 2012 ICD-10-CM and ICD-10-PCS code sets. All three individuals are AHIMA-approved ICD-10-CM/PCS trainers. The author recognizes and appreciates the contributors' valuable role in the development of this publication.

Linda Galocy, MS, RHIA

Linda Galocy, MS, RHIA is the clinical assistant professor of the Health Information Technology program at Indiana University Northwest, Gary, Indiana. She has been the clinical coordinator as well as instructor of a variety of HIM courses for the past seven years. She received her AHIMA-approved ICD-10-CM/PCS trainer status in July 2009 from AHIMA. She has held a variety of roles on the Indiana Health Information Management Association board of directors, including president, delegate, and chairman of e-HIM and Professional Development committees for several years. Linda has 20 years of experience in HIM, ranging from HIM department management in acute care, ambulatory and physician office consulting, and temporary coding staffing with a national consulting firm.

Marion Gentul, RHIA, CCS

Marion Gentul, RHIA, CCS is an independent consultant, employing her 30 years of health information management experience to provide coding and auditing and educational services to clients in New Jersey and surrounding states. She has been an AHIMA-approved ICD-10-CM/PCS trainer since 2009. Marion is a past president of the New Jersey Health Information Management Association. Marion is coauthor of two chapters in AHIMA's publication *Effective Management of Coding Services* and is a subject matter expert for MC Strategies' online coding education courses. Marion is a contributor to Elsevier's Davis/LaCour publication *Health Information Technology*. She has taught coding in the classroom for health information management technology, administration, and coding certificate programs. Marion received AHIMA's Triumph Mentor Award, was named a Distinguished Alumna by SUNY Downstate Medical Center, and is a recipient of the NJHIMA Distinguished Member Award. Marion has served on AHIMA's Community of Practice Advisory Committee and the 2012 Triumph Awards Committee.

Mari Petrik, MBA, RHIA, CCS, CCS-P

Mari Petrik, MBA, RHIA, CCS, CCS-P, is an associate professor in the Health Information Technology Program at Moraine Valley Community College, Palos Hills, Illinois. Mari is past president of the Chicago Area Health Information Management Association and an active volunteer for AHIMA activities. She has authored articles for her regional association newsletter and has contributed to practice briefs for the *Journal of AHIMA* on the topic of transitioning to ICD-10-CM/PCS in the academic setting. Mari has presented ICD-9-CM and ICD-10-CM coding workshops. Mari is an AHIMA-approved ICD-10-CM/PCS trainer and is a faculty member for the AHIMA Academy for ICD-10-CM/PCS.

From the Author

The publication *Clinical Coding Workout: Practice Exercises for Skill Development,* published by AHIMA Press, would be an excellent follow-up resource to this text, providing beginning to advanced coding opportunities for the student. The case studies in the book help new coders become adept at sorting through detail to prioritize and code diagnoses—skills that will be essential in their coding profession.

Preface

Developing the skills necessary to be effective and efficient in coding takes practice. Such additional coding practice is what the student will find in *Basic ICD-10-CM/PCS Coding Exercises, Fourth Edition,* which contains coding exercises related to each chapter of the *Basic ICD-10-CM/PCS Coding* book, also written by Lou Ann Schraffenberger and published by the American Health Information Management Association. The objective in designing these exercises was to provide the student with further ICD-10-CM coding practice opportunities.

The exercises are short case studies and operative descriptions of real-life patient encounters in healthcare. The case studies provide the student with opportunities to code clinical information, rather than coding one- or two-line diagnostic and procedural statements. Depending on whether the case study describes an inpatient hospital admission or an outpatient visit, the student must determine the appropriate diagnosis and procedure codes to be assigned and apply them in the appropriate sequence. For inpatient hospital admissions, the principal diagnosis is listed first; for outpatient encounters, the main reason for the visit is the first-listed diagnosis code. Students must also decide what information to include as secondary diagnoses according to the clinical information presented and to coding guidelines.

Not every case study will require a secondary diagnosis/diagnoses in addition to a principal or first-listed diagnosis. Not every case study will require a procedure code(s). This is true in real-life situations as well; the coder must develop strong problem-solving coding skills to correctly decide what clinical information should be coded.

The student must apply the Draft ICD-10-CM Official Guidelines for Coding and Reporting to accurately assign diagnosis codes for these exercises. The guidelines may be found at the website for the National Center for Health Statistics, Classifications of Diseases at http://www.cdc.gov/nchs/icd/icd10cm.htm. ICD-10-CM code book publishers include the guidelines in their publications.

The 2012 Official ICD-10-PCS Guidelines are included in the 2012 ICD-10-PCS files on the Centers for Medicare and Medicaid services website, which includes more information on the new procedure coding system, ICD-10-PCS, that is a replacement for ICD-9-CM, Volume 3. The guidelines were used to assign the ICD-10-PCS codes for the exercises. Another valuable tool for assigning ICD-10-PCS codes is the ICD-10-PCS Reference Manual, found on the following website:

http://www.cms.gov/Medicare/Coding/ICD10/2012-ICD-10-PCS.html.

The exercises must be used in conjunction with the 2012 draft ICD-10-CM and ICD-10-PCS code sets that are available online from the National Center for Health Statistics and the Centers for Medicare and Medicaid Services at:

http://www.cdc.gov/nchs/icd/icd10cm.htm and

http://www.cms.gov/Medicare/Coding/ICD10/index.html.

The print version of the 2012 draft ICD-10-CM and ICD-10-PCS, published by Ingenix and OPTUMInsight™, was also used to code the exercises.

Students (and teachers) will notice that these scenarios require the student to apply ICD-10-PCS procedure codes to inpatient admissions but not for the outpatient visits. In actual practice, CPT or HCPCS procedure codes are assigned for hospital outpatient visits and other ambulatory encounters, such as those in physician offices. The requirement for using the ICD-10 coding system, including the International Classification of Diseases, 10th Revision, (ICD-10-CM) for diagnosis coding and the International Classification of Diseases, 10th Revision, Procedure Coding System (ICD-10-PCS) for inpatient hospital procedure coding, as well as the Official ICD-10-CM and ICM-10-PCS Guidelines for Coding and Reporting, was published in the January 16, 2009, ICD-10-CM and ICD-10-PCS final rule (74 FR 3328 through 3362).

Comments from students and teachers using the *Basic ICD-10-CM/PCS Coding Exercises, Fourth Edition,* are most welcome. Please send your comments to the publisher at publications @ahima.org. The book will only improve with your input and feedback. Thank you.

Resources and Reference List

Websites

AHIMA ICD-10 Resources
http://www.ahima.org/ICD10/

Centers for Medicare and Medicaid Services ICD-10 Website
2012 Official ICD-10-PCS Coding Guidelines and ICD-10-PCS Reference Manual
http://www.cms.gov/Medicare/Coding/ICD10/index.htm

National Center for Health Statistics Website
ICD-10-CM Official Guidelines for Coding and Reporting 2012
http://www.cdc.gov/nchs/data/icd10/10cmguidelines2012.pdfl

National Center for Health Statistics Website
International Classification of Diseases, Tenth Edition, Clinical Modification
http://www.cdc.gov/nchs/icd/icd10cm.htm

Books

Barta A., K. DeVault, A. Zeisset, and M. Endicott. 2012. *ICD-10-PCS Coder Training Manual. 2012 Instructor's Edition*. Chicago: AHIMA.

Barta, A. 2012. *ICD-10-CM and ICD-10-PCS Preview Exercises,* 2nd Ed. Chicago: AHIMA.

Hazelwood, A. and C. Venable. 2009. *ICD-10-CM and ICD-10-PCS Preview*. Chicago: AHIMA.

Kuehn, L. and T. Jorwic. 2012. *ICD-10-PCS: An Applied Approach*. Chicago: AHIMA.

Schraffenberger, L.A. 2012. *Basic ICD-10-CM/PCS Coding*. Chicago: AHIMA.

Zeisset, A. and A. Barta. 2011. *Root Operations: Key to Procedure Coding in ICD-10-PCS*. Chicago: AHIMA.

Zeisset, A. and S. Bowman. 2011. *Pocket Guide Pocket Guide of ICD-10-CM and ICD-10-PCS*. Chicago: AHIMA.

Chapter 1

Certain Infectious and Parasitic Diseases

Coding Scenarios for *Basic ICD-10-CM/PCS Coding*

The following case studies are organized following the sequence of the chapters in the *ICD-10-CM and ICD-10-PCS* code books. The objective of this book is to provide the student with more detailed clinical information to code, rather than one- or two-line diagnosis and procedure statements. ICD-10-CM diagnosis codes are to be assigned to both the inpatient hospital admission and the outpatient visit case studies. In this book, the ICD-10-PCS procedure codes are to be assigned only to the inpatient hospital admission cases. In actual practice, outpatient cases are assigned CPT/HCPCS codes. The ICD-10-PCS codes are only required for inpatient procedures.

1

A 22-year-old woman presented to the Family Practice Clinic after being told she should see her physician because her partner had recently been treated for nongonococcal urethritis. The woman did not have any complaints other than some vague pelvic discomfort and vaginal discharge that she did not consider serious. A physical examination, pelvic examination, and Papanicolaou test (Pap smear) were performed. Based on her history and physical findings, the patient was diagnosed with acute chlamydial cervicitis and given a prescription for 2 weeks of antibiotic oral medications and an appointment for a follow-up examination in 3 weeks.

First-Listed Diagnosis: _____

Secondary Diagnoses: _____

2

A male patient, known to have acquired immune deficiency syndrome (AIDS), was admitted with a fever, shortness of breath, and a dry cough. The symptoms had been increasing in severity over the past several days. A chest x-ray showed extensive pulmonary infiltrates. A sputum culture was obtained, and the diagnosis of pneumocystic pneumonia was made based on the microscopic examination. The patient was told that his pneumonia was a result of having AIDS. During his hospital stay, he developed oral candidiasis, which was treated along with the pneumonia with a combination of medications administered intravenously and orally. The patient was discharged with an appointment to the HIV outpatient clinic in 1 month.

Principal Diagnosis: _____

Secondary Diagnoses: _____

Principal Procedure: _____

Secondary Procedure(s): _____

3

A 38-year-old man with known chronic viral hepatitis resulting from hepatitis B is seen in the outpatient infectious disease clinic to be evaluated for therapy. The patient also has cirrhosis of the liver with suspected early stages of liver failure. His liver disease continues to be monitored. The patient is a known heroin addict in remission and faithfully has been taking methadone on a long-term basis through a program at this university medical center. All of these factors were considered when a combination of antiviral agent interferon-alpha plus lamivudine treatment was chosen and will be initiated at his next visit, scheduled in 1 week.

First-Listed Diagnosis: _____

Secondary Diagnoses: _____

4

An 85-year-old woman who lived alone was found in her bed semi-conscious during a visiting nurse well-being check. The nurse immediately called the rescue squad to transport the patient to the nearest emergency department. The patient was able to tell the first-responders that she had been sick for a week with a fast heart beat, fever, chills, and difficulty breathing. She had been in bed for three days and was unable to get out of bed to answer the phone or the door. When she was taken to the emergency department, her vital signs were markedly abnormal with a temperature of over 39 degrees C, a heart rate of 100, and a respiratory rate of 22/min. She was admitted to the intensive care unit (ICU), with an admitting diagnosis of "sepsis" and was treated with antibiotics administered intravenously, stat. Within one day of admission, the infectious disease consulting physician described her condition as severe sepsis with resulting respiratory failure. Despite aggressive measures, after admission the patient required endotracheal intubation and mechanical ventilation for 36 hours to treat acute respiratory failure. The physicians sought to identify the underlying source of infection as well as to provide hemodynamic and respiratory support and were successful in avoiding septic shock in this patient. The patient's attending physician provided the diagnoses of severe gram-negative sepsis due to *Escherichia coli* [E. Coli] with acute respiratory failure.

Principal Diagnosis: _____

Secondary Diagnoses: _____

Principal Procedure: _____

Secondary Procedure(s): _____

5

A 62-year-old woman rushed to her primary care physician's office complaining of the abrupt onset of a fiery-red swelling of her face. The physician's physical examination found that the swelling covered nearly all of the right side of the woman's face with well-demarcated raised borders. Her face was erythematous and edematous on the right side and the patient had a slightly elevated temperature. The patient stated that her face felt hot but described feeling only mildly ill. An infectious disease physician's office was next door and he was asked to see this patient immediately, as her primary care physician had never seen this type of facial swelling and was concerned that her airway would eventually close. The infectious disease physician recognized the condition immediately as a superficial dermal and subcutaneous infection, usually caused by group A beta-hemolytic Streptococcus. He called the condition "acute erysipelas cellulitis" or "acute facial erysipelas" and advised immediate hospital admission for intravenous antibiotics. The patient was taken to the hospital by her family in a private car because her primary care physician ordered a direct admission.

First-Listed Diagnosis: _____

Secondary Diagnoses: _____

6

An 18-year-old woman, who attends a state university about 90 miles away from home, is brought to her family physician's office after her parents brought her home because of a mumps epidemic at the university. During the office visit, the patient complained of fever, malaise, myalgia, and anorexia. She also had an earache and, due to the swelling of her jaw, reported that it was difficult to chew and swallow. A physical examination found the classic findings of mumps. Both sides of the woman's face were swollen consistent with bilateral infectious parotitis. Given her recent exposure to other students diagnosed with mumps, the family physician concluded that the patient had mumps but could not find evidence of any complications in other body systems. The patient was sent home and was advised to avoid contact with people outside her family. The treatment included analgesics and warm compresses to the parotid area to relieve swelling and reduce symptoms. No medications are known to be effective in treating this viral infection.

First-Listed Diagnosis: _____

Secondary Diagnoses: _____

7

A 21-year-old male student came to the college health service center at this state university with complaints of urethral discharge, frequent urination, blood in the urine, and a stinging sensation during urination. The man, who admitted to several sexual partners, stated that these symptoms had become obvious in the past week. A physical examination confirmed the presence of a urethral discharge and swollen glands in the groin region. A urinalysis and urine culture were ordered. The patient noted that his symptoms were similar to a previous episode when he was told he had an acute gonococcal infection. An oral antibiotic was prescribed, and the patient was advised to stop all sexual activity until the treatment was completed and inform his sexual partners of his diagnosis so that they could be tested and treated as necessary. The patient was given an appointment to return in 14 days. The college health service physician wrote acute gonococcal urethritis and acute gonococcal cystitis on the outpatient encounter form.

First-Listed Diagnosis: _____

Secondary Diagnoses: _____

8

A 65-year-old semi-retired nurse came to her primary care physician's office with the following complaints: coughing, chest pain, shortness of breath, fatigue, fever, sweating at night, and a poor appetite. She recently returned from volunteering at a clinic in Southeast Asia where there were many patients diagnosed with pulmonary tuberculosis. The patient previously had tuberculin skin tests that were negative. The physician ordered a chest x-ray, and a tuberculin skin test was administered. Sputum was obtained and submitted for culture. The physician made the diagnosis of pulmonary tuberculosis based on the patient's symptoms and recent exposure to the disease. The patient was given a prescription for an oral medication, isoniazid, which would probably be required for 6 months to 1 year. The patient is also known to have essential hypertension and is one-year status post percutaneous coronary angioplasty for coronary artery disease. Her cardiovascular status was also assessed and prescriptions were renewed. A follow-up visit was scheduled for 2 weeks.

First-Listed Diagnosis: _____

Secondary Diagnoses: _____

9

A 60-year-old female patient was referred to the neurologist's office by her primary care physician because of a new onset of weakness, fatigue, and pain in her left leg. This leg had been affected by acute poliomyelitis (polio), which she had 50 years ago. She had atrophy of the muscles of the left leg since having polio as a child. She walks with a limp because of the weakened, slightly shortened leg. On this occasion, following examination, the neurologist concluded that her symptoms reflect postpolio syndrome, which includes a progressive dysfunction and loss of motor neurons that had been compensating for the neurons lost during the original infection. The patient did not have a new onset of the polio infection. The consultant's diagnosis was progressive atrophy of the leg muscles due to postpolio syndrome.

First-Listed Diagnosis: _____

Secondary Diagnoses: _____

10

A 9-year-old boy was brought to the emergency department by his father, who stated that the child had an acute onset of fever, chills, headache, neck stiffness, photophobia, and pain in his eyes. He also had some nausea and vomiting. Upon physical examination, the emergency department physician found meningismus—a constellation of signs and symptoms—suggestive of meningitis. The child was admitted to an isolation room in the pediatric intensive care unit, and a spinal tap was performed by inserting a needle percutaneously into the spinal canal in order to obtain spinal fluid. The examination of the cerebral spinal fluid and results of other tests led the physician to conclude the patient had coxsackie-virus meningitis. Because this is a viral illness, medical treatments are limited and are directed at relieving symptoms. The patient had an uncomplicated recovery and was discharged home for continued rest.

Principal Diagnosis: _____

Secondary Diagnoses: _____

Principal Procedure: _____

Secondary Procedure(s): _____

11

The patient is a 67-year-old female admitted to the hospital from the emergency room. She reported that she had nausea and vomiting and a fever for the last two days. She had been eating poorly for at least three days and within the last 12 hours started having chills, racing heart, and shortness of breath. She noticed a strong odor and dark color in her urine. The complete blood count (CBC) on admission had a result of 24,000 white cells with a shift to the left. Other laboratory tests confirmed an electrolyte imbalance, with hyponatremia and hypokalemia. The urinalysis showed too many white blood cells to count and many bacteria present. She was admitted for intravenous antibiotics and rehydration fluids to correct the electrolyte imbalance. The patient had been undergoing chemotherapy for recently diagnosed metastatic carcinoma in her axillary lymph nodes. The patient had breast cancer diagnosed and treated 5 years ago with surgery and chemotherapy. Her diagnosis on admission was acute sepsis with a suspected urinary tract infection as the cause. A urine culture and two blood cultures were positive for Klebsiella gram-negative organism. After the initiation of the IV fluids and antibiotics, the patient improved and was able to eat more and ambulate. She had no vomiting or diarrhea. The repeat urinalysis and blood counts showed values that were approaching a normal range. The oncologist examined the patient in the hospital and determined her next chemotherapy session would be delayed by two weeks to allow the patient to recover from this infection and regain her strength. Both the attending physician and the oncologist agreed that the patient's final diagnosis was sepsis due to underlying urinary tract infection, both due to Klebsiella gram-negative organism infection, hyponatremia, hypokalemia, and history of breast cancer with metastatic disease in the axillary lymph nodes. The patient was discharged home with home care nurses to visit the next day.

Principal Diagnosis: _____

Secondary Diagnoses: _____

Principal Procedure: _____

Secondary Procedure(s): _____

12

The mother of a 3-year-old female brought the child to the emergency department (ED) because of fast breathing, a fast heartbeat, and a generalized erythematous rash. The mother stated the child had been refusing food and drink and had not urinated much during the past 12 hours. The ED physician found the child, clinging to her mother, to be dehydrated, febrile, and lethargic. The child was started on an IV for rehydration and respiratory treatments of albuterol to improve her respiratory rate. Multiple chicken pox lesions were noted over the child's face, trunk, and legs, but the majority were crusted and nonvesiculating. The mother reported that her 6-year-old son had chicken pox recently. The physician also noted the child's abdomen to be distended. Examination of the ears showed a right otitis media with the left ear tympanic membrane normal. The chest exam demonstrated expiratory and inspiratory rhonchi with expiratory wheezes at the bases that were consistent with pneumonia. The child was placed into the pediatric observation unit. Over the next 12 hours the patient's symptoms improved after treatment. Amoxicillin medication was started for the ears. The child became more alert, smiling and happy, but still clinging to her mother. The mother was allowed to take the child home the next day with pediatric home care follow-up ordered. Discharge instructions included bed rest and continuation of albuterol suspension and amoxicillin. Discharge diagnoses were chicken pox complicated by pneumonia, dehydration, and acute nonsuppurative right otitis media.

First-Listed Diagnosis: _____

Secondary Diagnoses: _____

13

A 21-year-old male made an appointment with his optometrist because he thought he had a problem with his new contact lens. The patient complained of increasingly severe eye pain. When the optometrist questioned the patient on how he took care of his contacts, the patient described rinsing the lens in tap water at work (a sports/exercise facility) during the day and not always using the contact solution prescribed to store the lenses at night, again using tap water. The optometrist examined the patient and documented the patient had a mild to moderately severe case of acanthamoeba keratoconjunctivitis. The patient was told to throw out his current contacts, wear his glasses until his next doctor's appointment in one week, only use contact solution for rinsing and storage, and take nonsteroidal anti-inflammatory drugs to ease the eye pain.

First-Listed Diagnosis: _____

Secondary Diagnoses: _____

14

The patient is a 40-year-old female who is being seen today in the Transplant Clinic of the University Medical Center as part of her evaluation for a possible liver transplant. The patient is known to have chronic hepatitis C and autoimmune hepatitis. Her autoimmune hepatitis was diagnosed recently by antibody tests and a liver biopsy. The patient's symptoms from her disease have been significant, including fatigue, aching joints, jaundice, enlarged liver, and recurrent ascites. The patient's father and brother have died from "liver failure," and this patient's physician suspects there is a genetic factor in the family that leads to autoimmune hepatitis in which the patient's liver is attacked by the patient's immune system. The patient is on the liver transplant list and waiting for an orthotopic transplant to occur. The patient or her husband carries her transplant beeper at all times. The patient's diagnosis listed on the encounter form for this visit is (1) chronic hepatitis C, and (2) autoimmune hepatitis.

First-Listed Diagnosis: _____

Secondary Diagnoses: _____

15

On Monday evening, the parents of a 15-year-old female brought her to the Emergency Department (ED) and stated she had abdominal cramps, headache, muscle aches, chills, diarrhea, nausea, and vomiting for the past 12 hours. The family had been at a family picnic on Sunday with food served throughout the day, and the weather was hot. The teenager ate mostly raw foods and salads at the event. Today, the mother learned that other members of her extended family had similar symptoms, but her daughter appeared to be the most acutely ill. The patient was very lethargic and continued to have diarrhea and vomiting in the ED after she arrived. Immediate laboratory testing found her to be dehydrated, and intravenous fluids were promptly started. Based on her symptoms and history, the physician concluded the patient had acute gastroenteritis caused by salmonella food poisoning, complicated by severe dehydration. The patient remained in the ED for 6 hours, then was discharged to her parents' care.

First-Listed Diagnosis: _____

Secondary Diagnoses: _____

16

The patient is seen in the offices of an infectious disease specialist who treated her 1 year previously when she had Lyme disease. She complains of generalized joint pain and stiffness. Based on laboratory test results and physical examination, the physician concludes that the patient no longer has active Lyme disease. However, he concludes that her arthritis of multiple joints is the residual effect of the cured Lyme disease.

First-Listed Diagnosis: _____

Secondary Diagnoses: _____

Chapter 2

Neoplasms

Coding Scenarios for *Basic ICD-10-CM/PCS Coding*

The following case studies are organized following the sequence of the chapters in the *ICD-10-CM and ICD-10-PCS* code books. The objective of this book is to provide the student with more detailed clinical information to code, rather than one- or two-line diagnosis and procedure statements. ICD-10-CM diagnosis codes are to be assigned to both the inpatient hospital admission and the outpatient visit case studies. In this book, the ICD-10-PCS procedure codes are to be assigned only to the inpatient hospital admission cases. In actual practice, outpatient cases are assigned CPT/HCPCS codes. The ICD-10-PCS codes are only required for inpatient procedures.

1

A 63-year-old male patient, known to have emphysema, was advised by his physician to be admitted to the hospital to evaluate and treat his worsening lung condition. The patient quit smoking cigars 5 years ago, after he was told he had emphysema. The patient complained that his coughing and wheezing had become worse and his sputum was streaked with blood. A chest x-ray done on an outpatient basis the previous week showed a mass in the right main bronchus. After admission, a fiber optic bronchoscopy and excisional biopsy of the right main bronchial mass was performed. The pathologic diagnosis of the biopsy examination was small cell type bronchogenic carcinoma located in the right main bronchus. A nuclear medicine bone scan found areas of suspicious lesions that were determined to be bone metastasis. The diagnoses provided by the physician at discharge were bronchogenic, small cell carcinoma of the right main bronchus with metastatic disease in the bones, emphysema, and former nicotine dependence.

Principal Diagnosis: _____

Secondary Diagnoses: _____

Principal Procedure: _____

Secondary Procedure(s): _____

2

A 72-year-old man with a diagnosis of acute myeloid leukemia, M7, is admitted for the first scheduled chemotherapy infusion, which will last several days. The patient is given intravenous chemotherapy through the central venous catheter that had been placed during a previous hospital stay.

Principal Diagnosis: _____

Secondary Diagnoses: _____

Principal Procedure: _____

Secondary Procedure(s): _____

3

A patient with terminal carcinoma of the sigmoid colon with metastases to the liver was admitted to the hospital with hypotonic dehydration. The patient's hypotonic dehydration was the focus of the treatment with intravenous therapy, and the patient felt relief from his symptoms. Chemotherapy had been recently discontinued after discussions with the patient about its ineffectiveness in curing his disease and how sick the treatment made the patient feel. During the hospital stay, the patient and his family agreed to palliative care only, which was ordered along with an order to "do not resuscitate" (DNR). The patient was discharged to home hospice.

Principal Diagnosis: _____

Secondary Diagnoses: _____

Principal Procedure: _____

Secondary Procedure(s): _____

4

A 98-year-old man was brought to his primary care physician by his family for his regular check-up. The man, who was very alert and oriented for his age, stated that he was feeling increasingly tired with each day, causing him to sleep 10 to 12 hours a day. He also stated he had lost his appetite and felt slightly nauseated all the time. His physician, concerned by these symptoms present in a patient of advanced age, advised admission. The patient was admitted for probable dehydration, which was later confirmed by examination and laboratory findings. Intravenous hydration was started. Other laboratory tests showed evidence of chronic kidney disease (CKD) stage 4 and hypertension. Further workup revealed a mass at the head of the pancreas. The patient began to experience neoplasm-related pain and was given low doses of morphine. The patient, having lived a long life, refused surgery, chemotherapy, and all other treatments, preferring to return home to die in peace. The patient and his family consented to hospice care at home and the patient was discharged. The physician's final diagnoses included the statement "probable carcinoma of the pancreas, hypertensive CKD Stage 4, dehydration."

Principal Diagnosis: _____

Secondary Diagnoses: _____

Principal Procedure: _____

Secondary Procedure(s): _____

5

A 39-year-old woman with known cervical dysplasia had been seen in the outpatient surgery department the previous week for a colposcopy and biopsy. Pathologic exam of the biopsied tissue was inconclusive but suggested the possibility of a malignancy in the cervix. The patient returned to the outpatient surgery department for a conization of the cervix by loop electrosurgical excision (LEEP) using a colposcope for guidance in order to destroy the site of the possible malignancy. A portion of the cervix was submitted for histopathologic examination with the findings returned as carcinoma in situ of the uterine cervix. The patient will follow up in the office.

First-Listed Diagnosis: _____

Secondary Diagnoses: _____

6

This is a 56-year-old woman who has biopsy-proven malignant melanoma of the left upper arm on the shoulder. The pathology diagnosis was superficial spreading of malignant melanoma. The patient is brought to the hospital outpatient department for excision of the 2.5 × 1.5 cm lesion. She will be seen in the office in 14 days for suture removal and a discussion on what further treatment might be indicated.

First-Listed Diagnosis: _____

Secondary Diagnoses: _____

7

This is a 46-year-old woman who had biopsy-proven malignant melanoma and excision of the lesion on her forehead. Since the last visit the patient learned that her brother and possibly her father (who is now deceased) had lesions and moles removed that were skin cancer and, in her father's case, probably a melanoma. All three people shared the same history of growing up in a southern state with year-round extensive sun-related radiation exposure. The patient, her brother, and her father enjoyed fishing at the beach and rarely applied sunscreen lotion. On this occasion, she is brought back to the hospital outpatient department for a "wide excision" of the same location on her forehead where the lesion had previously been removed, 4 × 3 cm in area, at the site of the original excision. Because the affected area was her forehead, the patient asked for a plastic repair of the site. The surgeon agreed and documented that the plastic repair, which required the insertion of synthetic substitute, was not done for cosmetic reasons but done to avoid future possible painful scarring. The reason for the second excision was stated as "further excision as margins of initial excision showed evidence of remaining malignancy." The physician said this procedure was to "finish" the original excision to make certain the "margins are clean" and no malignant tissue remains. The pathology report states "normal tissues, margin clean, no evidence of remaining malignant melanoma." The patient will be seen in the office for suture removal and further treatment options are to be discussed.

First-Listed Diagnosis: _____

Secondary Diagnoses: _____

8

A 57-year-old male patient was admitted to the hospital with the known diagnosis of right ureteral obstruction caused by secondary neoplasm of the ureter. Known to have a primary malignancy of the stomach (body) that was surgically resected 6 months earlier, the patient was still receiving chemotherapy for the gastric malignancy. Outpatient testing showed evidence of minor ascites and right ureteral metastasis causing obstruction, resulting in right hydronephrosis. The patient was admitted for treatment of the hydronephrosis. The patient was taken to the radiation department where an interventional radiologist percutaneously inserted a nephrostomy tube directly into the right kidney for drainage. A percutaneous paracentesis was also performed for diagnostic purposes. Cytology examination of the peritoneal fluid showed evidence of peritoneal metastasis and malignant ascites. The patient did not want further aggressive therapy and was discharged home to consider using hospice services.

Principal Diagnosis: _____

Secondary Diagnoses: _____

Principal Procedure: _____

Secondary Procedure(s): _____

9

The patient is a 53-year-old woman with left breast cancer, metastatic to the bone and brain, all diagnosed in the past 6 months with continued management. The patient is seen in the hospital's outpatient oncology clinic for her next cycle of intravenous infusion, through a peripheral vein, of Aredia (pamidronate disodium), a chemotherapy drug used as palliative treatment for bone metastases. She does not receive treatment for the primary or other secondary malignancy.

First-Listed Diagnosis: _____

Secondary Diagnoses: _____

10

A 73-year-old man was seen in his physician's office with a variety of gastrointestinal complaints, including vague abdominal pain, diarrhea, urinary frequency, and flushing across his face, neck, and chest. Laboratory and radiology tests were inconclusive, but based on his continuing symptoms the physician suspected the patient might have a chronic form of appendicitis. Because of the uncertainty of the etiology of patient's symptomatology and his advanced age, an inpatient laparoscopic appendectomy was scheduled and performed. The entire appendix was excised. The final pathology report confirmed the frozen section diagnosis of malignant carcinoid tumor of the appendix. The surgeon was informed of this diagnosis, agreed with the pathologist, and documented malignant carcinoid tumor of the appendix as the final diagnosis. Additional testing performed during the inpatient encounter determined that the patient was experiencing a "carcinoid syndrome" because of this tumor, which explained many of his vague symptoms, including the flushing. The appendectomy is considered curative treatment for the appendiceal tumor. Upon discharge, the patient will be seen in the oncologist's office for further recommendations, especially to treat the carcinoid syndrome.

Principal Diagnosis: _____

Secondary Diagnoses: _____

Principal Procedure: _____

Secondary Procedure(s): _____

11

The patient is a 59-year-old woman who is admitted to the hospital after complaining of weakness, and also for her next cycle of chemotherapy. She has a primary malignancy of the transverse colon. On admission, bloodwork performed indicated severe anemia. The oncologist documented that the anemia was associated with malignancy. Chemotherapy was cancelled. The patient received a transfusion via a peripheral vein of (nonautologous) packed red blood cells and was discharged.

Principal Diagnosis: _____

Secondary Diagnoses: _____

Principal Procedure: _____

Secondary Procedure(s): _____

12

The patient is a 28-year-old man who was recently diagnosed with a seminoma and underwent an orchiectomy of his left testicle, which was normally descended. He has had several courses of retroperitoneal radiation therapy. Outpatient bloodwork scheduled before his next radiation therapy session indicated severe anemia. He was admitted for transfusion of nonautologous whole blood via a peripheral vein. Final diagnosis was stage I seminoma being treated with retroperitoneal radiation therapy, aplastic anemia due to adverse effect of radiotherapy.

Principal Diagnosis: _____

Secondary Diagnoses: _____

Principal Procedure: _____

Secondary Procedure(s): _____

13

The patient is a 49-year-old automotive mechanic who was working on his car at his home over the weekend when he developed what he called the "mother of all headaches" or the worst headache of his life. He had nausea but no vomiting. He later noticed visual disturbances and dizziness. Thinking the headache would go away, he went to bed but was unable to sleep all night because of the intensity of the headache pain, which was not relieved by Tylenol. He also felt some vague discomfort in his chest. He called his physician the next morning and was advised to go to the Emergency Department, and subsequently admitted. CT of the thorax and MRI scans of the head were performed. The MRI of the head found a three ring-enhancing lesion located in the parietal lobe of the brain associated with a large amount of edema extending into the occipital and temporal regions. The CT of the thorax found pulmonary lesions that seem to be cavitating in the right lung. The patient has been smoking cigarettes for the past 30 years. The patient consented to and underwent the following two procedures: (1) closed biopsy of the parietal lobe of the brain through a burr hole approach; and (2) bronchoscopic right lung biopsy. Based on the pathologic findings, the physician concluded the patient had a giant cell glioblastoma multiform of the parietal region with metastases to the lung. In addition to these diagnoses, the physician gave other final diagnoses of pre-diabetes and nicotine dependence. The patient was discharged home as he wished to seek a second opinion at a major university medical center. Copies of his records and radiology films in CD format were given to the patient for this purpose.

Note that at many facilities, inpatient coders are not required to assign codes for CTs or MRIs. These procedures are "hard coded" during the charge entry process using the charge-master.

Principal Diagnosis: _____

Secondary Diagnoses: _____

Principal Procedure: _____

Secondary Procedure(s): _____

14

The patient is a 69-year-old gravida 3, para 2, AB 1, female whose last menstrual period was in 1985. She originally came to the gynecologist's office complaining of postmenopausal bleeding. As an outpatient, she had an endometrial biopsy that revealed poorly differentiated adenocarcinoma with clear-cell features of the endometrium. Today the patient was admitted to the hospital for an open total abdominal hysterectomy and related surgery as deemed necessary by the surgeon during the hysterectomy. Her medical history includes ongoing treatment for hypertension, anxiety disorder, postsurgical hypothyroidism with a history of thyroid cancer, and type 2 diabetes mellitus. The surgery performed was a radical abdominal hysterectomy. The patient failed to mention that her fallopian tubes and ovaries were removed as a fail-safe method of birth control in the 1950s. There was no evidence of metastasis into other pelvic organs. A consultation with an oncologist was performed prior to discharge. The patient had an uneventful recovery from the surgery and was discharged on day three to follow up with her gynecologist and oncologist in the next two weeks.

Principal Diagnosis: _____

Secondary Diagnoses: _____

Principal Procedure: _____

Secondary Procedure(s): _____

15

The patient is a 37-year-old female who was diagnosed with breast cancer two years ago and had a partial mastectomy of her left breast. Her estrogen receptor status is positive. Her chemotherapy and radiation therapy treatments ended six months ago. She has had follow-up CT imaging, and there is no evidence of residual disease. The patient is in the doctor's office today to receive her first intravenous infusion of Herceptin (trastuzumab), which she will receive on a weekly schedule for the next five years if she can tolerate it and there are no side effects. The doctor reminds the patient that the drug is not an antineoplastic chemotherapy drug. It is an antineoplastic monoclonal antibody drug that attaches itself to cancer cells and signals the body's immune system to destroy them. It is antineoplastic in the sense that the drug decreases the risk of the cancer recurring in a patient like her with estrogen receptor positive status breast cancer. The drug is considered long-term therapy for consolidative treatment of her breast cancer.

First-Listed Diagnosis: _____

Secondary Diagnoses: _____

16

A 59-year-old woman was admitted to the hospital for a scheduled open total abdominal hysterectomy (TAH) with a bilateral salpingo-oophorectomy (BSO). The patient also had type 2 diabetes, which was well controlled by insulin. The patient first visited her gynecologist several months ago complaining of postmenopausal vaginal bleeding and abnormal vaginal discharge. An endometrial biopsy was taken in the office and was suggestive of uterine cancer. The TAH-BSO was performed, and the following postoperative diagnoses were recorded by the physician: Stage I endometrial adenocarcinoma (corpus uteri) and bilateral corpus luteum cysts of the ovaries, worse on the right side, fallopian tubes appeared normal. The patient continued to receive insulin while in the hospital.

Principal Diagnosis: _____

Secondary Diagnoses: _____

Principal Procedure: _____

Secondary Procedure(s): _____

17

HISTORY: A 55-year-old woman presented to the office with a right breast mass, approximately 2.0 cm × 2.0 cm, in the upper inner quadrant. There was no lymphadenopathy. She has a significant family history of breast cancer being diagnosed in her mother, maternal aunt, and older sister. Three days ago, a fine needle aspiration procedure demonstrated cells suspicious for malignancy. She was admitted to the hospital for definitive surgical treatment with a right breast lumpectomy.

OPERATIVE FINDINGS: A hard 2.0 × 2.0 cm mass in the upper inner quadrant of the right breast with no lymphadenopathy was confirmed. Pathology reports the specimen to be confirmed as carcinoma. The surgical margins on the mass excised were found to be normal. It is felt the entire lesion was removed.

DESCRIPTION OF PROCEDURE: After preoperative counseling, the patient was taken to the operating room and placed in a supine position on the table. The chest, right breast, and shoulder were prepped with Betadine scrub and paint and draped in the usual sterile fashion. The skin around the mass was anesthetized with 1% lidocaine solution. An elliptical incision was made, leaving a 1.5-cm margin around the mass in a circumferential fashion. The mass was sharply excised down to the pectoralis fascia, which was excised and sent with the specimen of the breast. The deep medial aspect of the specimen was marked with a long suture and the deep inferior margin marked with a short suture. The wound was left open until the pathologist returned the call that the margins were negative under frozen section. The wound was copiously irrigated. Hemostasis was achieved with Bovie cauterization and 3-0 Vicryl suture ligatures. The skin was closed with a running subcuticular 4-0 Vicryl, Benzoin, and steri-strips. A sterile dressing was applied. The patient was subsequently transferred to the recovery room in stable condition. She tolerated the procedure well and will be advised of the procedural findings when she is returned to her room.

Principal Diagnosis: _____

Secondary Diagnoses: _____

Principal Procedure: _____

Secondary Procedure(s): _____

18

HISTORY: The patient is a 62-year-old female who was admitted to the hospital for scheduled surgery to treat her recently diagnosed carcinoma of the rectosigmoid colon. She had noticed a change in her bowel habits about 6 to 7 months ago but did not seek medical care until two weeks ago when she went to her primary care physician. The patient was immediately scheduled for an outpatient colonoscopy, and a 10-cm tumor was found and biopsied, with carcinoma diagnosed. She has a long history of angina and had a percutaneous transluminal coronary angioplasty (PTCA) twice in the past 4 years, with two non drug-eluting stents in the right coronary artery. She also has a history of tobacco use. She was cleared for surgery by her cardiologist with the diagnoses of coronary artery disease with stable angina and hypercholesterolemia that continued to be managed with her usual medications while she was in the hospital. The patient was discharged home with home health services following an uneventful postoperative recovery. She has an appointment with her oncologist in 2 weeks to discuss the next treatment options.

OPERATIVE FINDINGS: During an anterior resection of the rectosigmoid colon, the patient was found to have a tumor that extended into the muscular wall but not through the muscular wall of the rectosigmoid colon. No tumor was found outside the rectosigmoid intestine. The pathologist identified the tumor as a primary infiltrating papillary adenocarcinoma of the colon, rectosigmoid junction, that extended focally into the outer muscular wall, with no evidence of metastasis to pericolonic lymph nodes. The tumor staging was T2 N0 M0. The colon specimen was a sessile round lesion about 12 cm in length with the tumor measuring 3 cm × 2.5 cm. The tumor was elevated about 0.8 cm above the surrounding mucosal surface.

DESCRIPTION OF PROCEDURE: The patient consented to an anterior resection of the sigmoid colon. Under endotracheal anesthesia, the abdomen was prepped and draped in the usual surgical manner. It was opened through a lower abdominal midline incision extending to the left of the umbilicus using a hot knife. Exploration of the abdominal cavity revealed a normal-feeling and appearing stomach, liver, gallbladder, and large and small bowels. The aorta and iliac vessels had some atheromatous plaque. Both kidneys appeared and felt normal. The Bookwalter retractor was used. The sigmoid colon was freed from its attachment in the pelvis on the right and left side by sharp dissection. The ureters were both identified and avoided. The blood supply of the rectosigmoid area was serially clamped, divided, and tied with 2-3 Ethibond sutures. The tumor was palpated just below the peritoneal reflection. The colon was freed below the peritoneal reflection. Again the blood supply was serially clamped, divided, and tied with 2-0 Ethibond sutures. Proximally, a portion of the sigmoid colon mesentery was serially clamped, divided, and tied as well. Satinsky clamps were placed proximally and distally, and the colon and specimen were removed. An end-to-end anastomosis was performed in a single layer with interrupted 3-0 silks. The wound was inspected for bleeding, and it was dry. A Penrose drain was placed down near the anastomosis from the stab wound in the left lower quadrant. The first sponge and needle count was correct. The peritoneum was closed with continuous 2-0 Vicryl, fascia with interrupted 2-0 Ethibond, subcutaneous with Vicryl, and the skin with skin clips. The drain was sutured in place. All sponge and needle counts were correct. The patient tolerated the procedure well and left the operating room in satisfactory condition.

Principal Diagnosis: _____

Secondary Diagnoses: _____

Principal Procedure: _____

Secondary Procedure(s): _____

Chapter 3

Diseases of Blood and Blood-forming Organs and Certain Disorders Involving the Immune Mechanism

Coding Scenarios for *Basic ICD-10-CM/PCS Coding*

The following case studies are organized following the sequence of the chapters in the *ICD-10-CM and ICD-10-PCS* code books. The objective of this book is to provide the student with more detailed clinical information to code, rather than one- or two-line diagnosis and procedure statements. ICD-10-CM diagnosis codes are to be assigned to both the inpatient hospital admission and the outpatient visit case studies. In this book, the ICD-10-PCS procedure codes are to be assigned only to the inpatient hospital admission cases. In actual practice, outpatient cases are assigned CPT/HCPCS codes. The ICD-10-PCS codes are only required for inpatient procedures.

1

A 20-year-old African-American man is admitted to the hospital from the emergency department with acute vaso-occlusive pain and pulmonary symptoms including shortness of breath, chills, and cough. He was known to have Hb-SE sickle-cell disease. A chest x-ray showed new pulmonary infiltrates. Treatment was focused on reducing the chest pain to improve breathing and treat the respiratory infection. The physician's discharge diagnosis was acute chest syndrome due to the sickle-cell crisis.

Principal Diagnosis: _____

Secondary Diagnoses: _____

Principal Procedure: _____

Secondary Procedure(s): _____

2

A severely anemic 75-year-old male patient with known inoperable carcinoma of the head of the pancreas is admitted to the hospital for nonautologous red blood cell transfusions, which were given through a catheter inserted into a peripheral vein in the left arm. The discharge diagnosis was anemia of chronic disease due to inoperable carcinoma of the pancreas.

Principal Diagnosis: _____

Secondary Diagnoses: _____

Principal Procedure: _____

Secondary Procedure(s): _____

3

While an inpatient in an acute care hospital, a 60-year-old woman was referred for consultation to a hematologist with a diagnosis of anemia. A bone marrow aspiration biopsy of the right iliac crest was performed. Pathologic analysis of the specimen concluded the patient had "hypercellular marrow with diminished iron consistent with iron deficiency anemia" with the iron deficiency anemia also documented by the consultant in a post-procedure note. The attending physician agreed with the pathologist's conclusion. Code only for the consultant's diagnosis and procedure performed.

Principal Diagnosis: _____

Secondary Diagnoses: _____

Principal Procedure: _____

Secondary Procedure(s): _____

4

An 80-year-old woman was seen by her family practice physician in the office for symptoms of fatigue, palpitations, and weakness. She had recently moved from her home of 50 years to an assisted living center. Although she likes the new residence, she feels the move has caused her to become ill. She has no appetite and was distressed over all she had to do prior to the move. Laboratory tests were ordered, including a CBC, a comprehensive metabolic profile, and an EKG and chest x-ray. Her hemoglobin and hematocrit were abnormal and, given her history, especially the lack of adequate nutrition, the diagnosis of nutritional anemia was made. The patient was encouraged to take advantage of the assisted living center's on-site dietitian to review her nutritional needs. The patient was scheduled to return to the physician in two weeks. If the blood count does not improve by then, the option of administering packed cells via transfusion will be discussed. The only other finding of her diagnostic studies was known chronic obstructive pulmonary disease (COPD) that is under treatment, and a healed myocardial infarction that occurred three years ago and is currently asymptomatic.

First-Listed Diagnosis: _____

Secondary Diagnoses: _____

5

The patient, a 40-year-old man, was diagnosed with acquired hemolytic anemia, auto-immune type with warm-reactive (IgG) antibodies (warm type), and had been treated with glucocorticoids (prednisone). The patient failed to respond to this medication. The patient is also under treatment for systemic lupus erythematosus. Given the aggressive nature of his anemia, he was advised to be admitted to the hospital and have a total splenectomy to eliminate the body's further destruction of red blood cells. The open, total splenectomy was performed without complications, and the patient was discharged to be followed in the physician's and surgeon's offices.

Principal Diagnosis: _____

Secondary Diagnoses: _____

Principal Procedure: _____

Secondary Procedure(s): _____

6

A 70-year-old man was admitted after seeing bright red blood in the toilet following a bowel movement. An esophagogastroduodenoscopy (EGD) revealed a chronic gastric ulcer with evidence of recent bleeding. The final diagnoses documented were acute blood loss anemia and chronic gastric ulcer with recent hemorrhage.

Principal Diagnosis: _____

Secondary Diagnoses: _____

Principal Procedure: _____

Secondary Procedure(s): _____

7

A 60-year-old woman was placed in the observation unit after complaining of chest pain. She was recently seen for a follow-up visit at the hematologist's office for recently diagnosed pernicious anemia. The patient is also known to have agammaglobulinemia that is frequently found in patients with pernicious anemia. The patient is also being treated for chronic atrophic gastritis that is a consequence of her pernicious anemia. The patient is treated with medications to replace the cobalamin deficiency of pernicious anemia. The chest pain was attributed to her chronic atrophic gastritis and she was discharged the same day.

First-Listed Diagnosis: _____

Secondary Diagnoses: _____

8

A 50-year-old woman is admitted directly from her hematologist-oncologist's office after a follow-up visit concerning drastically reduced blood counts as reported on recent laboratory tests. After workup, the attending physician diagnosed acquired aplastic anemia. The physician also refers to her aplastic anemia as "pancytopenia with hypocellular bone marrow." The patient has been undergoing aggressive cytotoxic chemotherapy for left ovarian carcinoma. No chemotherapy was administered during this visit. The patient was discharged and scheduled to report to the hospital outpatient transfusion center tomorrow for two units of red blood cells to be infused for the aplastic anemia, documented as an adverse effect of her chemotherapy.

Principal Diagnosis: _____

Secondary Diagnoses: _____

Principal Procedure: _____

Secondary Procedure(s): _____

9

The patient is a 20-year-old man who was born with factor VIII deficiency and diagnosed with hemophilia, type A. He has been receiving factor VIII replacement therapy with some response to treatment. The patient is admitted to the hospital on this occasion for his first course of plasmapheresis or extracorporeal immunoadsorption. The procedure is performed by drawing blood from an antecubital vein through a needle and returning it to another vein in the other arm. The access vein is connected to a primed blood processor. Blood is drawn into a cell separator. The plasma is passed to a monitor that controls continuous plasma flow through one of two ECI protein A columns. One column absorbs antibodies, and the other treats the remaining plasma. The treated plasma is returned to the blood processor, mixed with the patient's red blood cells, and reinfused back to the patient. This treatment took 4 hours 10 minutes. The patient was kept in the hospital overnight to observe for any possible complications. The patient is known to have "hemophilic arthritis" of the knees as a result of bleeding into these joints. This arthropathy caused by his hemophilia was evaluated by an orthopedic physician during his hospital stay. No complications of his immunoadsorption treatment were detected, and the patient was discharged, accompanied by his parents, for a follow-up visit in 1 week in the physician's office.

Principal Diagnosis: _____

Secondary Diagnoses: _____

Principal Procedure: _____

Secondary Procedure(s): _____

10

The patient is a 55-year-old woman with known chronic idiopathic thrombocytopenic purpura. The patient has been treated for this autoimmune disorder for approximately 1 year. The patient was previously seen in the office of her internal medicine specialist to discuss an elective splenectomy. The patient has failed to maintain a normal platelet count after a course of prednisone therapy. She also had major side effect reactions to the prednisone medication. After hearing of the risks and benefits of the splenectomy versus another course of steroid therapy, the patient is admitted and consents to the surgery, a laparoscopic partial splenectomy.

Principal Diagnosis: _____

Secondary Diagnoses: _____

Principal Procedure: _____

Secondary Procedure(s): _____

11

A 68-year-old woman was admitted to the hospital from a local nursing home because of severe anemia causing altered mental status. She has two large pressure ulcers on her sacrum and right hip. The sacral ulcer now appears to be oozing blood. The patient received one non-autologous red blood cell transfusion percutaneously through a peripheral vein, for her documented acute blood-loss anemia. The wound care physician and nurses treated her massive stage 3 sacral pressure ulcer and stage 2 right hip pressure ulcer. The patient was also treated for her well-controlled type 2 diabetes and hypertension. The patient also has chronic back pain from lumbar spinal osteoarthritis with radiculopathy. Given the size of the pressure ulcers, the intensive care necessary to manage the ulcers, her chronic back pain, and subsequent immobility, a surgical consultation was obtained to consider creating a diverting colostomy to alleviate the fecal incontinence that she had for the past several months that failed to respond to medical management. The fecal incontinence had done damage to her skin and affected her skin ulcers. After completion of the red blood cell transfusion, she was stable enough for the diversion colostomy open procedure of the descending colon. There were no postoperative complications, and after two days the patient was transferred to the skilled nursing facility for recovery from surgery and continued wound care.

Principal Diagnosis: _____

Secondary Diagnoses: _____

Principal Procedure: _____

Secondary Procedure(s): _____

12

A 70-year-old female patient with metastatic bone carcinoma from carcinoma of the right breast, still under treatment by chemotherapy and radiation therapy, is admitted with vague complaints of weakness. After workup, she was diagnosed as having aplastic anemia caused by her radiation therapy.

First-Listed Diagnosis: _____

Secondary Diagnoses: _____

13

A 60-year-old male patient with end-stage renal disease (ESRD) requiring dialysis is seen in his nephrologist's office for an evaluation of his known anemia due to ESRD. Up until now, the anemia was not severe. However, based on the patient's hemoglobin, transferrin saturation, and serum ferritin laboratory values, the physician concludes the patient will need to receive Epogen to treat the anemia and avoid the need for blood transfusions. The medication will be given intravenously 3 times a week at the dialysis center with the drug's dosage based on the patient's hemoglobin values and iron status. The patient will be monitored by the dialysis center physician and return to his nephrologist's office in 1 month.

First-Listed Diagnosis: _____

Secondary Diagnoses: _____

14

The patient, a 28-year-old female, is admitted with labor pains in her second trimester of pregnancy. She is expecting a boy. While in the hospital, she has a discussion of recent testing to determine her sickle-cell genetic status. The patient is married to a 29-year-old man who is known to carry the sickle-cell trait. The patient is informed she also is a carrier of the sickle-cell trait. The patient and her husband are anxious to begin a family. The physician informs the patient that the gene that causes sickle-cell anemia must be inherited from both parents to cause full-blown sickle cell anemia in a child. With both the father and mother carrying the sickle-cell trait, the couple has a 25 percent chance of having a child with the disease and a 50 percent chance of having a child who is a carrier. Otherwise, neither of the parents with the sickle-cell trait required treatment for the trait. She has a fetal ultrasound after the labor halted. The patient is discharged with the diagnoses false labor, sickle-cell trait.

Principal Diagnosis: _____

Secondary Diagnoses: _____

Principal Procedure: _____

Secondary Procedure(s): _____

15

A 40-year-old man of Mediterranean descent is admitted to the hospital after passing out. The patient has beta thalassemia major and requires blood transfusions every three to four weeks. On initial evaluation, the physician documents splenomegaly, which is unchanged. This sign, as well as the patient's reported fatigue and reduced appetite, are classic symptoms of this hereditary hemolytic anemia. Since his scheduled appointment for a blood transfusion of red blood cells coincides with the admission, he is transfused one unit of nonautologous red blood cells percutaneously through a peripheral vein. A neurologist is asked to see the patient. She does not believe that the patient passed out because of the beta thalassemia major, but cannot determine another cause. The final diagnosis is syncope, etiology unknown, beta thalassemia major.

Principal Diagnosis: _____

Secondary Diagnoses: _____

Principal Procedure: _____

Secondary Procedure(s): _____

Chapter 4

Endocrine, Nutritional, and Metabolic Diseases

Coding Scenarios for *Basic ICD-10-CM/PCS Coding*

The following case studies are organized following the sequence of the chapters in the *ICD-10-CM and ICD-10-PCS* code books. The objective of this book is to provide the student with more detailed clinical information to code, rather than one- or two-line diagnosis and procedure statements. ICD-10-CM diagnosis codes are to be assigned to both the inpatient hospital admission and the outpatient visit case studies. In this book, the ICD-10-PCS procedure codes are to be assigned only to the inpatient hospital admission cases. In actual practice, outpatient cases are assigned CPT/HCPCS codes. The ICD-10-PCS codes are only required for inpatient procedures.

1

A senior woman who lives alone was brought to the hospital Emergency Department by fire department ambulance after being discovered on the front porch by neighbors. She was in a semiconscious state. She was known to have type 1 diabetes mellitus, maintained on insulin. The doctors described her diabetes as very brittle with fluctuating blood sugar measurements during her hospital stay. A type and dosage of insulin was finally established. During her inpatient hospital stay the patient complained of vision problems. She was examined by an ophthalmologist and found to have mild nonproliferative diabetic retinopathy. The patient was able to be discharged home to be followed up in her doctors' offices, as well as by home health nurses. The discharge diagnosis was uncontrolled type 1 diabetes on insulin with mild nonproliferative retinopathy.

Principal Diagnosis: _____

Secondary Diagnoses: _____

Principal Procedure: _____

Secondary Procedure(s): _____

2

A 57-year-old female patient was sent to the hospital outpatient laboratory department by her physician with a written order for a blood glucose test. The patient has known type 2 diabetes mellitus with polyneuropathy and diabetic chronic kidney disease, stage 2; these diagnoses were documented on the order form as the reasons for the blood test.

First-Listed Diagnosis: _____

Secondary Diagnoses: _____

3

An 18-year-old female patient who has had type 1 diabetes for 10 years was admitted with ketoacidosis. She has an insulin pump. The pump was tested and found to have a breakdown; it was not pumping enough insulin, which is what caused the ketoacidosis. With intravenous hydration and insulin drip, the patient's ketones cleared quickly. The insulin pump was reset to the correct dosage.

Principal Diagnosis: _____

Secondary Diagnoses: _____

Principal Procedure: _____

Secondary Procedure(s): _____

4

A 36-year-old man is seen in his doctor's office for ongoing management of diabetes mellitus. As of this time, no obvious manifestations of diabetes are affecting any other body system. The patient takes insulin daily and has received a renewed prescription for insulin and needles. The patient noted that he was very satisfied with the new glucose monitoring device he was advised to use during his last visit. A follow-up appointment was made for 60 days following this visit.

First-Listed Diagnosis: _____

Secondary Diagnoses: _____

5

A 47-year-old woman was seen in her physician's office as a follow-up visit. Results for laboratory tests ordered during the previous visit revealed elevated calcium in the bloodstream. A second laboratory test found an excessive amount of parathyroid hormone in the bloodstream. Follow-up imaging studies confirmed the presence of a benign parathyroid adenoma. The patient is presently complaining of muscle weakness, fatigue, and some nausea and intermittent vomiting. Based on these findings, the doctor concludes that the patient is demonstrating primary hyperparathyroidism. The physician explains to the patient that the hyperparathyroidism can only be cured by surgical excision of the parathyroid adenoma. The patient refuses surgery. The physician agrees the need for surgery is not urgent at this time and orders a bone density radiologic examination to be done next week. The patient will have a follow-up appointment in one month and measurement of calcium levels and renal functions in six months. Symptoms of the primary hyperparathyroidism were treated at this time.

First-Listed Diagnosis: _____

Secondary Diagnoses: _____

6

A 52-year-old woman had been seen in her physician's office because of increasingly irritating symptomatology, including nervousness, irritability, increased perspiration, shakiness, and increased appetite with unexplained weight loss, increased heart rate, palpitations, sleeping difficulties, and other problems. The patient is returning to the office today to review her test results with her physician. The physician advised the patient of the following findings: The blood test for thyroid stimulating hormone had an elevated measurement, and a nuclear medicine scan of the thyroid found hyperactivity in the entire gland. Based on these findings, the diagnosis of hyperthyroidism in the absence of a goiter (rule out Graves disease) was made. The physician had eliminated a thyroid adenoma or a multi-nodular goiter as the cause of the hyperthyroidism. The patient was placed on an oral anti-thyroid medication to lower the level of thyroid hormones in the blood. Additional tests were ordered, and the patient was scheduled to return to the office in 10 days. Because the patient's heart palpitations were more pronounced than seen in other patients with hyperthyroidism, arrangements were made for her to have a consultation with a cardiologist tomorrow.

First-Listed Diagnosis: _____

Secondary Diagnoses: _____

7

The parents of a 16-year-old boy accompanied him to the hospital for admission for the insertion of a totally implantable insulin infusion pump and injection of insulin. The patient has had type 1 diabetes mellitus since the age of 11 years. The insertion of the pump into the subcutaneous tissue of his abdomen was successful. On numerous occasions during the admission, the patient's diabetes had been uncontrolled with various types and dosages of insulin that were administered through the pump. The patient was discharged and will return to the hospital's diabetic clinic in one week with his parents for insulin pump titration and training. For the next week the pump will run with saline.

Principal Diagnosis: _____

Secondary Diagnoses: _____

Principal Procedure: _____

Secondary Procedure(s): _____

8

The patient is a 42-year-old woman who is admitted for bariatric surgery for morbid obesity with alveolar hypoventilation. The patient, who has been obese since childhood, currently weighs 150 pounds more than her ideal body weight. The patient's BMI is 48.4. In the past 20 years, she has been treated for essential hypertension, hyperlipidemia, obstructive sleep apnea, insulin resistance, and primary osteoarthritis of the hips and knees. She has had repeated failures of other therapeutic approaches and various diets to lose weight and has been cleared by a psychiatrist who could find no psychopathology that would make her ineligible for this procedure. The patient underwent a laparoscopic Roux-en-Y gastric bypass (gastroenterostomy) procedure, consisting of the creation of a small gastric pouch connected to the jejunum. The procedure and postoperative course were uneventful, and the patient was discharged the following day. During this hospital stay, hypertension, hyperlipidemia, insulin resistance, and osteoarthritis of the multiple joints were also treated.

Principal Diagnosis: _____

Secondary Diagnoses: _____

Principal Procedure: _____

Secondary Procedure(s): _____

9

The patient is a 32-year-old man who is admitted for laparoscopic bariatric surgery for morbid obesity due to excess calories. The patient currently weighs 200 pounds more than his ideal body weight with a body mass index of 54. In the past 10 years he has lost and gained back more than 100 pounds, but now suffers from several major health conditions that require more aggressive management of his obesity. He has a strong family history of morbid obesity. It occurs in his parents, two sisters, and one brother. In the past 10 years, he has been treated for essential hypertension, dyslipidemia, obstructive sleep apnea, gallstone pancreatitis, type 2 diabetes with diabetic amyotrophy, and osteoarthritis localized to his knees for which he has had bilateral knee replacements. He has had repeated failures of other therapeutic approaches to losing weight and has been cleared by a psychiatrist who could find no psychopathology that would make him ineligible for this procedure. The patient underwent a laparoscopic gastric restrictive procedure with an adjustable gastric band and port insertion. The patient had an uneventful postoperative recovery in the hospital and was discharged for follow-up in the office. During this hospital stay, the conditions of hypertension, dyslipidemia, and type 2 diabetes were also treated.

Principal Diagnosis: _____

Secondary Diagnoses: _____

Principal Procedure: _____

Secondary Procedure(s): _____

10

A 35-year-old man is seen in his doctor's office for dietary counseling and ongoing surveillance of his familial hypercholesterolemia, low density lipoid type. He has been taking the HMG-CoA reductase inhibitor drug, lovastatin (Mevacor), as directed. He has no identifiable adverse effects from the medication. He recently quit smoking, having been nicotine dependent since his teenage years, and was counseled to maintain his smoke-free status. A follow-up appointment is made for a repeat visit in 3 months.

First-Listed Diagnosis: _____

Secondary Diagnoses: _____

11

The patient is a 57-year-old man who was seen in the office for a regular follow-up appointment for the management of secondary diabetes mellitus and his insulin dosage. The Accucheck performed in the office showed a result of 515. The patient stated his glucose is usually over 300 when he checks it at home. He reported feeling fairly well with a little more fatigue than usual. The patient is a retired truck driver and is fairly active, including helping his neighbors with yard work and snow shoveling. He has a history of pancreatic cysts treated surgically by partial pancreatectomy that has produced his secondary diabetes and hypoinsulinemia. Since it was noted that his blood glucose was at a critically high level, he was advised admission. He was admitted and seen by an endocrinologist, who carefully monitored his glucose levels and adjusted his insulin dosage until his glucose levels remained at normal levels. No other complications of his diabetes were found. The patient was discharged with instructions to follow up with the endocrinologist in one week, and to make an appointment for diabetic teaching in the diabetic clinic.

Principal Diagnosis: _____

Secondary Diagnoses: _____

Principal Procedure: _____

Secondary Procedure(s): _____

12

The patient was admitted to the hospital after outpatient laboratory testing revealed a potassium level of 6.3 with elevated creatinine. A nephrology consultation was obtained to evaluate his hyperkalemia. He was given Kayexalate, and his potassium levels improved. The consultant's report suggested that two issues may be contributing to his high potassium. He was taking medications for high blood pressure and a prophylactic anticoagulant, and he did not avoid high potassium foods as previously instructed. He was not always compliant in taking his medications as prescribed. The combination of medications and dietary indiscretion may have resulted in the inadvertent potassium intake excess. The attending physician and consultant took the opportunity of this hospital stay to evaluate the patient's many chronic conditions and encourage compliance with his medications and dietary restrictions. In addition to hyperkalemia, the physician included the following conditions in the discharge summary:

acute renal insufficiency, hypertension with chronic kidney disease stage 1, coronary artery disease, status post cardiac pacemaker, atrial fibrillation, and noncompliance with medications. He was seen by a dietician and provided with information about avoiding foods high in potassium. The patient was encouraged to return to the physician's office in two weeks.

Principal Diagnosis: _____

Secondary Diagnoses: _____

Principal Procedure: _____

Secondary Procedure(s): _____

13

The patient is a 70-year-old female who was a former office employee of her primary care physician. She had called the doctor's office three days prior to admission complaining of general weakness and nausea, and, according to her niece who checked in on her every few days, was apparently not able to get around her house very well. The physician advised her to come to the office, and she agreed but did not show up. The patient had often been noncompliant with medications and treatments recommended. When the doctor's office called her after she failed to show, she said she did not feel well enough to drive but her niece would drive her to the doctor's office the next day. The patient did not show up the next day either. On the third day, the doctor's office called her again. When she sounded less responsive on the telephone, one of the doctor's office staff nurses was given permission to go to the house to check on the patient. When the nurse got to the home, she found the front door unlocked and the patient in bed very lethargic, feverish, and not responding clearly to questions. An ambulance was called, and the patient was brought to the Emergency Department and admitted as an inpatient. The patient was known to have type 1 diabetes with several body systems affected. She was also known to have alcohol dependence, consuming a pint of vodka on a daily basis. Initial laboratory work showed a glucose level of 245, urinalysis with 3+ bacteria and greater than 150 white cells with 10-20 RBCs, a positive blood alcohol level indicating acute intoxication, and ketoacidosis. A urine culture grew E. coli bacteria. She was started on IV antibiotics. She improved steadily and described herself as feeling the best she had felt in a long time. She was watched closely for signs of alcohol withdrawal, but nothing obvious was noted. During her hospital stay, the following conditions were treated: diabetes mellitus, type 1, with ketoacidosis with coma; diabetes mellitus with worsening nephropathy; diabetic severe nonproliferative retinopathy and macular edema; E. coli urinary tract infection; history of UTIs; alcohol dependence; and noncompliance with medical care. The attending physician was queried and documented that the diabetic ketoacidosis best met the definition of principal diagnosis. A social work consultation was requested, and the patient and her niece were given information about assisted living centers to help the patient live safely with some medical supervision. However, the patient flatly refused to consider the option and was discharged home with home health services requested for medical management.

Principal Diagnosis: _____

Secondary Diagnoses: _____

Principal Procedure: _____

Secondary Procedure(s): _____

14

The patient is a 10-month-old female infant who was discharged from the hospital 48 hours ago after treatment for a community-acquired pneumonia and gastroenteritis. The child received IV antibiotics in the hospital. The fever and the diarrhea abated, and the child was discharged to her parents' care. However, early this morning the child's father called the doctor and said her fever and diarrhea had returned, she was increasingly lethargic, and was refusing to take fluids or food. The child was readmitted to the hospital for dehydration and hypokalemia. She was placed on IV fluids and medications to treat the dehydration and hypokalemia, and continued on antibiotics for resolving pneumonia. Within 24 hours the child was afebrile with no diarrhea and a good appetite. Electrolyte laboratory values were back in the normal ranges. The baby also had a diaper rash that was treated in the hospital with medication that was also given to the parents to take home. The patient was discharged to her parents' care with prescriptions given and a follow-up appointment made for 5 days later. The diagnoses listed by the physician in the discharge summary were (1) dehydration, (2) hypokalemia, (3) gastroenteritis, (4) resolving pneumonia, community-acquired, and (5) diaper rash.

Principal Diagnosis: _____

Secondary Diagnoses: _____

Principal Procedure: _____

Secondary Procedure(s): _____

15

A 30-month-old male toddler was admitted to the university hospital for investigation of a complex group of symptoms. The child and parents live four hours away from the hospital. The child was admitted so that the majority of the testing could be done at one time without repeated long trips back and forth to the hospital. The mother reported she noticed changes in the child's facial appearance starting about six months ago. She also noted a loss of previously acquired skills, including language, and observed new aggressive behavior. Upon examination, the doctor noted an enlarged liver and spleen with a distended abdomen and suspected there were cardiovascular complications as well. A series of laboratory tests were performed and an extensive medical history was taken from both parents. The physicians concluded the patient had a type of inherited metabolic disorder called mucopolysaccharidosis (MPS), specifically type MPS IIA, also known as Hunter Syndrome. The patient's problem is his body's inability to produce specific enzymes to carry out essential functions. The parents were told there is no cure for Hunter Syndrome at this time and treatment focuses on managing signs and symptoms of the disease to provide relief to the child as the disease progresses. Known life-threatening complications include cardiovascular, respiratory, brain, and nervous system, in addition to skeletal and connective tissue problems. Because this condition is known to be an X-linked recessive disease, the mother of the child was tested for the mutated gene known to cause Hunter Syndrome. It was determined the mother was a carrier of this disease because she had the X-linked recessive disorder with the mutated gene located on one of her X chromosomes and the normal gene on the other. The mother is unaffected by the disease but can pass it on to children, most often to a son. The parents were told that enzyme replacement therapy and other emerging therapies may offer their son more help in the future. The family was given a follow-up appointment to return in three months for possible hematopoietic stem cell transplant planning. The family was also made aware of the National MPS Society that provides support for families and research support.

Principal Diagnosis: _____

Secondary Diagnoses: _____

Principal Procedure: _____

Secondary Procedure(s): _____

16

A 7-year-old girl was admitted for dehydration due to gastroenteritis. The patient had been seen in the pediatrician's office and was treated for the gastroenteritis, but the patient's family brought her to the emergency department when she became increasingly lethargic and weak. Intravenous fluids were administered for rehydration, and the patient was admitted for treatment of the dehydration. During the two-day hospital stay, the patient's gastroenteritis was also treated, but the focus of her treatment was to correct her dehydrated status. The pediatrician noted that the patient would not have been admitted for treatment of the noninfectious gastroenteritis alone.

Principal Diagnosis: _____

Secondary Diagnoses: _____

Principal Procedure: _____

Secondary Procedure(s): _____

Chapter 5

Mental, Behavioral, and Neurodevelopmental Disorders

Coding Scenarios for *Basic ICD-10-CM/PCS Coding*

The following case studies are organized following the sequence of the chapters in the *ICD-10-CM and ICD-10-PCS* code books. The objective of this book is to provide the student with more detailed clinical information to code, rather than one- or two-line diagnosis and procedure statements. ICD-10-CM diagnosis codes are to be assigned to both the inpatient hospital admission and the outpatient visit case studies. In this book, the ICD-10-PCS procedure codes are to be assigned only to the inpatient hospital admission cases. In actual practice, outpatient cases are assigned CPT/HCPCS codes. The ICD-10-PCS codes are only required for inpatient procedures.

1

A 30-year-old man was brought to the emergency department by police who found him walking down the middle of a highway. The patient was obviously intoxicated and initially uncooperative, experiencing visual hallucinations. Based on the physical examination and laboratory work, with information later provided by the patient, the physician determined that the patient had impending delirium tremens that required admission. He was also monitored for nicotine withdrawal as he smoked two packs of cigarettes daily. He was given a nicotine patch and did not experience nicotine withdrawal. The patient's discharge diagnosis was delirium tremens and psychotic disorder/hallucinations due to alcohol dependence and nicotine dependence.

Principal Diagnosis: _____

Secondary Diagnoses: _____

Principal Procedure: _____

Secondary Procedure(s): _____

2

A 35-year-old woman was admitted to the hospital by the psychiatrist after being seen in the community mental health center for group therapy to deal with her escalating anxiety and depression. The patient also has agoraphobia with some panic disorder symptoms, so coming to the group meetings is often difficult for her and she stated that she would never return. During her admission she participated in group therapy with good results and felt able to return to the community mental health center for outpatient group therapy sessions.

Principal Diagnosis: _____

Secondary Diagnoses: _____

Principal Procedure: _____

Secondary Procedure(s): _____

3

After numerous drug possession arrests, a 40-year-old man was mandated to the substance abuse treatment unit of the hospital for admission to undergo detoxification for his cocaine addiction. He was suspected of criminal activity to support his cocaine dependence, but repeatedly denied breaking the law even though he had difficulties with his memory. He agreed to an administration of an intravenous barbiturate (narcosynthesis) in order to release any possible suppressed or repressed thoughts. It was then determined that he was telling the truth.

Principal Diagnosis: _____

Secondary Diagnoses: _____

Principal Procedure: _____

Secondary Procedure(s): _____

4

A patient with bipolar disorder, currently in a mild depressed state, was admitted to the hospital with side effects due to the prescription lithium carbonate she had been taking. According to her caregivers, the drug had been administered correctly, and there was no possibility of a drug overdose. The patient had been sleeping 20 hours a day and was diagnosed with hypersomnia as a result of lithium toxicity. A therapeutic drug level for the lithium carbonate was found to be increased. Her medication was monitored and the dosage was adjusted. The patient was able to be discharged back to the residential living center where she resided.

Principal Diagnosis: _____

Secondary Diagnoses: _____

Principal Procedure: _____

Secondary Procedure(s): _____

5

A 48-year-old male was brought to the emergency department after suffering an episode of syncope at a family picnic. The patient had been involved in a heated argument with several family members when he suddenly grabbed his chest and neck and collapsed to the ground. He awoke prior to the arrival of emergency medical personnel but was weak, diaphoretic, and confused, and brought to the hospital emergency department. Once in the emergency department, cardiovascular studies were performed, but no cardiovascular disease was immediately evident. There was no history of alcohol or substance abuse, and the patient had not consumed a large amount of alcohol at the party. After admission, the patient's private physician performed a comprehensive history and a physical examination. The patient admitted to a similar episode during a past business meeting, but this episode of syncope was more profound and disturbing to the patient. Upon questioning, it was learned that his mother had suffered similar attacks when the patient was a child, but he knew nothing of their causes and did not think she was ever treated by a physician for the attacks. Other diagnostic tests failed to reveal any cardiovascular or pulmonary pathology to account for the syncope or feelings of panic. A psychiatric consultation was obtained, and the patient was started on antidepressant medication and recommended to begin psychotherapeutic interventions with the psychiatrist in his office. The patient agreed and was discharged in improved condition on day three. The patient was much relieved that his problem was taken seriously and committed to ongoing treatment and management. The family physician agreed with the psychiatrist's conclusion of panic disorder without agoraphobia and added the secondary diagnosis of non-cardiac chest pain, resolved.

Principal Diagnosis: _____

Secondary Diagnoses: _____

Principal Procedure: _____

Secondary Procedure(s): _____

6

A 30-year-old woman, admitted with multiple and vague complaints of pain, is referred to a consultant psychiatrist for evaluation and continued management of her somatization disorder. The patient has a history of many physical complaints over the past 10 to 12 years and has suffered significant impairment in social, occupational, and other areas of normal functioning. The patient is receiving an antidepressant medication and this seems to be helping her. The medication is also helping with her obsessive ruminations associated with her obsessive-compulsive neurosis that were identified through psychotherapeutic interventions. After each investigation of her complaints, there has been no known medical condition to explain them. Her treatment of choice by this psychiatrist is behavior modification therapy as an attempt to control her access to other physicians for repeated physical investigations and to give her support that her psychological condition is treatable. The psychiatrist and attending physician agreed that the patient's complaints of pain were entirely due to her somatoform pain (psychologic) disorder.

Principal Diagnosis: _____

Secondary Diagnoses: _____

Principal Procedure: _____

Secondary Procedure(s): _____

7

A 38-year-old man was admitted to the drug treatment unit of the local hospital for detoxification from heroin, a drug he has been dependent on for several years. He is motivated for treatment because he is experiencing opioid-induced sexual dysfunction. In anticipation of expected withdrawal symptoms, the patient is managed medically, pharmacologically, and psychologically over the next 5 days. The patient suffers multiple symptoms of withdrawal but copes with the process appropriately. By day six, the patient is actively engaged in individual motivational counseling to help him reach his goal of an "opioid-free lifestyle." He has undergone drug detoxification in the past but appears much more committed during this hospital stay. The patient is discharged from the hospital on day eight to immediately enter a 21-day residential program at a local residential treatment facility. Long-term plans include a future stay at a drug-free recovery center and job training to enable the patient to improve his chances of recovery.

Principal Diagnosis: _____

Secondary Diagnoses: _____

Principal Procedure: _____

Secondary Procedure(s): _____

8

The patient is admitted to the psychiatric unit of the hospital after totally losing control of his emotions, verbally and physically lashing out at a coworker. He is known to have a borderline personality disorder. The patient has been faithfully taking his monoamine oxidase inhibitor (MAOI) medication and reports he feels it has helped him manage his impulsive, overly emotional, and erratic behavior up until he believed his coworker intentionally aggravated him. The patient is also a recovering cannabis addict whom the therapist describes as being "in remission." The patient will return next week for his scheduled appointment.

Principal Diagnosis: _____

Secondary Diagnoses: _____

Principal Procedure: _____

Secondary Procedure(s): _____

9

The patient was brought to the emergency department by city police after exhibiting extremely erratic behavior in jail after being arrested for a fight with the owner of a local restaurant in which he frequently dines. The business owner reports the man can be very nice and reasonable one day and completely "crazy" the next time he is in the restaurant. Today the patient got into a fight with another person in the restaurant, and the police were called. His family members arrived at the emergency department and informed the emergency department physician on duty that the patient is known to have paranoid-type schizophrenia and is under treatment by a physician at the VA Medical Center. The family also suspected the patient had not been taking his medications as he claimed he could not afford them, and had exhibited more paranoia recently, having been laid off from his job a month ago. The emergency department physician contacted the VA physician and arranged for an immediate transfer to the psychiatric unit at the VA Medical Center. Ambulance transfer was also approved. The emergency department physician used the diagnosis provided to him by the VA psychiatrist as paranoid schizophrenia.

First-Listed Diagnosis: _____

Secondary Diagnoses: _____

10

A 21-year-old woman is admitted to the eating disorders/psychiatric unit of the University Hospital for anorexia nervosa. The patient's current weight is less than 80% of her expected weight for height and age, and her body mass index (BMI) is 18.2. A thorough history, physical, and psychological examination is performed. It is determined the patient has a "restricting" subtype of anorexia nervosa, because she loses weight by use of caloric restriction accompanied by excessive exercise. The patient is also known to "fast" two days a week to "cleanse her system of food toxins." The patient is extremely reluctant to gain even a small amount of weight. Intensive medical and psychological support was given to the patient. Weight restoration to 90% of her predicted weight was her primary treatment goal. After admission, laboratory tests revealed a serious electrolyte imbalance, which was treated. Along with medical and psychological support, the patient established a positive relationship with a young female dietitian who gained the patient's trust and respect; this was extremely positive in helping the patient gain control of her disease. The patient was discharged on day eight with a small weight gain recorded. The patient was transferred to a residential treatment facility with a successful eating disorders management program for further care.

Principal Diagnosis: _____

Secondary Diagnoses: _____

Principal Procedure: _____

Secondary Procedure(s): _____

11

A 25-year-old man was brought to the hospital emergency department by fire department ambulance after being found by his father hanging from a rope in an attached garage at home. The father cut the rope, and the patient fell to the ground. When paramedics arrived on the scene, the patient was unconscious but became responsive after being administered oxygen. The patient complained of a sore neck and a "cold." The patient's past medical history includes methadone for heroin dependence and chronic pain syndrome as the result of an old back strain. The patient was taking the following medications: Xanax, lithium, methadone, Seroquel, and norco. The patient was first admitted to the medical floor for evaluation of possible injuries from his attempted suicide, and was also seen by the psychiatrist on-call for "depression." After evaluation on the medical unit, the patient consented to be transferred and admitted to the inpatient psychiatric unit. His psychiatric diagnosis was recurrent, severe major depressive disorder. He admitted to the suicide attempt and said it was impulsive after an argument with his parents and not planned ahead of time. He admits to depressive symptoms for the past 1–2 months, if not longer. While in the hospital he was diagnosed with pneumonitis and treated with antibiotics that were continued during his psychiatric stay. The orthopedic surgeon evaluated his neck and diagnosed an acute cervical strain, for which he received medications. The pain management physician, who knew the patient, evaluated the patient and agreed with the present medical management for chronic pain syndrome. The patient was discharged from psychiatric inpatient status on day 10 and was scheduled to begin outpatient therapy through the partial psychiatric hospitalization program the next day.

Assign the diagnosis codes for the inpatient psychiatric admission.

Principal Diagnosis: _____

Secondary Diagnoses: _____

Principal Procedure: _____

Secondary Procedure(s): _____

12

A middle-aged male patient was brought to the emergency department (ED) by fire department ambulance after being found unresponsive lying under a bench at a bus stop. Witnesses told the paramedics they saw the man sitting on the bench, and then having a "seizure" and fall under the bench. When they checked on him, they thought he had stopped breathing and died, and they called 911. When paramedics arrived, they found the patient breathing very shallowly and placed him on oxygen. The patient was not able to be aroused but reacted to painful stimuli. Blood and urine were obtained in the ED for laboratory testing, and the patient was placed on a cardiac monitor, which showed a slow but regular heart rhythm. The lab results returned with a very high blood alcohol level, 225 mg/100 mL. Based on the information in his wallet, his identity was determined, and his brother was called. The brother stated the patient had long suffered from chronic alcoholism but had been living independently and working part-time as a custodian cleaning office buildings at night. The brother promised to come to the hospital and pick up the patient when he got off work in about 8 hours.

The patient slept in the ED for several hours. When he woke up he was pleasant, cooperative, appreciative of the attention, and hungry. He was fed dinner and, later, a snack. His brother arrived to drive him home. The patient was given information about alcohol treatment programs and encouraged to consider it. The patient knew all about such programs and told the staff he would call his "sponsor" when he got home and return to Alcoholics Anonymous meetings to resume his recovery. His final diagnosis was acute alcoholic intoxication in a patient with chronic alcoholism.

First-Listed Diagnosis: _____

Secondary Diagnoses: _____

13

The patient is a 15-year-old male who was recently released from a long stay in an adolescent psychiatric therapeutic hospital. He is now in a weekday program to continue the management of his challenging behavioral health conditions. For many years he has had difficulties in school, which, along with major family conflicts and an encounter with the police, led to his recent hospitalization. He had been arrested on multiple occasions for battery but never convicted of the charges. He was first thought to be suffering from a conduct disorder and attention deficit hyperactivity disorder (ADHD), predominantly hyperactive, and these have been confirmed. As time passed, however, it became evident that the patient's main disability was chronic schizophrenia, schizophreniform type. Also, since the age of 4, the patient has been attracted to matches, lighters, and fires, and a diagnosis of pyromania was also established. The patient was raised in a chaotic household. His father has a long history of psychiatric disorders, and an older brother left home four years ago and had no contact with the family until recently, when the family learned he was incarcerated in a psychiatric prison. During the patient's recent hospital stay, his physicians were able to determine which medications were most beneficial to him. Since joining the day program, the patient has reported that his home life is more peaceful and he feels no urges to set anything on fire. He has been able to comply with his behavioral contract and reports that he has not had any flare-up of his auditory hallucinations and feels more in control of his hyperactivity disorder. The patient attributes his "success" to the medications, which he initially resisted because he didn't want to become an "addict" but realizes he must take them the rest of his life. He also recognizes the importance of continuing his behavioral therapy, family therapy, and group therapy. His current Axis I diagnoses are (1) schizophreniform disorder, schizophrenia, (2) conduct disorder, socialized, ADHD, pyromania. His current Axis II diagnosis is (1) learning disabilities. There are no Axis III disorders. His Axis IV is moderate to severe. Axis V is a GAF score of 40 upon discharge from the hospital.

First-Listed Diagnosis: _____

Secondary Diagnoses: _____

14

The patient is a 32-year-old male admitted to the hospital for medical detoxification for his cocaine dependence and cannabis dependence. He has been unable to quit using either drug on his own and now agrees to enter a residential treatment program for his drug addictions with the full support of his family and employer in order to save his marriage and his job. Prior to entering the residential program, the patient must complete at least a 48-hour detoxification program, and this is the reason he is admitted at this time. The patient was treated with chlorazepate for cocaine withdrawal. He received phenobarbital for cocaine-induced insomnia. He was also treated with thiamine hydrochloride and Allbee with vitamin C capsules. His admission drug screen was positive for cannabis and cocaine. For his persistent cocaine-induced insomnia, he received L-tryptophan. He was discharged on day four after a difficult detoxification experience to enter the predicted month or longer residential program. If successful, this stay is to be followed with transition to a very strong outpatient day hospital rehabilitation program and later phase into a full 2-year aftercare program and lifelong Narcotics Anonymous meetings.

Principal Diagnosis: _____

Secondary Diagnoses: _____

Principal Procedure: _____

Secondary Procedure(s): _____

15

The patient is a 28-year-old male veteran of the Iraq war who served two tours of duty. He was referred to a Veterans Affairs Medical Center for evaluation. He experienced combat and survived two improvised explosive device (IED) explosions while riding in military vehicles. Four fellow soldier friends were killed in the two vehicle explosions. After returning from Iraq two years ago, the patient began experiencing anxiety-like symptoms, including a pounding heart, sweating, and trouble breathing on occasions. He also reported bad dreams of his war experiences. He had difficulty falling and staying asleep. He also reported trouble getting along with his family members and coworkers in his civilian job because of his angry outbursts over relatively minor things. He describes himself as "emotionally numb" and admits to having thoughts of and plans for suicide. The patient is diagnosed with chronic posttraumatic stress disorder with suicide ideation. To fully evaluate the patient and begin therapy, the patient is admitted to an inpatient unit. Over the next five days, the patient is treated with supportive psychotherapy and cognitive-behavior therapy. At the time of discharge, the patient reported feeling better and is scheduled to continue receiving outpatient cognitive-behavior therapy.

Principal Diagnosis: _____

Secondary Diagnoses: _____

Principal Procedure: _____

Secondary Procedure(s): _____

Chapter 6

Diseases of the Nervous System

Coding Scenarios for *Basic ICD-10-CM/PCS Coding*

The following case studies are organized following the sequence of the chapters in the *ICD-10-CM and ICD-10-PCS* code books. The objective of this book is to provide the student with more detailed clinical information to code, rather than one- or two-line diagnosis and procedure statements. ICD-10-CM diagnosis codes are to be assigned to both the inpatient hospital admission and the outpatient visit case studies. In this book, the ICD-10-PCS procedure codes are to be assigned only to the inpatient hospital admission cases. In actual practice, outpatient cases are assigned CPT/HCPCS codes. The ICD-10-PCS codes are only required for inpatient procedures.

1

An 85-year-old woman was brought to the family physician's office by her family. She has severe dementia due to late onset Alzheimer disease. She is becoming increasingly difficult to manage at home. At times, she becomes aggressive and attempts to strike family members with household objects. She also has repeatedly wandered away from the home's backyard and has had to be located by calling police to assist in the search. The family members have refused to admit the patient to a long-term care facility. The family members will continue to care for the woman in their home. The physician's diagnosis is Alzheimer dementia with behavioral disturbances, specifically aggression and wandering.

First-Listed Diagnosis: _____

Secondary Diagnoses: _____

2

The patient is an 18-year-old male with spastic cerebral palsy with quadriplegia. He is brought to the Neurology Clinic for ongoing management. The patient also has recurrent seizures and asthma treated sporadically with an aerosol. He had a gastrostomy tube placed in 2006 and an intrathecal pump for baclofen inserted in 2011. The patient also had intermittent fecal impactions. During this examination the patient was found to be alert but could not answer questions, which is his normal state. He was not in any acute distress. The sites of the intrathecal pump and G-tube were clean and clear of infection. The patient has contracture deformities of his upper extremities with flexion of his elbows as well as clenching of his fingers. His skin was examined, especially on his back, buttocks, and legs, and was found to be free of any pressure sores. The patient was continued on his present medications: baclofen, Keppra, albuterol, and milk of magnesia and will return to clinic in six months or sooner if medically necessary.

First-Listed Diagnosis: _____

Secondary Diagnoses: _____

3

The patient is a 65-year-old man with a past medical history of progressive Parkinson's disease for the past several months with a history of Parkinson disease for the past 23 years. He was brought to the emergency room by his wife because of the patient's increasing rigidity, loss of speech, and a new development—his inability to walk and stand. The patient was admitted to inpatient status by his primary care physician. The patient was seen by his neurologist, who adjusted the patient's antiparkinson agent, carbidopa-levodopa, to 25 mg/200 mg. On physical examination a small abscess was noted over the left lower back area. The patient's wife stated it had been present for several months and was likely irritated by the transfer belt that had been used on the patient for gait stability, but the area was not as red at home as it appeared in the hospital. Over the next 3 days, the cutaneous abscess bloomed in size and began draining. The patient was recommended incision and drainage of the abscess while the patient was in the hospital because of the difficulty of bringing the patient back to the hospital as an outpatient for day surgery. A surgeon examined the patient and agreed with the plan. Because the patient was almost completely stiff and contracted, the surgeon recommended performing the surgery under general anesthesia for the patient's comfort. After general anesthesia induction in surgery, the patient was placed in the right lateral decubitus position, and the area was infiltrated with 0.5% plain Marcaine. An elliptical incision was made, and the cutaneous abscess was unroofed and drained. Aerobic culture was taken. The wound was irrigated and hemostasis obtained. The subcutaneous wound was packed with saline-soaked 2 × 2 gauze, and a pressure dressing was applied. The patient tolerated the procedure well and was taken to the recovery room in good condition. Postoperatively, the patient was placed on intravenous antibiotics for 48 hours and then discharged in good condition with prescriptions for his new antiparkinson agent and an oral antibiotic. He will be followed by home health nursing for postoperative wound care.

Principal Diagnosis: _____

Secondary Diagnoses: _____

Principal Procedure: _____

Secondary Procedure(s): _____

4

An 8-year-old boy was seen in the pediatric neurologist's office for his childhood absence epilepsy attacks. The mother reports two episodes of motor seizures over the past month that consisted of localized twitching of his right arm and leg. The patient has an older brother (age 18 years) who had the same type of epilepsy during childhood but has been seizure free for four years. The young patient has an electroencephalogram (EEG), during which electrodes were place on his scalp, to determine central nervous system electrical activity. He is prescribed mild antiseizure medications.

First-Listed Diagnosis: _____

Secondary Diagnoses: _____

5

The patient, a 75-year-old man, was brought to the Emergency Department with progressive deterioration of his overall mental and physical status, lethargy, and difficulty swallowing. The patient's family continued to try to feed the patient. The patient was found to be hypothermic with a temperature of 33.7°C and hypotensive with an initial pressure of 58/34 mm Hg that did not improve much with treatment. The patient was admitted to the intensive care unit, but his blood pressure and overall status did not improve with two liters of fluids, and he was started on Levophed and antibiotics. A chest x-ray showed a right lower lobe infiltrate consistent with aspiration pneumonia, probably due to food. The attending physician concluded that aspiration pneumonia was present. The patient was known to have Lewy body dementia, bed-bound status, and a stage III pressure ulcer of the sacrum. Upon admission the patient was diagnosed with severe sepsis with septic shock, acute renal failure, and acute hepatic failure. Given the patient's overall very poor prognosis, the patient was made DNR status by his physician after discussing the situation with the patient's family. On hospital day 2, the family decided to elect hospice care with no further aggressive care to be ordered. The patient was transferred to the inpatient hospice unit at the hospital.

Principal Diagnosis: _____

Secondary Diagnoses: _____

Principal Procedure: _____

Secondary Procedure(s): _____

6

A 42-year-old female patient was admitted to the hospital for surgery to correct her long-standing trigeminal neuralgia. She also had essential hypertension treated with atenolol medication. The patient has suffered from unremitting facial pain for the past eight months and has failed to respond to medical therapy. The patient was given the option of continued medical management with the drug carbamazepine, gamma knife radiosurgery, or open microvascular decompression to release the trigeminal nerve. She selected the open surgery to release the nerve. She was taken to surgery, and a right side suboccipital craniotomy was performed. Microvascular decompressive release of the trigeminal nerve was performed after clearly visualizing the trigeminal nerve. The patient was transferred to the intensive care unit for overnight monitoring. In the ICU she had serial neurologic monitoring, blood pressure control to minimize hypertensive-related bleeding, aggressive pulmonary toilet as well as stress gastritis prevention and mechanical DVT prophylaxis treatment. No complications were experienced. The patient was transferred to a surgical unit and was discharged in two days to be followed at home by intermittent nursing home health services.

Principal Diagnosis: _____

Secondary Diagnoses: _____

Principal Procedure: _____

Secondary Procedure(s): _____

7

The patient is a 60-year-old female who comes to her primary physician's office complaining of right-sided facial droop. She had decreased eye blinking on the right side and could not completely close her right eye. She was drooling out of the right side of her mouth. She also complained of a headache with throbbing. Based on these complaints and the physical exam, the physician diagnosed the patient with Bell, or seventh cranial nerve, palsy. The patient was placed on oral prednisone but must be watched carefully as the patient has type 2 diabetes and the prednisone could elevate the blood sugar. The patient takes glipizide orally for the diabetes. The patient was advised to wear gauze over the right eye at night to avoid drying out the eye and getting a corneal ulcer. She was also told to use artificial tears to moisten the eye. The patient is also a two-pack-a-day smoker and was, once again, strongly encouraged to quit smoking cigarettes. The patient was given a prescription for Zyban to take as the patient was trying to cut down on her smoking. The patient was sent to the outpatient laboratory after the office visit to have blood drawn for the Lyme titer and sedimentation rate that were ordered by the physician. An appointment was made for the patient to return to the office in 2 weeks.

First-Listed Diagnosis: _____

Secondary Diagnoses: _____

8

A 4-year-old boy was brought to the emergency department by his mother, who stated the child had become ill very rapidly over the course of 1 day. He had been treated for a right ear infection at the pediatric clinic last week. Upon physical examination, the emergency department physician noted a high fever, drowsiness, and stiffness in the neck. The mother reported the child had said his head hurt and also reported that he had vomited at home. The physician noted slight rash on the child's upper trunk and axilla bilaterally. Suspicious of meningitis, the physician requested and obtained a pediatric consult. The emergency department physician and pediatrician obtained consent for a diagnostic spinal tap, which was performed, and the child was admitted to the pediatric unit.

Over the next couple of days, the pediatrician made the diagnosis of bacterial meningitis with the causative organism of *haemophilus influenzae* (H. influenzae) based on the physical findings and the examination of the cerebrospinal fluid obtained by the spinal tap. The child is treated with intravenous antibiotics and other medications as well as supportive care. The pediatrician found the acute suppurative otitis media of the right ear still needed treatment. The child made a full recovery but will be followed closely as an outpatient to determine whether any effects of the meningitis, such as hearing loss, occur later. The child was discharged to the care of his mother.

Principal Diagnosis: _____

Secondary Diagnoses: _____

Principal Procedure: _____

Secondary Procedure(s): _____

9

A 2-year-old girl was brought to the emergency department by her mother, who stated the child had a cold, runny nose, congestion, and a mild fever. The patient then developed a dry, hacking cough that progressed to prolonged coughing spasms. Overnight the child became very ill. Upon physical examination, the emergency department physician noted a high fever and stiffness in the neck, and the child was very difficult to rouse. The mother reported the child had vomited at home. The child was admitted to the pediatric service. Infectious disease and pulmonary medicine specialists consulted with the attending pediatrician to make the diagnosis of whooping cough due to *Bordetella pertussis* with complicating pneumonia. The child was treated with intravenous antibiotics. The girl recovered from the bacterial illness and was discharged to the care of her mother with Home Health Agency nursing follow up.

Principal Diagnosis: _____

Secondary Diagnoses: _____

Principal Procedure: _____

Secondary Procedure(s): _____

10

A 75-year-old patient is admitted to the hospital with the acute onset of neurologic symptoms including double vision, speech difficulty, and loss of balance. Because the patient had a cerebral infarction 5 years previously, with residual hemiparesis on her left non-dominant side, the physician is concerned the patient is having another stroke. Physical and neurologic examination along with CT scanning and blood tests prove the patient has not had another stroke. The physician describes this episode of illness as a "TIA" or transient ischemic attack. The patient's symptoms completely resolve, but she is seen by a physical therapist for the residual hemiparesis on her left side that was the result of her previous cerebral infarction. The patient's essential hypertension is also treated. The stage II chronic kidney disease due to her type 2 diabetes mellitus was monitored and treated. The patient is discharged on the hospital day 3 for follow up in her physician's office in 1 week.

Principal Diagnosis: _____

Secondary Diagnoses: _____

Principal Procedure: _____

Secondary Procedure(s): _____

11

The patient is a 35-year-old female who was in an auto accident four months ago. She was treated in the emergency room of a local hospital as well as in this doctor's office following the accident and had been diagnosed with a concussion. The patient reported to her doctor during the current visit that she has had headaches almost every day since the accident. She stated that over-the-counter pain medication helps relieve the pain but she is concerned that the headaches are still present. The doctor examines the patient and makes the diagnosis of "chronic, intractable posttraumatic headaches due to post-concussion syndrome from her previous auto accident." The patient is referred to a neurologist for a consultation and will return to this doctor's office in 2 weeks to determine the next course of treatment if necessary.

First-Listed Diagnosis: _____

Secondary Diagnoses: _____

12

The patient is a 78-year-old man who was admitted to the hospital today for the implantation of a dual-chamber permanent pacemaker device. The patient had a several-month history of syncope that was investigated on a couple of encounters. Finally it was determined that the patient's neurocardiogenic syncope was caused by carotid sinus syndrome, which another physician referred to as carotid sinus hypersensitivity. The dual-chamber cardiac pacemaker was implanted into the subcutaneous tissue of the patient's chest, followed by insertion of leads into the right atrium and left ventricle via a percutaneous approach to treat the carotid sinus syndrome. The patient had no complications from the procedure and was discharged home with an appointment with his cardiologist in 10 days.

Principal Diagnosis: _____

Secondary Diagnoses: _____

Principal Procedure: _____

Secondary Procedure(s): _____

13

A 45-year-old man was admitted to the hospital for a decompressive laminectomy to treat his long-standing lumbar spinal stenosis. The back pain from the spinal stenosis has not been relieved by pain management treatment or physical therapy. The man has been off work for 3 months due to the chronic back pain and agreed to the spinal surgery as his last option to relieve the pain and support his family. The patient is healthy and has no other medical problems. The surgery was performed on the day of admission and involved removal of a small portion of a lumbar disc, open approach. During the surgery, a dural tear was noted as the result of an unintended durotomy. The tear was immediately repaired during the same procedure. The patient was informed of the unintended durotomy and the necessary repair. Otherwise the patient had no complications from the procedure and recovered well enough to go home in three days. The patient will be seen in his surgeon's office in one week.

Principal Diagnosis: _____

Secondary Diagnoses: _____

Principal Procedure: _____

Secondary Procedure(s): _____

14

The patient is a 60-year-old male farmer who was treated a month ago for the apparent toxic effects of herbicide chemicals (organophosphate compounds) that he was applying to his crops. Since that time the patient has had severe vertigo, headaches, nausea, and loss of sensations in his hands and feet. The patient was admitted to evaluate the relationship between his past toxic exposure and his current symptoms. The most recent toxicology studies indicated a moderate level of herbicides in the blood—less than one month ago when it was initially tested. The physician documented the final diagnosis as toxic polyneuropathy due to herbicide toxicity. Medications were prescribed to manage the symptoms the patient continued to experience, and the patient will return to the physician's office for additional blood tests in one month. In the interval, the patient is advised not to operate machinery or drive a car.

Principal Diagnosis: _____

Secondary Diagnoses: _____

Principal Procedure: _____

Secondary Procedure(s): _____

15

A 35-year-old male was admitted to the hospital. The admitting diagnosis documented on the history and physical examination report was "chronic pain syndrome and chronic lower back pain with exacerbation of lower back pain and lower extremity pain." Also included in the patient's history is the fact that the patient was injured in a serious automobile accident three years ago and has had back pain ever since that injury. However, the patient's pain has increased over the past three months and has become excruciating over the past week. The patient was admitted to the hospital specifically for pain management. The patient received intravenous and intramuscular pain medications as well a peripheral nerve block to manage his pain, which he reported as much improved at the time of discharge. The peripheral nerve block involved percutaneous injection of an anesthetic. The final diagnosis written by the physician was acute exacerbation of chronic pain due to trauma, chronic lower back pain, and lower extremity pain. The physician also wrote that the pain was likely the consequence of sympathetic lumbar nerve root damage from the injuries sustained in the automobile accident.

Principal Diagnosis: _____

Secondary Diagnoses: _____

Principal Procedure: _____

Secondary Procedure(s): _____

16

A 20-year-old male college student was brought to the emergency department complaining of a sudden onset headache, fever, and stiffness with pain in the neck. He had been treated in the college health service center for an ear infection in the past week. After admission, the patient also complained of chest pain, fatigue, cough, and nausea. A diagnostic lumbar puncture was performed and the findings were positive for meningitis. A chest x-ray revealed pneumonia. Sputum and spinal fluid cultures grew the pneumococcus organism (*Streptococcus pneumoniae*). The physical examination also confirmed the presence of acute otitis media of both ears. The patient was treated with intravenous antibiotics for the infections. The discharge diagnoses written by the physician were pneumococcal meningitis with pneumococcal pneumonia and acute suppurative otitis media.

Principal Diagnosis: _____

Secondary Diagnoses: _____

Principal Procedure: _____

Secondary Procedure(s): _____

17

The patient is admitted to the hospital with chronic postviral fatigue syndrome. The patient is known to have had infectious mononucleosis several months previously and has never felt well since that time. Laboratory tests and neurologic studies are used to evaluate the patient's condition and possible underlying cause. The physician concludes that the current condition is late effect of chronic Epstein-Barr infection. The patient was discharged home for rest and recovery.

Principal Diagnosis: _____

Secondary Diagnoses: _____

Principal Procedure: _____

Secondary Procedure(s): _____

Chapter 7

Diseases of the Eye and Adnexa

Coding Scenarios for *Basic ICD-10-CM/PCS Coding*

The following case studies are organized following the sequence of the chapters in the *ICD-10-CM and ICD-10-PCS* code books. The objective of this book is to provide the student with more detailed clinical information to code, rather than one- or two-line diagnosis and procedure statements. ICD-10-CM diagnosis codes are to be assigned to both the inpatient hospital admission and the outpatient visit case studies. In this book, the ICD-10-PCS procedure codes are to be assigned only to the inpatient hospital admission cases. In actual practice, outpatient cases are assigned CPT/HCPCS codes. The ICD-10-PCS codes are only required for inpatient procedures.

1

A patient is seen in the eye clinic at the University Medical Center. After taking a thorough history and conducting an extensive physical eye examination, the physician orders several tests to be done over the next week. At the conclusion of the visit, the physician writes the diagnosis of "bilateral primary low-tension open angle glaucoma."

First-Listed Diagnosis: _____

Secondary Diagnoses: _____

2

The patient is an 88-year-old woman who was living with her grandson, an Army captain, until he was deployed overseas. She now lives alone and has no other relatives in the area. The type of procedure planned for the patient could usually be performed on an outpatient basis, but because of her living situation the patient's procedure is scheduled as an inpatient procedure. The patient was diagnosed with retinal detachment, single break, right eye. The patient has vision of 20/400 in the right eye. She is status post cataract extraction in the left eye. The procedure performed was a retina repair by pars plana vitrectomy, gas/fluid exchange with autologous serum injection, and C#3/F#8 gas injection, which are components of the procedure of cryoretinopexy of the right eye. The procedure was performed percutaneously to repair the detached retina. The procedure was performed with intravenous moderate sedation. At the conclusion of the procedure, injections of dexamethasone and gentamicin were given subconjunctivally as part of the procedure. The patient was kept in the hospital overnight. The next day a neighbor picked up the patient and visiting nurse services were initiated.

Principal Diagnosis: _____

Secondary Diagnoses: _____

Principal Procedure: _____

Secondary Procedure(s): _____

3

A 40-year-old woman came to the ophthalmologist's office last week complaining of a fleshy fold of tissue that appeared in the corner of her left eye near her nose and started growing toward the center of her eye. She reported that it had begun to obstruct her vision. Upon examination, the physician found a progressive peripheral pterygium that starts in the conjunctiva and attaches to the cornea as it grows. The patient was scheduled for an excision of the pterygium of the left eye, with a corneal graft (nonautologous tissue substitute) to be performed next week at the outpatient surgery center.

First-Listed Diagnosis: _____

Secondary Diagnoses: _____

4

A 3-year-old female was admitted to the hospital for strabismus surgery on her left eye. The physician states her condition is monocular concomitant convergent strabismus, or early acquired esotropia, monocular. The physician described the deviation as 25 prism diopters and stable. The child was otherwise healthy and able to receive general anesthesia. Surgery was recommended to reestablish binocular vision. The open approach extraocular muscle surgery performed was a unilateral 6-mm left lateral rectus muscle (extraocular muscle) resection on the affected eye. The child was discharged in the care of her parents on the day after surgery.

Principal Diagnosis: _____

Secondary Diagnoses: _____

Principal Procedure: _____

Secondary Procedure(s): _____

5

A 50-year-old man, who has had type 2 diabetes mellitus for more than 10 years, complains of vision problems, worse in his left eye. He is seen in the ophthalmologist's office upon the recommendation of his family physician. The patient's diabetes is treated with oral medications and diet. After examining the patient, the physician concludes that the patient has moderate nonproliferative diabetic retinopathy, as a result of his type 2 diabetes mellitus.

First-Listed Diagnosis: _____

Secondary Diagnoses: _____

6

The patient is a 30-year-old man who has chronic allergic conjunctivitis, which causes him to rub his eyes continually. He had bilateral entropion repair four years ago and did well for at least 3 years. Over the last few months, he has had problems with rubbing of his right eye and with discharge from it. On examination by the ophthalmologist in her office, he was noted to have significant right upper eyelid laxity, or floppy eye syndrome. He also has inversion of his right lower lashes. Surgical correction of his right lower lid entropion and right upper lid exotropia were discussed. The patient agreed to the proposed procedure. The doctor's nurse will schedule the procedure and call the patient with the date and time of the procedure to be performed in the ambulatory surgery center in the next week. The doctor also provided recommendations on how to relieve the irritation from the chronic allergic conjunctivitis.

First-Listed Diagnosis: _____

Secondary Diagnoses: _____

7

The patient is a 40-year-old female with Down syndrome who was admitted to the hospital for a repeat penetrating keratoplasty (corneal transplant). The patient lives 120 miles away from the hospital with elderly parents and, because of the distance to be traveled, was being admitted instead of having an outpatient procedure. The patient had a penetrating keratoplasty on the left eye in the past. She developed a corneal ulcer and perforation, requiring a repeat penetrating keratoplasty via percutaneous approach in the left eye. The patient did understand the procedure and agreed to it but the consent form was signed by her father. At the time of the corneal transplant it was noted again that her eye was soft and appeared to be perforated with a flat anterior chamber. The donor cornea was prepared. The previous donor cornea was removed from the patient's eye. Four interrupted 10-0 nylon cardinal sutures were placed to secure the new donor tissue to the host, and a symmetrical rhomboid crease on the donor was noted. A total of 12 more interrupted 10-0 nylon sutures were placed equally distant from each other to secure the donor to the host, and the chamber was intermittently formed. The wound was checked for leaks, and none were seen. Subtenon injections of 80 mg Depo-Medrol and 40 mg gentamicin were given as part of the procedure. Vigamox eye drops were placed in the eye. A bandage contact lens was placed in the eye with a shield on top. The patient was awakened and transferred to the recovery room. She stayed in the hospital overnight for pain control and management. She was examined the next morning by the ophthalmic surgeon and discharged to the care of her adult brother and parents to be driven home.

Principal Diagnosis: _____

Secondary Diagnoses: _____

Principal Procedure: _____

Secondary Procedure(s): _____

8

The patient is a 35-year-old male who is a construction worker who suffered a traumatic intraocular foreign body and secondary cataract formation about one year ago. The eye condition was successfully surgically repaired after the injury. However, he is intolerant of contact lens wear and spectacle correction of his aphakia primarily because of his occupation and the safety equipment he must wear. His visual acuity with a contact lens in place is about 20/40. Without his glasses or contact lens his visual acuity is 20/400. During this office visit, the physician recommended another surgical procedure—a capsulectomy and sector iridectomy and secondary sulcus intraocular lens placement. The patient was undecided about more surgery but agreed to think it over and will call the office if he decides to proceed with surgery. The doctor listed traumatic aphakia with pupillary membranes, left eye with status post cataract extraction as the diagnoses on the encounter form.

First-Listed Diagnosis: _____

Secondary Diagnoses: _____

9

The patient is a 68-year-old man with a visually significant nuclear sclerotic cataract in addition to chronic angle closure glaucoma (severe stage) in his right eye that requires multiple glaucoma medications, including pills and drops. After discussion with his ophthalmologist in her office, the patient agreed to have surgery, specifically the cataract extraction with a trabeculectomy with mitomycin-C. The procedure was scheduled for the following week at the free-standing ambulatory surgery center near the patient's home.

First-Listed Diagnosis: _____

Secondary Diagnoses: _____

10

A 50-year-old woman had a malignant skin tumor removed from her left upper eyelid about one year ago followed by lid reconstruction surgery. Due to scarring of the left upper eyelid, the patient was examined in the ophthalmologist office. The physician found the patient to have a cicatricial entropion, cicatricial ectropion, exposure keratoconjunctivitis, and scarring from the previous surgery, all on the left upper eyelid. The physician proposed an excision and repair of the eyelid with adjacent tissue transfer, correction of the lid retraction, and possibly a full-thickness graft to repair the eyelid completely. The doctor explained that further reconstruction may also be necessary. The patient agreed to read the educational material provided by the physician and call the doctor's physician assistant to schedule the procedure if she decides to proceed.

First-Listed Diagnosis: _____

Secondary Diagnoses: _____

11

The patient, a 45-year-old male, was seen in the Intensive Care Unit by the ophthalmologist in consultation. The patient was acutely ill with sepsis and infected joints. The patient was noted to have a very red swollen eye. The consultant concluded the patient had acute panophthalmitis and received consent from the patient's wife to perform a sclerotomy and drainage of the right eye vitreous as well as an intra-vitreal injection of anti-infective agents into the eye. The patient was taken to surgery and the eye was examined again. There was significant pus in the anterior chamber with layered hypopyon inferiorly. No view of the posterior segment was possible. An ultrasound of the eye showed the retina to be flat. A lid speculum was placed in the right eye and Betadine dripped on the conjunctival surface. A needle was placed through the temporal pars plana into the mid vitreous cavity and 0.5 cc of liquid vitreous was aspirated without difficulty. Vancomycin 1 mg in 0.1 cc and ceftazidime 2 mg in 0.1 cc were each injected into the mid-vitreous by way of the temporal pars plana without difficulty. The vitreous sample was sent for culture. The eye was protected with a dressing for surgical recovery.

Code only for the eye condition and procedure.

Ophthalmology Diagnosis: _____

Ophthalmology Procedure(s): _____

12

The patient is a 75-year-old woman who has experienced increasingly hooded lateral vision due to dermatochalasis. This was interfering with her driving her car. She also had left eyebrow and upper eyelid ptosis due to Bell palsy. The patient was seen in the ophthalmologist's office upon recommendation of her primary care physician. The doctor explained the proposed blepharoplasty to treat the bilateral dermatochalasis, which was worse on the left, and the procedure to repair the paralytic ptosis of the left upper eyelid. The patient signed the consent for surgery and agreed to a surgery date two weeks later at a local hospital for the outpatient procedure.

First-Listed Diagnosis: _____

Secondary Diagnoses: _____

13

The patient is a 26-year-old man seen in the ophthalmologist's office upon request of his primary care physician. The patient sustained a chemical burn to the right eye several months ago. The burn has healed, but the patient has increased intraocular pressure in the right eye. This moderate stage glaucoma is the sequela of the chemical burn trauma. The intraocular pressure is not controlled with conventional medications. Therefore the recommendation was made by the ophthalmologist to place an Ahmed valve in the eye to reduce the pressure. The patient consented to the procedure and agreed to meet the physician the next morning at the outpatient surgery center for the procedure.

First-Listed Diagnosis: _____

Secondary Diagnoses: _____

14

The patient is a 75-year-old male who had a right penetrating keratoplasty (corneal transplant) recently for a previous infectious keratitis. He was seen today in the Corneal Clinic and found to have ruptured descemetocele in the right eye. This problem is a mechanical complication due to the corneal graft. The patient had a prior temporary tarsorrhaphy with sutures pulling through. The patient agreed to the recommended surgery of a more prominent tarsorrhaphy to prevent potential exposure keratopathy. The patient will meet the physician later the same day at the outpatient surgery center to have the procedure performed.

First-Listed Diagnosis: _____

Secondary Diagnoses: _____

15

The patient is an 80-year-old woman who has been treated at the University Medical Center Glaucoma Clinic for many years. She has been seen several times in the past few months with increasing right eye pain. The patient's chronic eye pain exists in a visually useless eye. The severe eye pain is the result of long-standing glaucoma, which is now considered absolute glaucoma. The patient is requiring increasing amounts of pain medications and is very tired of the constant eye pain. Surgical options were discussed with the patient and her daughter. The patient agreed with the recommendation of evisceration of the ocular contents with placement of an ocular implant. The procedure will be performed in four days in the University's outpatient surgical center.

First-Listed Diagnosis: _____

Secondary Diagnoses: _____

Chapter 8

Diseases of the Ear and Mastoid Process

Coding Scenarios for *Basic ICD-10-CM/PCS Coding*

The following case studies are organized following the sequence of the chapters in the *ICD-10-CM and ICD-10-PCS* code books. The objective of this book is to provide the student with more detailed clinical information to code, rather than one- or two-line diagnosis and procedure statements. ICD-10-CM diagnosis codes are to be assigned to both the inpatient hospital admission and the outpatient visit case studies. In this book, the ICD-10-PCS procedure codes are to be assigned only to the inpatient hospital admission cases. In actual practice, outpatient cases are assigned CPT/HCPCS codes. The ICD-10-PCS codes are only required for inpatient procedures.

1

A 30-year-old man who is a member of a well-known musical band is seen in the "Performing Arts Clinic" at the University Medical Center. The musician complained of ringing, buzzing, and clicking in his ears and hearing loss, especially on the right side. The musician said he was told by other musicians that he had "rock and roll deafness." Upon examination and audiometric testing consisting of auditory processing using a computer, the physician diagnosed the patient as having sensorineural hearing loss of the right ear as a result of acoustic trauma from performing loud music over the past 12 years. His left ear was fine. The patient was advised to return for further evaluation and possible hearing aid fitting because this type of sensorineural deafness is likely to be permanent.

First-Listed Diagnosis: _____

Secondary Diagnoses: _____

2

The patient is a 60-year-old male who is seen in his primary care physician's office complaining of a buzzing and hissing sound in his right ear. The sounds also make hearing difficult out of the same ear. The patient thinks sometimes the sounds are in both ears but definitely worse in the right ear. An extensive history is taken from the patient and it was determined the patient has not had any ear infections, wax in the ears, or foreign body in the ear. Medically the patient did not have a history of cardiovascular disease, anemia, or hypothyroidism that can have a relationship to tinnitus. Other risk factors discovered were that the patient is a farmer who is around noisy equipment and he had a head injury 5 years ago when he fell down a long flight of stairs. The patient agreed to go to the local hospital for a comprehensive audiologic assessment and a CT scan of the temporal bone. Depending on the findings, an MRI scan of the head may be ordered later. The doctor advised the patient that treatment for tinnitus is usually directed to the underlying disease. If an underlying disease is not found, the patient may find that a hearing aid suppresses the tinnitus. The patient agrees to a follow-up appointment in one week after completion of the outpatient tests ordered. Doctor's diagnosis for the encounter is right ear tinnitus.

First-Listed Diagnosis: _____

Secondary Diagnoses: _____

3

An 82-year-old woman is seen in the ENT physician's office upon request of her primary care physician. The patient is complaining of short episodes of dizziness that occur when the patient turns over in bed or attempts to get out of bed or out of her recliner chair. She also feels lightheaded and nauseous, but all except the dizziness passes if she sits still for a few minutes before attempting to ambulate. The patient had the same symptoms a year ago but they disappeared as suddenly as they occurred. Prior to coming to the ENT doctor's office, the patient had outpatient testing completed, specifically, hearing tests and tests of the vestibular system and a MRI scan of the brain. Upon considering all the facts of the case and the test results, the doctor concluded the patient had benign paroxysmal positional vertigo. Various physical maneuvers and exercises were prescribed by the physician to relieve symptoms. The patient has a follow-up appointment with her primary care physician in two weeks.

First-Listed Diagnosis: _____

Secondary Diagnoses: _____

4

A 70-year-old man was seen in his primary care physician's office with complaints of not being able to hear out of both ears, but the right ear seemed to be worse. He said his ears felt "plugged." Several years ago a different physician cleaned wax out of the patient's ears. Upon physical examination, the doctor found the patient had bilateral hard impacted ear wax in both ears. The doctor's nurse gently worked to soften and remove the ear wax out of both ears. Afterward, the patient commented on how much better his ears felt and how his hearing had improved. The patient and his wife were counseled on how to use over-the-counter ear drops to soften ear wax. The patient was encouraged to come back to the office if he felt that his ears were plugged in the future. The diagnosis for this encounter was documented as cerumen, both ears.

First-Listed Diagnosis: _____

Secondary Diagnoses: _____

5

The patient is a 25-year-old male who came to the emergency department on his own complaining that he was deaf in his left ear. When he was questioned, the patient was vague about his recent activities or illnesses or whether he suffered any trauma to his head. He claimed he did not have any trauma to his ear or any other medical problems. Upon examination, the physician found a small central perforation of the tympanic membrane of the left ear with some discharge in the ear canal. The right ear appeared normal. The patient did not have a primary care physician or health insurance. The patient was advised that the perforation was small and would probably heal on its own but he was strongly encouraged to keep the appointment made for him at the local public health clinic. He was also advised to avoid getting water in his ear and to avoid any potential for trauma to his head because if the perforation did not heal he could have permanent hearing loss. The discharge diagnosis documented on the emergency department record was small central perforation of the left tympanic membrane.

First-Listed Diagnosis: _____

Secondary Diagnoses: _____

6

The patient is a 28-year-old woman who has a complicated otologic history. She had recent surgery by another otorhinolaryngologist where a myringotomy tube was placed with difficulty. The patient noticed significant hearing loss in her left ear after the procedure and presented to this ENT doctor in his office for evaluation. Upon examination it was noted that the patient had a retained myringotomy tube and possible perforation of the tympanic membrane. There was also marked crusting of the tympanic membrane. The patient's hearing was tested, and she was found to have significant mixed hearing loss as well as a drop in sensorineural hearing in the higher frequencies. The diagnoses written by the physician in the patient's record were (1) Left side only sensorineural hearing loss, (2) chronic serous otitis media, and (3) possible perforation of tympanic membrane. The patient consented to a left exploratory tympanotomy with removal of the myringotomy tube and possible placement of a paper patch on the tympanic membrane. The procedure will be performed in two days at the ambulatory surgery center.

First-Listed Diagnosis: _____

Secondary Diagnoses: _____

7

The patient is a 20-year-old man who has a long history of left chronic otitis media. The patient has failed numerous medical treatments. During the examination in the ENT physician's office, he was found to have a large cholesteatoma filling up the left auditory canal. The left external canal was also filled with pus. This physician has treated the patient for several years and suspects there may be destruction of the incus, malleus, stapes, and stapes footplate as a result of the long-term ear infections. For diagnoses the doctor wrote in the office record cholesteatoma left external ear and left chronic otitis media. The patient and his mother agreed to a future admission in the hospital for a left mastoidectomy and possible total ossicular replacement procedure (TORP).

First-Listed Diagnosis: _____

Secondary Diagnoses: _____

8

Brought to the Emergency Department (ED) by her husband, the patient is a 28-year-old female who had just returned from her honeymoon complaining of severe bilateral ear pain and difficulty hearing. The couple came directly to the hospital from the airport after a long flight home. The couple had gone deep-sea diving several times during the past week. The husband had no ear pain or other symptoms. The patient, however, had an acute upper respiratory tract infection when she left on the trip but had fewer symptoms of it today. Upon examination, the physician saw possible bleeding in the ear with swelling and possibly a ruptured ear drum on the right side. The ED staff arranged for the patient to see an otolaryngologist tomorrow morning in his office. The final diagnoses entered in the ED record by the physician were (1) bilateral ear pain, (2) acute upper respiratory infection, (3) possible otitic barotrauma, and (4) possible perforated ear drum.

First-Listed Diagnosis: _____

Secondary Diagnoses: _____

9

The mother of an 18-month-old male child brought her son to the pediatric Emergency Department (ED) at 2200 hours. The mother stated the child has been very irritable this evening, pulling on his left ear, crying, and unable to go to sleep. The child has been diagnosed with acute suppurative otitis media on another occasion in the past 6 months. When the physician examined the child, she saw an erythematous bulging tympanic membrane in the left ear but did not see a perforation. The right ear did not appear to have an infection. There is no smoking in the household or at day care. The child's pediatrician was phoned and asked the

ED physician to prescribe the same antibiotics the child received during the last ear infection that resolved the condition. The final diagnosis on the ED record was recorded as recurrent acute suppurative otitis media, left.

First-Listed Diagnosis: _____

Secondary Diagnoses: _____

10

A 22-year-old female came to the neighborhood health center complaining of tenderness, redness, and swelling over the mastoid area. The patient said she started having ear pain about two weeks ago and thinks she has a fever and some drainage out of her right ear. Due to the fact neither the patient nor her parents had health insurance, she did not go to a doctor's office or the Emergency Department of the local hospital. The physician was certain the patient had acute right mastoiditis as a result of her untreated acute otitis media on the right side that was still present. An initial antibiotic was prescribed and a sample of the otorrhea was taken for culture. The patient was referred to the university medical center's ENT clinic for follow-up in one week. The diagnosis written by the health center doctor on the referral form was "acute right-sided mastoiditis and acute purulent right otitis media."

First-Listed Diagnosis: _____

Secondary Diagnoses: _____

11

A 80-year-old man returned to his physician's office to review the findings of the tests that were performed in the past week. The patient had been in his physician's office a week ago complaining of severe unrelenting ear pain, a temporal headache, purulent discharge from his ears, dysphagia, and hoarseness. These conditions were still present. The physical exam again demonstrated marked tenderness in the soft tissue between the mandible ramus and the mastoid tip. The tympanic membrane was intact in both ears. The physician reviewed the results of the chemistry tests and cultures and bone scan. A minimal amount of osteomyelitis was found. The patient had type 2 diabetes and it was not always well controlled. The patient was informed that he had malignant externa otitis of the right ear and type 2 diabetes with hyperglycemia. The management of his condition was proposed to be meticulous glucose control and aural toilet with systemic and ototopic antimicrobial medications. The patient was given a follow-up appointment in three weeks with a repeat bone scan to be performed prior to that visit.

First-Listed Diagnosis: _____

Secondary Diagnoses: _____

12

The mother of a 14-year-old male brought him to the emergency department. When interviewed, the young man said he had severe pain, itchiness, and a feeling of fullness in both ears. On physical examination and gentle otoscopic inspection, the physician found otorrhea, diffuse external ear canal edema and erythema, and tenderness of both ears, particularly the pinna and tragus. He was unable to visualize the tympanic membranes due to the swelling. The young man was a competitive swimmer and spent hours practicing in his school's pool. The physician informed the patient and his parent and documented in the record that the patient had "swimmer's ear, bilaterally." A prescription was given to the patient for medicated ear drops and he was advised to discontinue swimming practice and avoid getting water in his ears. The mother agreed to make an appointment with the primary care physician in 2 days to recheck the patient, especially to visualize the ear drums to ensure there was no perforation.

First-Listed Diagnosis: _____

Secondary Diagnoses: _____

13

The patient was a 60-year-old female known to have Meniere disease. On this visit to her primary care physician's office, the patient reported she was having a familiar "attack" of this condition. She was experiencing fluctuating hearing loss, whirling vertigo, and a low, roaring tinnitus. The patient had been investigated numerous times in the past to find an underlying reason for this disorder of the inner ear, and none had been found. The patient again was treated for her symptoms. A repeat audiometry test was ordered to compare her perceived hearing loss to her baseline test of 2 years ago. The patient was given prescriptions again for Antivert for the vertigo and a diuretic to reduce the fluid in the inner ears and was advised to continue her salt-restricted diet and to avoid caffeine and alcohol, which were suspected to be triggers of her symptoms. The patient's condition, Meniere disease, was again documented in her health record for this visit.

First-Listed Diagnosis: _____

Secondary Diagnoses: _____

14

The father of a 6-year-old male child brought him to the pediatrician's office for a follow-up visit to reexamine him for the acute otitis with effusion in his left ear that was diagnosed three days before this visit. Once again the physician noted fluid present in the middle ear but this time found no evidence of infection in the left ear. The tympanic membrane was intact. No evidence of fluid was obvious in the right ear. The physician advised the parent that an appointment will be made for the child with an otolaryngologist to determine if a myringotomy with insertion of a ventilating tube will be necessary.

First-Listed Diagnosis: _____

Secondary Diagnoses: _____

15

A 19-year-old female was seen in the otolaryngology consultant's office one week after an Emergency Department visit because of severe vertigo with repeated nausea and vomiting. There was persistent nystagmus as well. The condition is minimally better as the nausea and vomiting have stopped. The patient had also seen her primary care physician in the prior week and completed outpatient testing including an audiologic assessment and MRI of the head. Based on the test results and the physician's examination of the patient, including a detailed history interview, the physician concluded the patient had bilateral vestibular neuronitis and documented the diagnosis in the health record and in the report returned to the primary care physician. The physician explained to the patient that the disease is considered to be a neuronitis affecting the 8th cranial nerve and suspected to be viral in origin. The patient was advised that some patients only have one attack such as the one she suffered, while other individuals have repeated episodes over a period of one year or more.

First-Listed Diagnosis: _____

Secondary Diagnoses: _____

Chapter 9

Diseases of the Circulatory System

Coding Scenarios for *Basic ICD-10-CM/PCS Coding*

The following case studies are organized following the sequence of the chapters in the *ICD-10-CM and ICD-10-PCS* code books. The objective of this book is to provide the student with more detailed clinical information to code, rather than one- or two-line diagnosis and procedure statements. ICD-10-CM diagnosis codes are to be assigned to both the inpatient hospital admission and the outpatient visit case studies. In this book, the ICD-10-PCS procedure codes are to be assigned only to the inpatient hospital admission cases. In actual practice, outpatient cases are assigned CPT/HCPCS codes. The ICD-10-PCS codes are only required for inpatient procedures.

1

A 50-year-old man was admitted to the hospital complaining of chest pain that was determined to be a result of an acute inferior wall myocardial infarction (MI). The patient was treated for the acute MI. In addition, a right and left heart catheterization was performed with a Judkins fluoroscopic coronary angiography of multiple coronary arteries, and a right and left angiocardiography was performed using a low osmolar contrast dye. The patient was found to have coronary arteriosclerosis due to lipid-rich plaque. The patient was also treated for preexisting atrial fibrillation and discharged on day 5 in stable condition.

Principal Diagnosis: _____

Secondary Diagnoses: _____

Principal Procedure: _____

Secondary Procedure(s): _____

2

A 59-year-old male patient with coronary artery disease of the native arteries was admitted to the hospital for scheduled four vessel aortocoronary artery bypass grafts using the left leg's greater saphenous vein grafts (harvested by an open approach) performed under cardiopulmonary bypass. Postoperatively, the patient developed pulmonary emboli that were treated successfully with no catastrophic consequences. After 3 days in the surgical ICU, the patient was transferred to a surgical floor and monitored closely. Phase I of cardiac rehabilitation was started on day 4, and the patient was able to be discharged on day 7. The patient will be seen in the surgeon's office 7 days later and is scheduled to begin Phase II cardiac rehabilitation within the next month.

Principal Diagnosis: _____

Secondary Diagnoses: _____

Principal Procedure: _____

Secondary Procedure(s): _____

3

An 80-year-old woman was seen in her physician's office as a follow-up visit. Six months previously she had a cerebrovascular accident (CVA) for which she was admitted to the hospital at that time. As a consequence of her CVA, she has right-side (dominant) hemiparesis and dysphasia. She has been receiving outpatient physical therapy and has made good progress. She also is being treated for essential benign hypertension and atrial fibrillation. The patient's prescription medications were renewed, and she will be seen in the office in 6 months. She was advised to call her physician if she does not feel well or if new problems develop.

First-Listed Diagnosis: _____

Secondary Diagnoses: _____

4

The patient, a 75-year-old man, collapsed at home and was brought to the emergency department by fire department ambulance and admitted to the hospital. A CT scan of the brain using low osmolar contrast showed an acute cerebral embolus of the right middle cerebral artery with cerebral infarction. Dysphagia and left hemiparesis were present on admission. The patient is right-handed. The patient is also under treatment for hypertension. At the time of discharge, the dysphagia had cleared, but the hemiparesis was still present. The patient was transferred to a rehabilitation facility.

Principal Diagnosis: _____

Secondary Diagnoses: _____

Principal Procedure: _____

Secondary Procedure(s): _____

5

A 65-year-old retired man collapsed in the driveway of his residence, a single family house, after shoveling heavy, wet snow. Fire department ambulance brought the man to the nearest hospital in full cardiac arrest. Family members stated the patient had cardiomegaly and had been on prescription medication for hypertensive heart disease in the past but had not seen a doctor for over one year. Cardiopulmonary resuscitation was initiated but was unsuccessful, and the man was pronounced dead 50 minutes after arriving at the hospital. The patient was never admitted to the hospital with all of his medical care received in the emergency department. The emergency department physician's conclusion in the emergency department record was "Cardiac arrest, probably due to acute myocardial infarction triggered by strenuous exertion. Hypertensive heart disease."

First-Listed Diagnosis: _____

Secondary Diagnoses: _____

6

A 70-year-old woman was seen in her physician's office for ongoing management of several medical conditions. The patient has congestive heart failure as a result of hypertension, chronic kidney disease, stage 2, and long-standing type 2 diabetes with polyneuropathy. Her main reason for being at the doctor's office today is to renew medication for her heart failure.

First-Listed Diagnosis: _____

Secondary Diagnoses: _____

7

The patient is a 70-year-old man who was admitted by his cardiologist with the diagnosis of acute coronary syndrome. The patient had not had coronary angioplasty or coronary bypass surgery in the past. The patient consented to and underwent a diagnostic left heart cardiac catheterization and fluoroscopic coronary arteriography of multiple arteries with low osmolar contrast by Judkin technique, which showed extensive arteriosclerotic coronary occlusion of the left anterior descending (LAD). Other vessels also had minor coronary artery disease. Prior to the procedure, the patient understood there was the possibility that he would require a coronary stent placement, to which he also consented. Following completion of the diagnostic catheterization, the physician performed a coronary angioplasty of the LAD with the insertion of one nondrug-eluting coronary stent into the LAD. A platelet inhibitor drug (Integrilin) was also infused intravenously. The physician's final diagnosis was "acute coronary syndrome due to arteriosclerotic coronary artery disease." The patient was discharged for follow-up evaluation and possible cardiac rehabilitation therapy.

Principal Diagnosis: _____

Secondary Diagnoses: _____

Principal Procedure: _____

Secondary Procedure(s): _____

8

A 72-year-old retired family practice physician called an ambulance from his home to take him to the hospital in which he had practiced medicine for 40 years. En route to the hospital, he asked the paramedics to call the interventional radiologist at the hospital to meet him in the emergency department. The radiologist was waiting for the physician-patient when the ambulance arrived in the driveway. The physician-patient described his symptoms to the emergency department physician and radiologist and said "I'm certain I have an abdominal aortic aneurysm." The symptoms he experienced—abdominal pulsatile mass, abdominal pain and tenderness, rigidity, lower back pain, rapid pulse, paleness, nausea, clammy skin, sweating—were classic symptoms of what physicians call a "triple A." The patient was admitted and taken immediately to the interventional radiology suite. Based on a quick physical examination and intravascular ultrasound of the abdominal aorta, an aneurysm was found. The patient consented to a repair by the interventional radiologist, and within 1 hour of arrival the following procedure was started: Endovascular implantation of a synthetic graft into the abdominal aorta to reinforce the vessel to prevent a ruptured aneurysm. After the procedure, the patient was taken to the ICU for postoperative monitoring. The patient was also treated for long-standing essential hypertension, as well as for chronic gouty arthritis of the right hip that was current. The patient had an uneventful recovery and was able to leave the hospital within 1 week for further recovery at home.

Principal Diagnosis: _____

Secondary Diagnoses: _____

Principal Procedure: _____

Secondary Procedure(s): _____

9

The patient, a 68-year-old woman known to have congestive heart failure currently controlled by medication, is admitted to the hospital by her physician because of posterior calf pain with warmth and swelling of the proximal right lower leg. A duplex venous ultrasonography with pulse-wave Doppler detected a thrombus of the right popliteal vein intravascularly. Anticoagulant therapy was started to prevent pulmonary embolism or further venous embolization. The patient was stabilized and was able to be discharged home. Home health nurse services were arranged to take blood samples for ongoing prothrombin time (PT) laboratory tests to ensure the therapeutic level of the anticoagulant therapy in the blood. The patient was also treated for her compensated congestive heart failure while in the hospital.

Principal Diagnosis: _____

Secondary Diagnoses: _____

Principal Procedure: _____

Secondary Procedure(s): _____

10

The same patient described in question 9, a 68-year-old woman known to have congestive heart failure, was readmitted to the hospital 3 months later with fatigue, shortness of breath, and swelling of the legs, especially the right leg. Upon questioning, the patient admitted to excess foods that were not on her low-fat, low-salt diet over the past week, and her symptoms returned. Intravenous medications, including diuretic and cardiotonic drugs, were started, and the patient's heart function improved. The patient was still receiving maintenance warfarin sodium (Coumadin) to prevent recurrence of the right leg deep vein thrombosis she experienced 3 months previously. Doctor described this condition in the progress notes as DVT and history of DVT. A duplex intravascular venous ultrasonography with pulse-wave Doppler did not detect a recurrent thrombus in the right leg. The patient was stabilized and was able to be discharged home. Home health nurses were arranged to take blood samples for ongoing prothrombin time (PT) laboratory tests to ensure the therapeutic level of the anticoagulant therapy in the blood. The patient was also treated for compensated congestive heart failure while in the hospital.

Principal Diagnosis: _____

Secondary Diagnoses: _____

Principal Procedure: _____

Secondary Procedure(s): _____

11

The patient is a 100-year-old woman (a retired teacher) who was admitted to the hospital for further management of her congestive heart failure. The patient, who lives with her 82-year-old son in a single family home, has been remarkably well in spite of her advanced age. Six months ago she was admitted to the hospital, was found to be in congestive heart failure with chronic respiratory failure, and became oxygen dependent. The heart failure was described as chronic combined systolic and diastolic type. These conditions continue to be present. Her son states that the patient has been sleeping more and has less energy. A couple of days ago she fell while getting up from the bedside commode in her bedroom but insisted she was fine. Her son noticed her left wrist was slightly swollen and bruised. The patient has been treated for hypertension for many years and has a history of urinary tract infections. During this admission, she was found to have another urinary tract infection and was treated for it. She was continued on oxygen, and her hypertension and congestive heart failure medications were adjusted. An x-ray of the wrist showed a minimally angulated fracture involving the left distal radius. The wrist was placed in a splint for support. On day 2 of the hospital stay, the patient was noticeably weaker, in mild respiratory distress, and sleeping almost continually. Whenever she was attended to by the nurses, doctors, or her son, she asked them to "just let me be." The patient and her son were offered the services of hospice care and accepted. Within 48 hours of receiving supportive and comfort care, the patient died peacefully in her sleep.

Principal Diagnosis: _____

Secondary Diagnoses: _____

Principal Procedure: _____

Secondary Procedure(s): _____

12

The patient is a 35-year-old man who drove himself to the Emergency Room early in the morning because he had chest pain. The patient had been gambling in a casino overnight, drinking alcohol, and snorting cocaine as well as smoking cigarettes. As the night progressed, the patient became aware of chest discomfort that advanced to chest pain. He had had chest pain on previous occasions, but this time it lasted longer and was more severe. He became scared and came to the ER. The patient does not have a family physician but does see a psychiatrist intermittently for his bipolar I disorder and is taking Lamictal 100 mg daily for this condition. The patient was admitted after the EKG was found to be abnormal and the patient's troponin lab values were found to be elevated. The admitting diagnosis was rule out myocardial infarction. Cardiology consultation was obtained. During his hospital stay the patient was monitored on cardiac telemetry, and the myocardial infarction was ruled out. A chest x-ray showed evidence of bilateral basilar pneumonia. He did have subsequent episodes of chest pain but refused further cardiac workup and insisted on being discharged on day 3. The family practice physician assigned to the patient provided the following final diagnoses: Angina, cocaine addiction, alcohol abuse, tobacco dependence, pneumonia, and bipolar I disorder. The patient was given instructions to call the physician's office for an appointment within 1 week.

Principal Diagnosis: _____

Secondary Diagnoses: _____

Principal Procedure: _____

Secondary Procedure(s): _____

13

The physician went to the nursing home to see his 83-year-old male patient who was complaining of difficulty breathing and fatigue. The patient was known to have congestive heart failure. The physician diagnosed the patient as having chronic congestive diastolic heart failure and ordered new medications. He instructed the nurses at the nursing home to closely monitor the patient and notify him if the patient's symptoms worsened because the patient may have to be admitted to the hospital for treatment if that occurred.

Principal (Nursing Home) Diagnosis: _____

Secondary Diagnoses: _____

14

The same patient described in question 13, an 83-year-old male resident of a nursing home, developed more significant shortness of breath, increased edema in his legs, and chest pain during the two days after the physician had evaluated the patient in the nursing home. The patient was admitted to the hospital and treated for acute on chronic congestive diastolic heart failure. In addition, the patient continued to receive treatment for his hypertension and type 2 diabetes with peripheral neuropathy. The patient improved with treatments and was transferred to a skilled nursing facility for further recovery.

Principal Diagnosis: _____

Secondary Diagnoses: _____

Principal Procedure: _____

Secondary Procedure(s): _____

15

The patient is a 62-year-old man who was initially admitted to Hospital A and diagnosed with an acute ST elevation anterolateral wall myocardial infarction (STEMI). He had a cardiac catheterization done at Hospital A with the findings of native vessel coronary artery disease in four vessels. The patient's condition was stabilized, and the patient elected to be transferred to a larger hospital for recommended angioplasty and coronary artery stenting. Records and films were transferred with the patient directly to Hospital B for admission. At Hospital B, the patient had percutaneous transluminal angioplasty of three vessels with coronary artery disease. In addition, two non-drug-eluting stents were inserted into two coronary arteries. The patient had an uncomplicated recovery and was scheduled to begin the cardiac rehabilitation program in four weeks. Code for Hospital B.

Principal Diagnosis: _____

Secondary Diagnoses: _____

Principal Procedure: _____

Secondary Procedure(s): _____

16

A 65-year-old man with a history of hypertension was admitted to the hospital through the emergency department with progressive episodes of angina while watching political talk shows on the television. His admission diagnoses were severe angina pectoris, rule out both myocardial infarction and coronary artery disease. His History and Physical report noted that he had experienced episodes of angina pectoris in the past but always refused any diagnostic cardiology workup or procedure, consenting only to an EKG that was performed last year in his physician's office. The EKG showed no abnormalities. He was compliant with taking medication for essential hypertension. The workup in this hospital for this encounter did not reveal a myocardial infarction, but because of the severity of his anginal symptoms the patient was advised to have a cardiac catheterization and possible angioplasty, to which he consented. The patient was taken to the cardiac catheterization laboratory, where he had a left heart catheterization, left ventriculogram, and arteriography of multiple coronary arteries performed using the double catheter technique (Judkins) under fluoroscopy using high osmolar contrast.

He was found to have severe three-vessel coronary artery disease as the etiology of his angina pectoris. Because of the extent of the patient's coronary artery disease, angioplasty was not performed, and the patient was transferred to another hospital for possible coronary artery bypass graft surgery.

Principal Diagnosis: _____

Secondary Diagnoses: _____

Principal Procedure: _____

Secondary Procedure(s): _____

17

HISTORY: The patient is a 50-year-old female who was transferred for admission to this academic medical center from a community hospital. She was admitted to the community hospital for a coronary angiogram. The angiogram findings noted an ejection fraction of 30–35% with global dyskinesia. The echocardiogram revealed severe aortic valve stenosis and moderate mitral valve regurgitation. The patient is also known to have hypertensive kidney disease with end-stage renal disease (ESRD) requiring dialysis. She also has anemia of chronic disease (ESRD) and dyslipidemia. The patient also has a history of hepatitis C. Because the aortic stenosis and mitral regurgitation has caused significant chronic diastolic heart failure and congestive heart failure, the patient agreed to open heart surgery. The procedures performed at the academic medical center are aortic valve replacement with 19-mm tissue valve, mitral valve annuloplasty with 3-mm annuloplasty ring, left radial artery cutdown for arterial line insertion, Swan-Ganz catheter insertion, and cardiopulmonary bypass.

DESCRIPTION OF PROCEDURE: After detailed and informed consent was signed, the patient was brought to the operating room and placed supine on the operating table. General anesthesia was initiated and endotracheal intubation performed. Left radial artery cutdown was performed. She was prepped and draped in the usual sterile fashion. A Swan-Ganz catheter was placed via the left subclavian vein. A sternotomy was performed. The patient was heparinized. A standard cannulation was performed with arterial cannula in the ascending aorta and a single dual-stage venous cannula via the right atrial appendage. Antegrade cardioplegia catheter was inserted. Aortic cross clamp was applied, she was placed on the bypass pump, and the heart arrested. The aorta was opened. The patient had a calcified tricuspid valve. The aortic valve leaflets were excised and passed off the field. We then opened the left atrium. The echo had shown a central jet. The mitral valve sized to a 30-mm ring, and a 30-mm CG annuloplasty ring was sewn in place. The area was closed with running 4-0 Prolene. We then sized the aorta (valve) annulus to 19 mm and a Magna bioprosthesis tissue graft valve was sewn in with interrupted simple sutures. Once the valve was in, the aortotomy was closed with running 2 layers of 4-0 Prolene. De-airing was performed through this aortotomy. The aortic cross clamp was removed. Once the patient was warmed, ventricular pacing wires were placed. Ventilation was begun, and the patient was weaned from bypass. Protamine was administered. All cannulae were removed and hemostasis ensured. Two 32-French chest tubes were placed. The sternum was closed with four figure-of-8 sternal wires, and the soft tissue was closed in 3 layers. The patient was taken to the adult cardiovascular intensive care unit in stable condition.

Principal Diagnosis: _____

Secondary Diagnoses: _____

Principal Procedure: _____

Secondary Procedure(s): _____

18

A 82-year-old man was admitted to inpatient care through the emergency department with severe heart failure after complaining of fatigue and increasing difficulty in breathing. He also had type 2 diabetes mellitus that had been controlled by oral medications. During his stay, he was given insulin to control his blood sugar during this severe illness. He also had hypertension that was monitored and treated with oral medications. The physician described the type of heart failure this patient has as "acute on chronic systolic heart failure."

Principal Diagnosis: _____

Secondary Diagnoses: _____

Principal Procedure: _____

Secondary Procedure(s): _____

19

A 55-year-old female patient was admitted to her local community hospital with pre-infarction angina. She underwent a combined right and left heart cardiac catheterization with coronary angiography, Judkins technique, and was determined to have significant atherosclerotic heart disease. Triple coronary artery bypass graft (CABG) surgery was recommended for the 80% to 90% occlusion found in three native coronary vessels. The patient was an active cigarette smoker, documented as nicotine dependent. With counseling and upon consent, the patient was transferred to a medical center licensed to perform open heart surgery, and scheduled for the CABG. A triple coronary artery bypass graft, using the left greater saphenous vein harvested through an open approach, was performed on the left anterior descending, the circumflex, and the diagonal arteries. The origin of the bypass was the aorta. This was done using extracorporeal circulation while the patient was placed on cardiopulmonary bypass for the duration of the procedure, six hours. The final diagnosis documented by the provider at the medical center was triple vessel coronary artery disease, unstable angina, no myocardial infarction. Smoking cessation was strongly advised.

Principal Diagnosis: _____

Secondary Diagnoses: _____

Principal Procedure: _____

Secondary Procedure(s): _____

20

This 85-year-old man was brought to the emergency department by his family because of right-sided temporary blindness that lasted only a few minutes on one day but then occurred two more times on different days. The patient was admitted with a diagnosis of transient monocular blindness. The physician described his condition as a unilateral temporary blindness, also known as amaurosis fugax. After study, the physician documented that the underlying cause of the amaurosis fugax was carotid artery stenosis. As documented in the record, the physician explained to the patient that transient ischemia resulting from carotid artery disease affects the optic nerve and the retina and causes blindness. This may be seen as a warning of internal carotid disease. Carotid arteriography (plain radiography, no contrast) confirmed the presence of carotid artery stenosis and occlusion of both carotid arteries. The left carotid stenosis and occlusion was minor. The right carotid stenosis and occlusion was significant and thought to be the cause of the patient's symptoms. The patient consented to a percutaneous endoscopic right internal carotid endarterectomy and was discharged the next day in good condition.

Principal Diagnosis: _____

Secondary Diagnoses: _____

Principal Procedure: _____

Secondary Procedure(s): _____

21

The 80-year-old female patient is seen in the neurology clinic at the request of her family physician for assessment of her aphasia due to her past stroke. The patient has facial weakness due to her past stroke that is also evaluated during the visit.

First-Listed Diagnosis: _____

Secondary Diagnoses: _____

22

The 57-year-old male patient is a resident of a long-term care facility after suffering a stroke 2 months previously, with bilateral quadriplegia as a result. The patient is being discharged from this facility to be readmitted to another long-term care facility that specializes in the type of care the patient requires for his paralytic syndrome.

Principal (Nursing Home) Diagnosis: _____

Secondary Diagnoses: _____

Principal Procedure: _____

Secondary Procedure(s): _____

23

The patient is a 77-year-old female who is a resident of a nursing home. She had a stroke 10 months ago and since that time has had several seizures that have been determined to be a consequence of her stroke. None of the seizures has been very significant, but the patient has been placed on anticonvulsant medication. Her doctor wrote in the last progress note documenting his visit the diagnosis of "Patient stable, seizure disorder over the last 9 months, due to her previous stroke."

Principal (Nursing Home) Diagnosis: _____

Secondary Diagnoses: _____

Principal Procedure: _____

Secondary Procedure(s): _____

24

A patient who had a stroke seven months ago was admitted to the hospital for a surgical tendon transfer on his left hand. The patient acquired a contracture of the left hand as a result of the stroke. Otherwise the patient had recovered well from the stroke. During the hospital stay the orthopedic surgeon performed an open hand tendon transfer with no complications, and the patient was discharged from the hospital on the day after surgery. The patient also had two chronic conditions managed while in the hospital: essential hypertension and simple chronic bronchitis. The patient was discharged with instructions for postoperative care including a follow-up appointment in the orthopedic surgeon's office in 5 days.

Principal Diagnosis: _____

Secondary Diagnoses: _____

Principal Procedure: _____

Secondary Procedure(s): _____

Chapter 10

Diseases of the Respiratory System

Coding Scenarios for *Basic ICD-10-CM/PCS Coding*

The following case studies are organized following the sequence of the chapters in the *ICD-10-CM and ICD-10-PCS* code books. The objective of this book is to provide the student with more detailed clinical information to code, rather than one- or two-line diagnosis and procedure statements. ICD-10-CM diagnosis codes are to be assigned to both the inpatient hospital admission and the outpatient visit case studies. In this book, the ICD-10-PCS procedure codes are to be assigned only to the inpatient hospital admission cases. In actual practice, outpatient cases are assigned CPT/HCPCS codes. The ICD-10-PCS codes are only required for inpatient procedures.

1

A 70-year-old male patient with long-standing chronic obstructive pulmonary disease (COPD) was admitted through the emergency department with increasing shortness of breath, weakness, and fatigue. His admitting diagnosis was acute respiratory insufficiency. Treatment included respiratory therapy and medications. It was confirmed with the patient that he has not resumed his 50-year history of smoking, and he was encouraged to remain smoke-free. The final diagnoses written by the physician was acute respiratory insufficiency due to acute exacerbation of COPD. History of smoking.

Principal Diagnosis: _____

Secondary Diagnoses: _____

Principal Procedure: _____

Secondary Procedure(s): _____

2

An 80-year-old female patient from a nursing home was admitted to the hospital with symptoms of weakness, coughing, shortness of breath, and mental status changes. Swallowing studies revealed she had difficulty swallowing and easily aspirated particles into her respiratory tract. It was determined that she suffered from aspiration pneumonia. She also was found to have a superimposed bacterial pneumonia. Both conditions were treated with intravenous antibiotics, and the patient's condition improved. She was transferred back to the long-term care facility for care.

Principal Diagnosis: _____

Secondary Diagnoses: _____ .

Principal Procedure: _____

Secondary Procedure(s): _____

3

A 10-year-old boy was treated in the allergist's office for childhood asthma. He was treated for his allergic rhinitis due to pollen and animal dander with his asthma. The patient's conditions were well controlled with his current medications.

First-Listed Diagnosis: _____

Secondary Diagnoses: _____

4

A bilateral tonsillectomy and adenoidectomy was performed on a 9-year-old patient to resolve his recurring infections due to adenotonsillar hyperplasia. No infection was present at the time of the surgery. The patient was admitted as an inpatient for an overnight stay.

Principal Diagnosis: _____

Secondary Diagnoses: _____

Principal Procedure: _____

Secondary Procedure(s): _____

5

The patient is a 65-year-old man who is receiving chemotherapy for multiple myeloma from an oncologist on staff at this hospital. The patient came to the emergency department stating he had a cough, fever, chills, and felt extremely weak. The patient was admitted. The chest x-ray at the time of admission showed evidence of pneumonia in the left lower lobe. During the hospitalization, the patient received respiratory therapy treatments, intravenous antibiotics, and supportive care. His chemistry profiles showed an abnormal BUN and glucose. Cultures of the sputum showed no pathologic organism. Blood cultures were negative. The patient's hemogram was abnormal with a hemoglobin of 9.3, hematocrit of 27, white blood cell count of 3,200 and platelets 126,000. A repeat CBC showed the hemogram had dropped to 7.5 with the hematocrit at 22. There was no evidence of GI or other source of bleeding. His oncologist also followed his care during the hospital stay and determined the pancytopenia shown on the CBC was a result of the chemotherapy the patient was receiving. For this reason, the patient was given two units of nonautologous packed red blood cells via the patient's existing IV line in his peripheral vein. Follow-up CBC test showed hemoglobin at 9.6 and hematocrit at 28.

Follow-up chest x-ray showed significant clearing of the pneumonic process. The patient was switched to oral antibiotics at the time of discharge and given a prescription to continue taking both antibiotics for another week. The patient appeared significantly depressed, and this was discussed with him. A psychiatric consultation and possible medications were recommended, which the patient refused. The patient has a follow-up appointment with his oncologist and with the private physician within the next 10 days.

Principal Diagnosis: _____

Secondary Diagnoses: _____

Principal Procedure: _____

Secondary Procedure(s): _____

6

The patient is a 45-year-old man who comes to the physician's office for his 3-month follow-up visit for asthma. He is using a bronchodilator and steroid for control of his asthma. He is having no problems with the asthma at this time. He denies a change in cough and reports no increase in shortness of breath, no fluid retention, and no increase in wheezing. He is taking his medication regularly and not missing any doses. Upon physical examination, the lungs are clear with decreased breath sounds in both lung fields, heart is regular rhythm with no murmurs, and extremities are free of edema. Oximetry and pulmonary function tests have not changed since the last visit. The patient's diagnosis is stable asthma, on long-term systemic steroid therapy. The patient was advised to continue his present medications and return for a follow-up visit in 3 months.

First-Listed Diagnosis: _____

Secondary Diagnoses: _____

7

The patient is a 19-year-old man who comes to the physician's office complaining of a sore throat with fever for the past 4 days with pain in his right ear. He has difficulty swallowing and has been taking Tylenol for fever and throat lozenges for the sore throat. He feels weaker today. He has no known allergies. Physical examination showed the tonsillar arch reddened with tonsillar exudates. There are enlarged anterior cervical lymph nodes. The examination of the ears showed acute suppurative otitis media in both ears, but worse in the right ear.

A rapid strep screening test was positive. The diagnoses given were (1) possible early tonsillar abscess, (2) strep pharyngitis, and (3) acute suppurative otitis media. The patient was given an injection of antibiotics and a prescription for an antibiotic to be taken for the next 10 days.

First-Listed Diagnosis: _____

Secondary Diagnoses: _____

8

A physician in private practice admitted this patient to the hospital. The patient is a 78-year-old woman who has coronary artery disease and is status post coronary artery bypass graft 8 years ago. She is also under treatment for hypertension and mild congestive heart failure. The patient was admitted at this time for shortness of breath starting 2 days prior to admission and worse on the day of admission. She complained of wheezing and cough productive of white sputum. She thought she had a mild fever this morning but was afebrile on admission. She had no chills, nausea, or vomiting. Her paroxysmal nocturnal dyspnea and orthopnea remain unchanged. Physical examination showed the patient to be in mild distress but alert and oriented. Her blood pressure was 150/70 mm Hg, heart rate 70, and respiratory rate 16. Cardiovascular system examination revealed regular rate and rhythm. Lungs had poor air entry, and patient was wheezing. Abdomen was soft, nontender. The extremities were 2+ edema bilaterally. Neurologically, her left upper extremity and left lower extremity have weakness as the result of a CVA 2 years ago. The patient was admitted with COPD acute exacerbation. She responded well to respiratory therapy treatments and intravenous medications. She was discharged home with the following prescriptions: Prednisone, aspirin enteric-coated tablet, Albuterol inhaler, Persantine, Captopril, Theophylline, Diltiazem, Nitro paste, Lasix, and Digoxin. She will be seen in the office in 5 days. Discharge diagnoses are acute and chronic bronchitis/COPD, hypertension, CAD, status post CABG, CHF, old CVA with weakness/hemiparesis, left side in a right-handed woman.

Principal Diagnosis: _____

Secondary Diagnoses: _____

Principal Procedure: _____

Secondary Procedure(s): _____

9

The patient is a 9-year-old boy who is brought to the pediatrician's office by his mother because of the following: runny nose, fever, yellow discharge from the nose, swelling around the eyes, and tenderness in the cheeks. The child is snoring during sleep. The mother had given the child Children's Tylenol. Physical examination confirmed most of the subjective complaints and detected fluid in the sinuses. A prescription was given for 14-day oral antibiotic treatment and the doctor recommended continued use of Children's Tylenol for fever. The doctor concluded the child had acute sinusitis in the frontal and maxillary sinuses.

First-Listed Diagnosis: _____

Secondary Diagnoses: _____

10

A 62-year-old woman, on disability because of emphysema, is brought to the emergency department from home by fire department ambulance. The patient complained of sudden sharp chest pain, shortness of breath, and a nonproductive hacking cough. The patient has been under treatment for COPD and emphysema for more than 5 years and is dependent on oxygen. The patient described the pain as being on the left side with referred pain up to the shoulder. The patient was cautious when moving to protect her chest and shoulder. In the emergency department a chest x-ray and continuous pulse oximetry was ordered. Pulse oximetry showed low oxygen saturation. Physical examination revealed diminished breath sounds bilaterally, but significantly worse on the left side. The chest x-ray revealed a collapsed lung on the left side and fluid in the pleural space. The patient was admitted. A chest tube was inserted for pleural drainage and aspirate air and re-expand the lung. Follow-up chest x-ray showed the lung had re-expanded to its normal size, and the pleural effusion's fluid appeared to be reabsorbed and resolved. The physician's discharge diagnoses were COPD and emphysema with left side secondary spontaneous pneumothorax and pleural effusion.

Principal Diagnosis: _____

Secondary Diagnoses: _____

Principal Procedure: _____

Secondary Procedure(s): _____

11

The patient is a 50-year-old female with known systemic lupus erythematosus with nephritis. Her renal function has been worsening over the past several months. Today the patient came to the emergency room complaining of pain in her chest that was worse when she coughed or took a deep breath. The ER physician heard a "friction rub," but a chest x-ray did not show any pleural effusion. The patient was admitted to the hospital. It was determined that the patient had pleurisy, but it was uncertain if it was related to her lupus. The patient also had diarrhea, dehydration with hyponatremia, hypokalemia, and azotemia. Intravenous fluids and medications were administered to correct her metabolic disorders, diarrhea, relieve the pain of the pleurisy, and treat her worsening renal function.

Principal Diagnosis: _____

Secondary Diagnoses: _____

Principal Procedure: _____

Secondary Procedure(s): _____

12

The patient is an 89-year-old man with advanced COPD who was admitted to the hospital complaining of cough, shortness of breath, and fever. It was determined that he was suffering from COPD with acute bronchitis. He is supplemental oxygen dependent and also has cor pulmonale. He was treated with bronchodilators, antibiotics, and a tapering dose of steroids. The patient was on "do not resuscitate" (DNR) status. The patient was becoming progressively weaker with more respiratory distress. During this hospital stay, the family members decided to initiate comfort care measures after speaking with the physician about the patient's prognosis. The family elected to receive hospice care and took the patient home to receive home end-of-life and comfort care.

Principal Diagnosis: _____

Secondary Diagnoses: _____

Principal Procedure: _____

Secondary Procedure(s): _____

13

A 5-year-old male was brought to the emergency room by his mother who gave the patient's history of having a 2-day history of increasing lethargy, decreased appetite, and vomiting. The mother stated the child's sister had similar symptoms and was seen in the doctor's office and diagnosed with viral syndrome during the past week. A physical examination and laboratory tests were performed on the 5-year-old male that showed evidence of dehydration and decreased breath sounds. A chest x-ray showed some diffuse areas in the right lower lobe possibly involving pneumonia. The patient was admitted with an admitting diagnosis of dehydration and possible pneumonia of a viral or bacterial type. During the hospital stay the child received IV antibiotics and fluids to treat the infection and dehydration. Within 12 hours the child became alert, active, and back to normal per his mother. He was given a clear liquid diet and later wanted more to eat, with no vomiting reported. Repeat chemistry, hematology, and urinalysis lab tests were repeated the following morning and showed results back to normal. The child was discharged to his mother's care on day 2 with a follow-up appointment made in the primary care physician's office for day 5. The physician's conclusion on the discharge summary written the day of discharge was "pneumonia, possibly viral origin, complicated by dehydration."

Principal Diagnosis: _____

Secondary Diagnoses: _____

Principal Procedure: _____

Secondary Procedure(s): _____

14

The patient was a 59-year-old man brought to the emergency room by ambulance with increasing shortness of breath and worsening color. The patient was mottled below the knees. Due to shortness of breath, the patient was not able to give any history in the emergency room before his family arrived. When they arrived, his family reported that he had become more lethargic at home over the past 24 hours. The patient had been a smoker for 45 years and had continued to smoke until one week ago. He had chronic obstructive asthma that was steroid dependent for many years and developed steroid-induced diabetes in the past 5 years. He was diagnosed with status asthmaticus upon admission. He was able to work up until the age of 55, when he received disability retirement benefits from his company and Social Security because of his poor health. Since his retirement he was also diagnosed with congestive heart failure. A month ago he was found to have a large left chest mass when a chest CT exam was performed because of an increasing cough. After this finding was described to him, he refused any further workup and signed an advance directive that specified no heroic efforts in his final days. After admission, an order was written for "no code" per his advance directive, but the patient did allow respiratory therapy and intravenous medications for his heart and lung disease. Over the next 24 hours he seemed to improve with the breathing treatments of Solu-Medrol and Lasix, but his pulse oximetry was rarely above 80% without an oxygen mask. A portable chest x-ray showed his left lower lobe obstructing mass, larger than imaged one month ago, and pneumonia. Testing proved it to be pneumonia due to pseudomonas aeruginosa. His blood sugars improved, and he appeared to be stabilizing much to the surprise of his family and physicians. He had brief periods of alertness and was able to converse with his family and eat small meals. However, the evening before his passing, palliative care orders were written to make him as comfortable as possible, as his lung function was worsening again. Early in the morning of the third day he became unresponsive and then was noted to be without respirations or pulse at 0130. His wife and son were at his bedside when he was pronounced dead by the hospitalist on duty. His final diagnoses included pneumonia due to pseudomonas, systemic therapy steroid-dependent asthma in status asthmaticus, steroid-induced diabetes, large left lung mass, congestive heart failure, and respiratory failure—all probably related to his tobacco dependence. No autopsy was performed.

Principal Diagnosis: _____

Secondary Diagnoses: _____

Principal Procedure: _____

Secondary Procedure(s): _____

15

The patient, a 60-year-old man, was taken to the emergency room of a local hospital from a wedding reception after he developed symptoms of shortness of breath and chest pain. He also reported that he felt very tired after traveling to this city for the wedding and has learned he cannot tolerate as much walking as he had even one month ago. The patient knew he had lung cancer. The ER physician contacted his family physician, who told him the patient had small cell carcinoma of the left upper lobe of the lung, diagnosed 14 months ago, and he had been followed for possible malignant pleural effusion that resolved without treatment 3 months ago. The patient was admitted to the hospital and examined by an oncologist and cardiologist. After several tests were performed, it was determined the patient had exudative pleural effusion, which the oncologist referred to as "malignant pleural effusion of the left lung." The cardiologist performed a therapeutic thoracentesis that provided immediate relief. The patient rested in the hospital for one more day and was discharged to the care of his family. The physicians advised the patient to rest at least 2 more days in this city before driving 250 miles with his family back to his hometown. Records were given to the patient to take to his oncologist at home.

Principal Diagnosis: _____

Secondary Diagnoses: _____

Principal Procedure: _____

Secondary Procedure(s): _____

16

HISTORY: The patient is a 75-year-old man with stage IV gastroesophageal junction carcinoma. He developed severe respiratory distress and was brought to the hospital emergency department and admitted. A large left pleural effusion was noted on CT scan and chest x-ray. His condition progressed to acute hypoxic respiratory failure, and he required intubation and mechanical ventilation for 25 hours. A chest tube insertion was recommended to relieve the patient's hypoxic respiratory failure caused by the left pleural effusion, and the patient consented to the procedure.

DESCRIPTION OF PROCEDURE: The patient was placed in the supine position in the medical intensive care unit on propofol drip. His left anterior chest was prepped and draped. One percent plain Xylocaine was given, and a small incision was made. Using the hemostat, the chest cavity was entered and fluid was returned. Then, using the trocar, the chest tube was placed in the superior portion of the left upper lobe. There was approximately 1,000 mL of fluid returned. The patient tolerated the procedure well, and the chest tube was sewn in place. A follow-up chest x-ray confirmed good positioning of the tube, and a decrease in the amount of pleural effusion was noted. Cytology examination of the pleural fluid did not show malignant cells.

Principal Diagnosis: _____

Secondary Diagnoses: _____

Principal Procedure: _____

Secondary Procedure(s): _____

17

An 80-year-old man who has been a long-term nursing home resident with chronic obstructive pulmonary disease (COPD) was admitted to the hospital by his primary care physician with shortness of breath, elevated white blood count, and bibasilar infiltrates. A pulmonary disease consultant agreed with the attending physician that the patient had aspiration pneumonia and acute respiratory failure, both present on admission. In addition, the pulmonologist describes the man's COPD as obstructive chronic bronchitis with exacerbation. The patient had an Advance Directive that indicated he did not want to be placed on a ventilator. Intravenous antibiotics were administered, and the patient agreed to be placed on intermittent positive airway pressure for 48 hours. Fortunately, appropriate treatment was able to control the conditions quickly, and the patient was taken to a skilled nursing facility for extended recovery from the aspiration pneumonia and respiratory failure.

Given the fact that the patient had symptoms of three conditions (chronic lung disease, aspiration pneumonia, and respiratory failure) all present on admission, and any could have been the reason after study for the admission to the hospital, the coder asked the attending physician's assistance in identifying the principal diagnosis as determined by the circumstances of admission, the diagnostic workup, and/or therapy provided. The physician chose the aspiration pneumonia as patient's principal diagnosis, as it was one of the main reasons for the admission and required the greatest intensity of care and use of resources. According to the doctor, the respiratory failure was suspected to have resulted from either the aspiration pneumonia or the worsening chronic lung disease affected by the aspiration pneumonia.

Principal Diagnosis: _____

Secondary Diagnoses: _____

Principal Procedure: _____

Secondary Procedure(s): _____

18

This was the first admission to a long-term acute care hospital (LTACH) for the 45-year-old male patient who was unconscious and respiratory dependent because of his chronic respiratory failure. He acquired the respiratory failure after suffering a multi-drug overdose 2 weeks ago. According to his family, it was believed the patient was addicted to multiple illegal drugs but exactly which drugs was unknown. The patient had a tracheostomy in place for connection to the mechanical ventilator. The patient is admitted to the LTACH for managing his respiratory failure and possibly weaning from mechanical ventilation. All attempts to wean the patient from the ventilator were unsuccessful. After 30 days in the LTACH, the patient was transferred to a long-term care ventilator unit at a skilled nursing facility for further care. His final diagnoses were noted to be chronic respiratory failure from multiple drug overdose, polysubstance dependence, ventilator dependency, and tracheostomy status. He remained on the ventilator the entire time he was in the LTACH.

Principal Diagnosis: _____

Secondary Diagnoses: _____

Principal Procedure: _____

Secondary Procedure(s): _____

Chapter 11

Diseases of the Digestive System

Coding Scenarios for *Basic ICD-10-CM/PCS Coding*

The following case studies are organized following the sequence of the chapters in the *ICD-10-CM and ICD-10-PCS* code books. The objective of this book is to provide the student with more detailed clinical information to code, rather than one- or two-line diagnosis and procedure statements. ICD-10-CM diagnosis codes are to be assigned to both the inpatient hospital admission and the outpatient visit case studies. In this book, the ICD-10-PCS procedure codes are to be assigned only to the inpatient hospital admission cases. In actual practice, outpatient cases are assigned CPT/HCPCS codes. The ICD-10-PCS codes are only required for inpatient procedures.

1

A 40-year-old woman has been treated for symptoms of gallstones without improvement. The patient also was known to have chronic cholecystitis. She was admitted for a laparoscopic cholecystectomy. After the laparoscopy procedure was started, the physician stated the gallbladder could be visualized but could not be removed. The procedure was converted to an open procedure and the gallbladder was removed. The pathology report confirmed the preoperative diagnosis of chronic cholecystitis with cholelithiasis.

Principal Diagnosis: _____

Secondary Diagnoses: _____

Principal Procedure: _____

Secondary Procedure(s): _____

2

A 30-year-old woman has been treated for Crohn disease of the small intestine since 18 years of age. She has had several exacerbations of the disease over the past years. At this time, the patient comes to the emergency department in extreme pain. A small bowel x-ray shows a small bowel obstruction. The patient was admitted to the hospital. Later the obstruction was found to be a result of mural thickening. The patient is taken to surgery and a partial resection of the terminal ileum is performed to release the obstruction. An end-to-end anastomosis is performed to close the small intestine. The patient was also noted to have flat, firm, hot, and red painful small lumps on the shins of both legs. Consultation with the wound-care physician determined the ulcers to be erythema nodosum, a known complication of Crohn disease. The wound care physician prescribed oral and topical medications.

Principal Diagnosis: _____

Secondary Diagnoses: _____

Principal Procedure: _____

Secondary Procedure(s): _____

3

A 68-year-old man was admitted to the hospital for an inguinal hernia repair that could not be done on an outpatient basis because of anticipated extended recovery time required due to his other medical conditions. After being prepared for surgery and taken to the operating room, the patient complained of precordial chest pain. The surgery was cancelled, and the patient was returned to his room. Cardiac studies failed to find a reason for the chest pain, which resolved the same day. The patient's medications for his hypertension and COPD were also given.

Principal Diagnosis: _____

Secondary Diagnoses: _____

Principal Procedure: _____

Secondary Procedure(s): _____

4

A 70-year-old man who lives in another city and was visiting relatives in the area was brought to the emergency department by family members. The patient complained of vomiting blood and having very dark stools that appeared to have blood in them as well. The patient had gone out to dinner with relatives for a prime rib dinner. After he came home, he started vomiting and having diarrhea and blamed it on the large meal. He continued to have these symptoms overnight, and his family members insisted he come to the emergency department. The patient was admitted. The patient is taking Prinivil, Lanoxin, and Lasix for congestive heart failure and atrial fibrillation, and these medications were continued during the hospital stay. The gastroenterologist was called for a consultation and saw the patient. The patient agreed to an upper and lower GI endoscopic examination. The esophagogastroduodenoscopy (EGD) examination included a biopsy and cauterization of a gastric polyp and a biopsy of a pyloric ulcer. The findings of the EGD, confirmed by pathologic studies, were hiatal hernia, acute gastritis with bacteria determined to be helicobacter, gastric polyp, and a chronic deep pyloric ulceration. Hemorrhage was noted in the stomach, coming from the gastritis and the ulcer. The colonoscopy included a cecal polyp at 80 cm that was removed with a hot biopsy forceps. Extensive diverticulosis was present but no areas of bleeding were seen. The attending physician agreed with the findings of the endoscopic examination as reasonable explanations for the patient's symptoms. The serial blood counts did not find any significant anemia. The patient was discharged and given prescriptions and copies of his medical records to take home for his private physician to review.

Principal Diagnosis: _____

Secondary Diagnoses: _____

Principal Procedure: _____

Secondary Procedure(s): _____

5

The patient is an 81-year-old woman who was admitted to the hospital for intractable emesis, near syncope, and extreme weakness and fatigue. The patient had been in the hospital 2 weeks previously for pneumonia, which was treated at that time. A visit in the physician's office 5 days ago revealed the pneumonia to be resolving. During this hospital stay it was determined the patient had a nonspecific form of gastroenteritis with resulting dehydration. Because the patient had multiple conditions, the physician was queried as to what was the main reason for admission after study, and she stated it was the gastroenteritis. The patient is also known to have a hiatal hernia and reflux esophagitis, which were treated with her usual medications. A chest x-ray still showed the pneumonia to be present, and she was continued on oral antibiotics. The patient was discharged home to continue taking oral antibiotics and usual other medications.

Principal Diagnosis: _____

Secondary Diagnoses: _____

Principal Procedure: _____

Secondary Procedure(s): _____

6

A 75-year-old man was admitted to the hospital after coming to the emergency department after having a black melanotic stool the day before and on the day of admission. He had no pain, nausea, or vomiting but felt a little "light-headed." Testing in the emergency department found grossly guaiac positive stools. His admitting diagnosis was gastrointestinal bleeding. The patient has an extensive past medical and surgical history including:

1. Coronary artery bypass graft 7 years ago after a myocardial infarction with no symptoms today, but takes one baby aspirin a day

2. Recurrent deep vein thrombosis of lower extremity and recurrent pulmonary emboli; currently taking Coumadin to prevent recurrence

3. History of congestive heart failure; currently taking Lanoxin and Dyazide

4. History of arthritis; currently taking Tolectin

5. History of hyperlipidemia; currently taking Lescol

6. Suspected carcinoma of the pancreas with an exploratory laparotomy 5 years ago that only proved pancreatitis to be present, no malignancy

7. Appendectomy, colon resection done years before for what sounds like a bowel obstruction and stomach surgery for what the patient calls a "blockage"

8. Large ventral hernia related to his left upper quadrant abdominal incision from past surgery, which is of no consequence at this time

During this hospital stay, he was given intravenous medications, vitamin K injection, and two units of nonautologous, fresh plasma through his IV via the peripheral vein to reverse the effects of the Coumadin. Serial CBCs were done, which showed marginally low hemoglobin and hematocrit but nothing requiring treatment for anemia. An EGD was performed by the gastroenterologist, who documented a hiatal hernia with reflux esophagitis, a bleeding proximal jejunal ulcer, and evidence of a past gastrojejunostomy. The EGD was simply diagnostic; no biopsies were taken. The private physician used the diagnoses from the EGD and from the past medical and surgical history as the final diagnoses for the case. The patient continued to receive all of his medications while in the hospital and was discharged home for follow-up in the physician's office in 1 week.

Principal Diagnosis: _____

Secondary Diagnoses: _____

Principal Procedure: _____

Secondary Procedure(s): _____

7

A 60-year-old man was acutely ill when admitted to the hospital for hematemesis. After study, the upper gastrointestinal (GI) bleeding was found to be due to a gastric varix that was caused by alcoholic cirrhosis of the liver and acute alcoholic hepatitis. The patient was known to have long-term chronic alcoholism with which he continues to struggle. The patient was also found to have esophageal varices, but these were not bleeding at this time. The surgery performed was the creation of a transjugular intrahepatic portosystemic (venous) shunt (TIPS) performed in the radiology suite. A shunt was passed down via the jugular vein and was inserted between the portal and hepatic veins within the liver to establish communication between these two veins.

The patient was discharged to a skilled nursing facility for surgical recovery and ongoing management of his serious GI diseases.

Principal Diagnosis: _____

Secondary Diagnoses: _____

Principal Procedure: _____

Secondary Procedure(s): _____

8

A 55-year-old man was admitted to the hospital through the emergency department for suspected gallstone pancreatitis. After study it was found the patient had acute pancreatitis, radiologic evidence of gallstones, and possibly stones in the common bile duct. The patient was taken to surgery for an open cholecystectomy and common duct exploration. It was confirmed the patient had chronic cholecystitis with cholelithiasis and choledocholithiasis with obstruction of the biliary system. The physician stated the acute pancreatitis was a consequence of the bile duct stones, but the main reason for the patient's admission to the hospital and the need for surgery were the gallstones and the bile duct stones. The patient had a slow but steady recovery from surgery and was able to return home for further convalescence.

Principal Diagnosis: _____

Secondary Diagnoses: _____

Principal Procedure: _____

Secondary Procedure(s): _____

9

A 40-year-old man was admitted to the hospital through the emergency department for acute abdominal pain. The patient appeared to have alcoholic intoxication. He was treated with nasogastric suction, IV fluids, and pain medications. The patient stated he was told by another physician at another hospital that he had chronic pancreatitis. The diagnosis of acute and chronic pancreatitis was made based on physical findings and laboratory and radiology test results. The patient stated he was supposed to take Dilantin for a "seizure disorder" but stopped taking them because his prescription ran out. He said he had not had a seizure in more than 1 year. A neurologist was consulted but declined to prescribe the Dilantin again, as the patient had no evidence of seizures while in the hospital. It was determined the patient did have chronic alcoholism. To prevent withdrawal, the patient was given multiple vitamins and mild tranquilizers and the patient did not experience alcohol withdrawal symptoms during his hospital stay. The patient was discharged and requested to come to the physician's office for follow-up in 5 days. The patient was advised to stop drinking and was referred to the outpatient substance abuse treatment center run by the hospital for counseling after discharge, which he agreed to visit.

Principal Diagnosis: _____

Secondary Diagnoses: _____

Principal Procedure: _____

Secondary Procedure(s): _____

10

The patient is a 25-year-old woman with moderate mental retardation who needs dental extractions for dental caries on the chewing surface of the tooth penetrating into the pulp and chronic apical periodontitis in three upper right teeth and three lower right teeth. Prior to surgery, the patient was instructed to stop the anticoagulant drug, Coumadin, she is taking and begin taking Lovenox instead. The patient has a history of mitral valve and aortic valve replacements and needs subacute bacterial endocarditis prophylaxis before the surgery. She is taking the anticoagulation therapy because of her past heart surgery. Because the patient needed to be monitored for therapeutic anticoagulant drug levels prior to surgery, she was admitted to the hospital. Management of the anticoagulation was completed in 2 days, and the patient had the surgical dental extractions of all six diseased teeth on day 3. The patient was allowed to return home on day 5 after the Coumadin was restarted on day 4 with no ill effects. The patient has follow-up appointments with the oral surgeon and the family physician in the next week.

Principal Diagnosis: _____

Secondary Diagnoses: _____

Principal Procedure: _____

Secondary Procedure(s): _____

11

The patient is an 84-year-old woman who was brought to the emergency department by her family upon the advice of the family physician. The patient said she had increasing abdominal pain, nausea, and some vomiting. This condition started 2–3 days ago, and the patient could not eat due to the nausea. Prior to this episode of illness, the patient had been reasonably well, receiving medications for hypertension and hypothyroidism. The patient was admitted. Overnight the patient appeared to become more acutely ill, developed respiratory distress, and the rapid response team evaluated her and obtained her physician's order to transfer her to the ICU. Soon after, the patient required intubation and mechanical ventilation for acute respiratory failure. The patient had signs and symptoms of septicemia and sepsis, possibly with an intra-abdominal source. Blood cultures grew E. coli. She was taken to the operating room, where she underwent an exploratory laparotomy. The surgeons found acute bowel ischemia and gangrene involving 100% of the small bowel and the right colon. This was an inoperable condition, and the laparotomy site was closed. The family was advised of the patient's very poor prognosis and offered hospice care, which they accepted. The mechanical ventilation was discontinued after 24 hours in place, and the patient was extubated. She was kept as comfortable as possible overnight and expired in the early morning hours of hospital day 4. The physician's final diagnoses were acute ischemic and gangrenous intestine, acute respiratory failure, E. coli septicemia, hypertension, and hypothyroidism.

Principal Diagnosis: _____

Secondary Diagnoses: _____

Principal Procedure: _____

Secondary Procedure(s): _____

12

A 39-year-old female patient was transferred from the long-term acute care hospital to the university hospital for admission. The patient had a four-day history of diffuse and worsening abdominal pain. The patient is ventilator dependent, with a tracheostomy in place for chronic respiratory failure, resulting from her severe dermatopolymyositis. She had evidence of sepsis and was later found to have E. coli septicemia with sepsis. She was taken to surgery with the preoperative diagnosis of acute abdomen with free intraperitoneal air. She was found to have a perforated transverse colon with intra-abdominal abscess. The tracheostomy was malfunctioning, too. The surgery performed was an exploratory laparotomy, an entire transverse colectomy with primary end-to-end anastomosis, loop ileostomy, drainage of the intra-abdominal (mesentery) abscess, and open revision of the tracheostomy. After a long stay in the intensive care unit and on the medical-surgical floor, the patient slowly recovered from this major illness. The patient remained on the ventilator for the entire 14-day hospital stay. She was transferred back to the long-term acute care hospital for extended recovery time.

Principal Diagnosis: _____

Secondary Diagnoses: _____

Principal Procedure: _____

Secondary Procedure(s): _____

13

The patient is a 59-year-old male who was referred to the gastroenterologist by his primary care physician for evaluation of abdominal pain and black stools. The patient said he had acid indigestion and heartburn for many years and took Tums and Pepto-Bismol on a daily basis. Over the past several days, he had been experiencing burning and cramping epigastric pain that was not relieved by the usual medications. He also had noted black tarry stools, which was a new problem for him. His primary care physician had placed the patient on Pepcid. The patient's mother had a history of peptic ulcer disease, but there were no other major illnesses in the family. The gastroenterologist recommended the patient have an upper GI endoscopy to further evaluate the source of the problem, and the patient consented. On an outpatient basis, the physician performed an esophagogastroduodenoscopy at the hospital. The findings included a normal-appearing esophagus. There was a large hiatal hernia pouch extending about 4 cm below the junction to the diaphragmatic closure. The stomach body, angulus, and antrum were normal. The pyloric channel was normal. There was one solitary erosion measuring 3–4 mm in the duodenal bulb, but there was no evidence of recent bleeding. The descending duodenum was normal. No biopsies were taken. The physician's conclusion at the end of the examination was (1) gastroesophageal reflux, (2) hiatal hernia, and (3) small chronic duodenal ulcer. The physician recommended to the patient that he continue to take the Pepcid but discontinue the use of Pepto-Bismol because it possibly could cause the black tarry stools. The patient was to return to the gastroenterologist's office in one month and if symptoms continue and consider an abdominal ultrasound and workup of the large bowel.

First-Listed Diagnosis: _____

Secondary Diagnoses: _____

14

The patient is a 74-year-old male who was admitted for a chronic bleeding duodenal ulcer. Because of significantly abnormal laboratory results, additional studies were performed and it was determined he had obstructive jaundice due to a suspected common bile duct stone. The patient was seen by the gastroenterologist in the hospital and scheduled for an endoscopic retrograde cholangiopancreatography (ERCP). An ERCP with low osmolar contrast was performed with an Olympus video gastroduodenoscope. The duodenum was easily accessed. The ampulla was erythematous and widely patent. The catheter was placed into the pancreatic duct, and a pancreatogram was obtained. The catheter was repositioned into the common bile duct, and a guide wire was passed into the liver. The cholangiogram showed a filling defect within the common bile duct. A double channel papillotome was placed in the common bile duct and a 1 cm sphincterotomy was performed for drainage. The common bile duct was dilated and with an 11-mm balloon, the physician removed a large, hard, yellow stone without difficulty. Using contrast dye injected into the edges of the cut wound, hemostasis was achieved, and the scope was removed. The postoperative diagnoses for the procedure titled ERCP with sphincterotomy and stone extraction were (1) common duct stone obstructed, and (2) chronic duodenal ulcer under treatment.

Principal Diagnosis: _____

Secondary Diagnoses: _____

Principal Procedure: _____

Secondary Procedure(s): _____

15

The patient is a 55-year-old man with a 35-year history of alcohol abuse. He came to the hospital emergency room after having one melenic stool at home. While in the ER he had another melenic stool. He is known to have esophageal varices secondary to alcoholic liver cirrhosis. He has had sclerotherapy for the varices in the past, but it was noted to be a failure. The patient had attempted to complete alcoholic rehabilitation on three occasions but has been unsuccessful and continues to drink—according to the patient, "only a couple of beers every day." The patient is also known to have thrombocytopenia that may be the result of bone marrow suppressive effect of alcohol but has not been proven, and serial blood counts were performed during this admission. He has had gastrointestinal bleeding investigated during two previous admissions. The patient was admitted and was seen in consultation by a gastroenterologist and a psychiatrist. The day after admission, the patient became increasingly tremulous and anxious, with anticipated alcohol withdrawal occurring. The withdrawal was successfully managed with medications, and the patient stayed in the hospital after threatening to leave against medical advice the evening of day 2. An upper GI endoscopy (EGD) was performed three days after admission. The findings of the exam were two small grade 1 distal esophageal varices 1 cm in length without stigmata. There were no gastric varices. The fundus and body of the stomach were within normal limits. There was mild peripyloric edema but no ulcers in the pylorus or duodenum. No sclerotherapy of the esophageal varices was necessary. It was suspected the GI bleeding had come from the esophageal varices, as there was no other source of bleeding found. The patient was given strong encouragement to continue to work toward his sobriety, especially given the fact he had detoxification therapy while in the hospital to manage his withdrawal. He acknowledged it was a good time to return to Alcoholics Anonymous, which he acknowledged was a good program for him in the past, and take advantage of other community support systems for recovering alcoholics that the psychiatrist informed him about during this hospital stay, including two visits from gentlemen from the community program. The discharge summary prepared by his attending physician included the final diagnoses and procedures of bleeding esophageal varices in alcoholic liver cirrhosis disease, continuous alcoholism, alcoholic withdrawal, thrombocytopenia, EGD, and alcohol withdrawal treatment.

Principal Diagnosis: _____

Secondary Diagnoses: _____

Principal Procedure: _____

Secondary Procedure(s): _____

16

A 65-year-old patient had experienced blood in his stools, or melena, for the past several days. Over the past 12 hours, the bleeding had increased, and the patient felt very weak and dizzy. He was admitted to the hospital by his physician. The patient was known to have diverticulosis of the colon, and his physician's first impression was that the bleeding was a result of diverticulitis. The patient was advised to have a colonoscopy and an upper GI endoscopy (EGD), to which he agreed. The colonoscopy was performed, and the patient was found to have diverticulosis, but no inflammation was seen. However, an area of erosion, ulceration, and bleeding was seen in the duodenum during the EGD examination. A biopsy of the duodenum was taken during the EGD. The physician's diagnosis was acute duodenal ulceration with hemorrhage; diverticulosis of colon.

Principal Diagnosis: _____

Secondary Diagnoses: _____

Principal Procedure: _____

Secondary Procedure(s): _____

17

HISTORY: This patient is a 35-year-old man with a recurrent, reducible right inguinal hernia, noted on examination. He had undergone surgical repair of a right inguinal hernia 2 years ago, so he was familiar with the symptoms and called this surgeon's office for an appointment. The young man works in a health club as a personal trainer of body builders and, therefore, does heavy lifting on a daily basis. Otherwise, he is healthy, well-nourished, and well-built with no other surgical history and no other evident medical problems. Preoperative testing, including a chest x-ray, EKG, and usual laboratory work, were all within normal limits. He is admitted to the hospital for this procedure because it is a recurrent hernia, and the procedure will require that he have highly limited mobility for the next 36–48 hours. He will also stay in the hospital for a short recovery period. He will then be placed on work-related disability and advised to avoid working for a minimum of 4 weeks.

OPERATIVE FINDINGS: A recurrent, reducible right inguinal hernia, direct and indirect, was found. There was no strangulation or gangrene. A right inguinal hernia repair (Bassini) with high ligation was performed.

DESCRIPTION OF PROCEDURE: The patient was taken to the operating room and placed in a supine position on the table. After satisfactory general anesthesia was administered, the right groin was prepped with Betadine scrub and paint and draped in the usual sterile fashion. The skin overlying the groin was incised through the external inguinal ring, exposing the spermatic cord. The cord was then mobilized and a Penrose drain passed around it at the level of the pubic tubercle. The cord was skeletonized proximally, revealing a very small indirect inguinal hernia sac. The sac was dissected away from the remainder of the cord structure, which was left free of injury. The sac was opened and found to contain no contents. There was also a direct inguinal hernia noted but no femoral hernia noted. The sac was twisted and ligated with 3-0 silk suture ligature. The remainder of the sac was amputated. A floor repair was performed as described by Bassini with interrupted 0 Ethibond sutures between the transversalis fascia and the shelving edge of the inguinal ligament. The internal inguinal ring was left to the size of the tip of an adult finger, and the initial suture medially was from the transversalis fascia into the aponeurosis over the pubic tubercle. Upon completion, hemostasis was adequate, and no relaxing incision was necessary. Spermatic cord was returned to the inguinal canal. The ilioinguinal nerve was blocked prior to this procedure and reblocked again with 0.5% Marcaine and epinephrine solution. The pubic tubercle, inguinal ligament, and subcutaneous tissue were also anesthetized with 0.5% Marcaine and epinephrine solution. The external oblique was then closed with running 3-0 Vicryl. The wound was copiously irrigated and the skin closed with skin clips. A sterile dressing was applied. Gentle traction was placed on the right testicle to fully return it to the scrotum. The patient was transferred to the recovery room in stable condition.

Principal Diagnosis: _____

Secondary Diagnoses: _____

Principal Procedure: _____

Secondary Procedure(s): _____

18

HISTORY: This is a 72-year-old man who presented with a history of epigastric pain for several months. This lasts 3–4 hours each time and has been occurring every 2–3 days. He has been nauseated, although there was no vomiting. He has had the urge to go to the bathroom for frequent bowel movements after meals. He has tried to avoid greasy food and has been placed on a prescription antacid, but this only helped to some extent. An ultrasound was performed on the gallbladder, and gallstones were found. An upper GI x-ray showed mild esophageal motility problems with a hiatal hernia. He gets a screening prostate specific antigen (PSA) every year and has had a colonoscopy, which was normal. He consented to a laparoscopic cholecystectomy and was admitted to the hospital.

OPERATIVE FINDINGS: The laparoscopic examination revealed evidence of inflammation of a chronic nature of the gallbladder along with gallstones. There was also a nodule on the liver on the inferior surface on the right lateral aspect of the gallbladder fossa. The rest of the visualized viscera were unremarkable. After pathologic examination, the postoperative diagnoses documented by the provider are cholelithiasis with chronic cholecystitis with a benign right intrahepatic bile duct adenoma.

DESCRIPTION OF PROCEDURE: The patient was prepared and draped in the usual fashion. An umbilical incision was made. A Veress needle was introduced with a sheath, and pneumoperitoneum was established with the usual precautions. Then an 11-mm port was placed. A laparoscope was introduced. Under direct vision, an operative port in the right upper quadrant and two 5-mm lateral ports were placed. A laparoscopic examination revealed evidence of inflammation of a chronic nature of the gallbladder with gallstones. There was also a nodule in the liver. The rest of the viscera visualized were normal. The cholecystectomy was done by gently grasping the fundus. Adhesions were taken down. The neck was then grasped. The Calot's Triangle was then exposed. The anatomy was carefully defined. The cystic duct and the cystic artery were traced up to the neck of the gallbladder. Herein it was secured with hemoclips, divided, and closed to the neck of the gallbladder. Then it was dissected off of the gallbladder bed and retrieved in an Endopouch and removed. Irrigation was carried out. Excellent hemostasis was ascertained. Following this, an evaluation of the nodule was carried out using a hook cautery. The surrounding borders of this nodule, in the area of the right inferior surface of the lobe of the liver, were cauterized. Then a small wedge biopsy of this tissue was taken. The base was cauterized. This tissue was then sent, with the gallbladder tissue, for histopathological analysis. At this point, having ascertained good hemostasis, all the ports were removed under direct vision. The fascia was closed with 0 Vicryl sutures. Subcutaneous tissue was closed with 0 Vicryl sutures. The skin was closed with 4-0 Monocryl. Marcaine 0.5% with epinephrine was injected to achieve postoperative analgesia. The patient tolerated the procedure well and was stable at the end of the procedure and taken to recovery.

Principal Diagnosis: _____

Secondary Diagnoses: _____

Principal Procedure: _____

Secondary Procedure(s): _____

19

HISTORY: The patient is an 85-year-old woman who lives independently with her husband in their own home. She has been treated for hypothyroidism, hypertension, and dyslipidemia in the past. Medications for these conditions were continued during her hospital stay. Early this morning she awoke with acute onset of right flank pain. Her husband called 911, and she was brought to the hospital's emergency department. On examination she was found to be in acute pain with a palpable mass in her abdominal area. Radiologic examination found dilated loops of small bowel trapped between the abdominal wall and the ascending colon and cecum. She was admitted and taken emergently to the operating room for a suspected small bowel obstruction. The patient was found to have elevated blood pressure, which was proven to be due to her acute stress reaction about her condition and impending surgery.

OPERATIVE FINDINGS: The procedure performed was an exploratory laparotomy and release of acute closed loop small bowel obstruction due to adhesions, by lysis of adhesions. Fortunately the bowel was viable and did not have to be resected.

DESCRIPTION OF PROCEDURE: After routine preparation, the patient was taken to the operating room. A midline incision was made through the scar of previous surgery, which was a hysterectomy. Supraumbilical extension of the scar was performed. Once these minor non-obstructing adhesions were taken down, the abdominal cavity was entered. One loop of small bowel was almost completely obstructed by dense adhesions. These adhesions were carefully lysed, releasing the small bowel from obstruction. The entire small bowel was mobilized and explored from the ligament of Treitz all the way to the ileocecal valve. The wound was irrigated. Hemostasis was obtained after lysis of adhesions that released the acute small bowel obstruction. Lap count and instrument count were correct. Seprafilm adhesion barrier substance was placed in the peritoneal cavity prior to closure. The fascia was closed with PDS loop. The skin was closed with a skin stapler. A dressing was applied. The patient tolerated the procedure well under general anesthesia and was taken to the post-anesthesia recovery area in good condition.

Principal Diagnosis: _____

Secondary Diagnoses: _____

Principal Procedure: _____

Secondary Procedure(s): _____

20

A 63-year-old man was brought to the emergency department by a fire department ambulance with his family, who reported that he was found unconscious on his front porch. The patient was admitted with a blood alcohol level of 115 mg/100 mL, indicating acute intoxication and intoxication delirium, documented by the emergency department physician. The family and later the patient confirmed that the man suffered from chronic continuous alcoholism. The diagnostic workup also found evidence of alcoholic liver cirrhosis. The immediate concern was the life-threatening hepatic encephalopathy, which required intensive treatment. The liver cirrhosis was evaluated and treated but will remain a continuing problem for the patient. He recovered from his extreme condition, however, and was able to be discharged. He was strongly advised to stop drinking, and he agreed to attend Alcoholics Anonymous meetings, as he realized the seriousness of his alcoholism.

Principal Diagnosis: _____

Secondary Diagnoses: _____

Principal Procedure: _____

Secondary Procedure(s): _____

21

The patient was a 45-year-old man who was admitted to the hospital by his private physician after vomiting bright red blood during a visit in the office the same day. A consultation with a gastroenterologist was requested. The gastroenterologist recommended an immediate esophagogastroduodenoscopy (EGD) to determine and control the source of the bleeding. The patient consented to the EGD, which revealed an acute, hemorrhaging duodenal ulcer. The bleeding points were controlled endoscopically by cautery. It was also noted that the patient had a sliding hiatal hernia. The patient recovered from the procedure well, suffered no further episodes of vomiting or bleeding, and was discharged with medications. Follow-up appointments with his physicians were scheduled.

Principal Diagnosis: _____

Secondary Diagnoses: _____

Principal Procedure: _____

Secondary Procedure(s): _____

Chapter 12

Diseases of the Skin and Subcutaneous Tissue

Coding Scenarios for *Basic ICD-10-CM/PCS Coding*

The following case studies are organized following the sequence of the chapters in the *ICD-10-CM and ICD-10-PCS* code books. The objective of this book is to provide the student with more detailed clinical information to code, rather than one- or two-line diagnosis and procedure statements. ICD-10-CM diagnosis codes are to be assigned to both the inpatient hospital admission and the outpatient visit case studies. In this book, the ICD-10-PCS procedure codes are to be assigned only to the inpatient hospital admission cases. In actual practice, outpatient cases are assigned CPT/HCPCS codes. The ICD-10-PCS codes are only required for inpatient procedures.

1

A 90-year-old woman, a resident of a long-term care facility, was admitted to the hospital with a severe decubitus ulcer on the right buttock described as a stage III pressure ulcer. The patient also had a small chronic ulcer on the right heel, currently limited to the skin. The patient also has generalized atherosclerosis of both extremities. Treatments of the skin conditions were an excisional debridement of the skin of the heel and an excisional debridement into the muscle of the buttock. The wound care nurse closely monitored the patient after surgery and gave detailed instructions to the nurses at the long-term care facility who would be taking care of the patient after discharge. The patient was transferred back to the long-term care facility. The wound care physician and nurse would visit the patient in the long-term care facility within 1 week to monitor the healing of the pressure and chronic ulcers.

Principal Diagnosis: _____

Secondary Diagnoses: _____

Principal Procedure: _____

Secondary Procedure(s): _____

2

A 20-year-old woman was admitted for a procedure to treat a pilonidal cyst that had become abscessed. The procedure performed was an incision and drainage of the pilonidal sinus. The patient will continue to take oral antibiotics to resolve the infection. The patient was discharged home with a follow-up appointment in 7 days with the surgeon who performed the procedure.

Principal Diagnosis: _____

Secondary Diagnoses: _____

Principal Procedure: _____

Secondary Procedure(s): _____

3

A 19-year-old woman was seen in the dermatologist's office with extensive inflammation and irritation of the skin on her eyelids and under her eyebrows that was spreading to her temples and forehead. Upon questioning the patient, the physician learned that she had recently used new eye cosmetics. The physician had examined the patient during a prior visit for cystic acne. During this visit, the physician also examined the patient's cystic acne on her forehead and jawline. He advised her to continue to use the medication he had prescribed previously. The physician's diagnosis was contact dermatitis due to cosmetics and cystic acne. He advised the patient to immediately discontinue use of any makeup on the face until the next follow-up visit. The patient was given a topical medication to resolve the inflammation.

First-Listed Diagnosis: _____

Secondary Diagnoses: _____

4

A 50-year-old woman was seen in her primary care physician's office complaining of warmth and redness of her left anterior lower leg. Last weekend she was doing yard work and received a small puncture wound on the same area of her leg. She did not think she had a foreign body in the wound. Over the next couple of days the area became red and began to show slight swelling. Upon physical examination, the physician found a tiny puncture point with obvious cellulitis tracking down her leg from below the knee almost to the ankle. The wound itself required no treatment. The physician recommended the patient take a short-term course of antibiotics and return for a follow-up visit in 5 days. The diagnosis written on the encounter form was puncture wound resulting in cellulitis of the lower leg.

First-Listed Diagnosis: _____

Secondary Diagnoses: _____

5

A 60-year-old man was seen by a dermatologist at the request of his primary care physician while hospitalized for other medical conditions. The patient states he spends a lot of time outdoors as a mailman and golfing every weekend. The patient expresses the concern that he may have skin cancer. He remembers that his father, a farmer, had many of these same kind of lesions on his arms and neck through the years. After performing a thorough skin examination, the physician finds multiple brown annular keratotic lesions on the patient's arms and lower legs with patchy dry areas around them. The physician performs a skin biopsy of a lesion on his right lower arm and examines the lesion microscopically. No cancer type cells are seen. Given the patient's history of the same lesions in the family and his frequent exposure to ultraviolet sunlight, the physician explains to the patient that he has what is referred to as DSAP or disseminated superficial actinic porokeratosis. Further, he explains there is no treatment to prevent these lesions from returning once removed. The patient elects not to have any lesions removed at this time but will consider it and make an appointment in the future if he decides to have them removed.

Code only the reason for the consultation and the procedure performed as result of the consultation.

Dermatology Diagnosis: _____

Secondary Dermatology Diagnoses: _____

Dermatology Procedure: _____

Secondary Dermatology Procedures: _____

6

The 25-year-old patient is seen in the dermatologist's office upon the advice of the family practice physician with the complaint of excessive sweating in particular areas of her body, such as her underarms, soles of her feet, and the palms of her hands. The patient notes that the excessive sweating started when she was a young teenager. She describes this condition as very embarrassing and difficult to manage because nearly every day, she has to take extra clothing with her in order to change her blouse at work. The physician takes a complete history and cannot find any medical condition that might be causing this problem. The physical examination confirms, however, excessive moisture under the arms and on her hands and feet. The physician is certain the patient suffers from primary focal hyperhidrosis. Her primary care physician had given her a prescription for a certain antiperspirant designed for this condition. The patient had tried the antiperspirant but found it to be ineffective as well as irritating to her underarm skin. The dermatologist recommends injections of botulinum toxin at the sites where excessive sweating is occurring. The drug promptly freezes the nerve that would normally stimulate the sweat gland. He had used this therapy for other patients who were pleased with the results. The patient immediately wants the procedure. The physician injects both axillae with the "botox" under sterile technique. The patient is to return in 4 weeks to report on the results or sooner if problems are detected. The physician states that if the patient has a positive response, the injections will need to be repeated every 6 to 9 months.

First-Listed Diagnosis: _____

Secondary Diagnoses: _____

7

Upon the advice of his family physician, the patient made an appointment with a dermatologist to evaluate an itching, red, blistering condition that recently appeared on his lower arms and lower legs. The patient is a 26-year-old man who works as a salesman in a computer store. The dermatologist asks the patient questions about his recent contact with new soaps, detergents, chemicals, fabrics, fragrances, and outdoor or indoor plants, but the patient reports he has had no new experiences with these items. Upon further questioning, the doctor learns the patient had a new roommate move in 1 month ago with a dog that had taken a strong liking to the patient and followed him everywhere. The physician is then certain the patient's condition is a contact dermatitis resulting from exposure to animal dander. The physician gives the patient samples of a topical ointment and a prescription for a topical corticosteroid medication to reduce the inflammation and relieve the itching. The patient is told this condition is likely to continue as long as the animal resides with him. The patient is advised to return in 2 weeks for a follow-up visit.

First-Listed Diagnosis: _____

Secondary Diagnoses: _____

8

The patient is a 54-year-old woman who has suffered from left-side chronic ulcerative colitis for many years. Today she is seen in her physician's office for a follow-up visit. Of most concern to the patient today are the "red bumps" that are present on her right lower leg. The patient has had similar lesions before now, but the lesions have recently returned and are larger in size than previously. The physician recognizes the lesions as a recurrence of erythema nodosum, which is a complication of her underlying systemic condition. The tender red nodules appear to be coinciding with the worsening of her colitis. The patient thinks she might have bumped her leg against a grocery cart the previous week and blamed that for the tender nodules that appeared first. A topical ointment is prescribed, and the physician advises the patient that the nodules will probably heal as her colitis becomes more controlled with the medication she is currently receiving. The physician treats both the colitis and the erythema nodosum during the visit today.

First-Listed Diagnosis: _____

Secondary Diagnoses: _____

9

A 60-year-old man returns to the Wound Care Clinic today for a follow-up visit for treatment of his diabetic right heel foot ulcer. The ulcer was present with skin breakdown only. The patient is a type 1 diabetic with an ulcer on the heel of his right foot that is attributed to his diabetes. The wound was infected when the patient was first seen in the Wound Care Clinic, but today the ulcer is much smaller in size and is no longer infected. Close surveillance, wound dressings, and the appropriate use of antibiotics were successful in treating this man's foot ulcer and prevented it from becoming gangrenous. The patient receives ongoing education about proper skin and foot care because his diabetic condition makes him at risk for more ulcers. The patient will return in 2 weeks for a follow-up visit.

First-Listed Diagnosis: _____

Secondary Diagnoses: _____

10

The patient is a 47-year-old woman who returns to her dermatologist's office after a 1-year absence with pityriasis rosea, a condition she has had several times before. Usually in the spring of the year, the patient suffers from this skin condition. She explains to the physician that she first noticed a 3–4 cm annular or ring-shaped lesion on her trunk that was followed a few days later with many smaller ring-shaped and pustular lesions parallel to the skin folds on her chest and abdomen. The physician notes the red and brown lesions with a trailing scale. Once again, the patient describes the condition as extremely itchy and is seeking another prescription for the topical glucocorticoid cream the physician prescribed in the past. The physician is agreeable to renewing the prescription and offers the patient the option of UV B (ultraviolet light) phototherapy, as the outbreak seems to be more severe this year. The patient states she will try the cream first and make another appointment for the phototherapy if there is no improvement.

First-Listed Diagnosis: _____

Secondary Diagnoses: _____

11

The patient was admitted to the hospital for other medical conditions. The patient was seen in consultation by a dermatologic surgeon at the request of his primary care physician.

The 53-year-old man had two lesions on his scalp. One lesion was 1.2 cm × 1.3 cm × 1.0 cm on the posterior scalp and was slightly raised and slightly erythematous. After injection of local anesthesia in the center of the lesion, a 3-mm punch biopsy was performed. The biopsied tissue was then removed and sent for frozen section to pathology. The frozen section was positive for basal cell carcinoma. A 5-0 Prolene stitch was used to close the defect. The patient had a second lesion about 2 cm away from the first lesion and measuring 0.5 cm × 0.2 cm. The lesion was excised by using a sharpened scalpel to penetrate the skin and dermis on both sides. This lesion was then removed and sent to pathology. The second lesion was reported to be an actinic keratosis and removed in its entirety. It was closed with a 5-0 Prolene stitch times two. Steri-strips were applied. We informed the patient that we will refer him to a plastic surgeon for removal of the basal cell carcinoma, as this may require significant undermining and wound closure may be problematic because of the size of the lesion. There is quite a bit of tension on the patient's scalp, and the excision of the basal cell carcinoma will require the skills of a plastic surgeon. The patient will be seen for follow up in this surgeon's office in 7 days and was given the name and phone number of the plastic surgeon to call for an appointment within the next 2 weeks.

Code the diagnosis and procedure performed as a result of the consultation.

Dermatology Diagnosis: _____

Secondary Dermatology Diagnoses: _____

Dermatology Procedure: _____

Secondary Dermatology Procedures: _____

12

The patient is a 56-year-old woman admitted to the hospital after being seen in the physician's office for two large draining abscesses on her back. One was on the left-upper back and the other on the right-lower back skin. Both lesions were large, actively draining, and showed some necrotic features to the surrounding tissue. These areas on the back were warm to the touch and tender. Because of the size of the lesions, the patient was admitted as an inpatient for surgery. The surgeon performed an incision and drainage on two areas of the back. The right-lower back actually had two areas of abscess with necrotic tissue present. The cavity was widely opened with an incision that connected the two abscesses. Another incision was made in this area because the fluctuance had penetrated deeper down, and the entire area required drainage and copious irrigation. A Penrose drain was placed to keep the tracks open. The left-upper back had an area of fluctuance of 3 cm × 5 cm. A transverse incision was made deep into the subcutaneous cavity, and all the purulent material was removed from the widely opened area. It was copiously irrigated. Specimens were collected from all these areas for cultures. The fluid cultures grew Methicillin-resistant staphylococcus aureus susceptible to Clindamycin. While in the hospital, the patient received intravenous antibiotics. The patient was continued on this antibiotic orally for one more week. The drain was left in for the surgeon to remove about 3 days after discharge. The patient was known to have hypertension, and it was treated during the hospital stay. The patient had two fasting glucose tests performed in the hospital, and both were significantly elevated at 160 and 180. A hemoglobin A1c was performed with a finding of 9.5. The patient was informed that she had type 2 diabetes, poorly controlled. She had a dietary consultation in the hospital and will attend diabetic education classes after discharge. She was discharged with a glucose monitoring kit and a prescription for oral diabetic medication. She will be seen in the primary care physician's office in 1 week.

Principal Diagnosis: _____

Secondary Diagnoses: _____

Principal Procedure: _____

Secondary Procedure(s): _____

13

The patient was a 69-year-old man who had many previous admissions for cellulitis and alcoholic cirrhosis of the liver proven by biopsy. He had hepatic encephalopathy on several occasions and hepatorenal failure two times when he was previously hospitalized. He also has marked exogenous obesity. On this occasion he was admitted for an abrupt elevation of temperature with diaphoresis on the night of admission following a dinner party. His lower abdominal area was the site of marked reddening and induration at the fold of his panniculus adiposis. His admitting diagnosis was cellulitis of abdominal tissues, and he was started on intravenous antibiotics. He was seen in consultation by an infectious disease physician and a nephrologist. It appeared his cellulitis this time was triggered by edema of the extremities. His abdominal cellulitis responded virtually overnight to the intravenous cephazolin. He also had stasis dermatitis and cellulitis of his legs, but the legs were less red and indurated than his lower abdomen. He was also proven to be hypoalbuminemic. Blood cultures were drawn and pseudomonas aeruginosa was found in his blood. This organism was not susceptible to the antibiotic he received for the first four days of his hospitalization. Because the antibiotics he was receiving would not have been expected to kill the pseudomonas, it was speculated that the process involving the lower abdominal wall was due to gram-positive coccal organisms such as staphylococcus or streptococcus, which is why the abdominal cellulitis responded so quickly to the cephalosporin antibiotics. The organism causing the abdominal cellulitis was not proven. But it was not surprising to find the pseudomonas in his blood by virtue of his anatomic problems as well as his poor hepatic function, which leaves him prone to bacteremia. However, the bacteremia produced no symptoms in this patient with a well-established history of cirrhosis. He was anicteric and did not have any evidence of encephalopathy. He was continued on treatment with the best antipseudomonal agent and continued with gentle diuresis to remove the edema fluid in both lower extremities that produce the leg cellulitis. His liver function studies were not any worse than previously noted, but the doctors again encouraged the patient to completely eliminate alcohol consumption. Because the patient travels extensively for business and pleasure, the doctors emphasized the need to take all of his medications faithfully in order to maintain his apparent resilience in the knowledge of his extensive liver disease and to carry antibiotics with him so that any early onset of cellulitis might be aborted by early treatment. The patient agreed and was discharged after an 11-day hospital stay. His discharge diagnoses were documented as cellulitis, anterior abdominal wall, gram-negative bacteremia (pseudomonas), stasis dermatitis and cellulitis bilateral lower extremities, advanced alcoholic liver cirrhosis with hypoalbuminemia, and morbid obesity.

Principal Diagnosis: _____

Secondary Diagnoses: _____

Principal Procedure: _____

Secondary Procedure(s): _____

14

The 4-year-old female was admitted to the hospital directly from her pediatrician's office because of symmetrical raised red skin lesions over 20% of her body. She also has edema of her upper and lower eyelids. The child had been treated with a penicillin-type drug for an upper respiratory infection, and it was suspected the child was having a reaction to that drug. A pediatric infectious disease specialist examined the patient immediately. After reviewing laboratory results, the consultant concluded the patient had Stevens-Johnson syndrome, which is a toxic epidermal necrolysis that produces the skin lesions seen on this child. The consultant attributed the edema of the eyelids to the same syndrome. The patient received a 4-day treatment of intravenous immunoglobulin drugs and made an excellent recovery. The consultant stated the 20–25% exfoliation of her skin surface caused by the Stevens-Johnson syndrome was an adverse effect of the penicillin this child received for the respiratory infection. The child was discharged home to her parents' care with pediatric home health nursing follow-up.

Principal Diagnosis: _____

Secondary Diagnoses: _____

Principal Procedure: _____

Secondary Procedure(s): _____

15

The patient is an 89-year-old female admitted to the hospital from the nursing home for surgical treatment of her stage IV pressure ulcer of the coccyx. The patient was taken to surgery, and the physician dictated an operative report that described a debridement of the coccyx wound with sharp excision down to the fascia and the bone. The patient was transferred back to the nursing home two days later to be visited by the surgeon and the wound care clinical nurse specialist in one week. While the patient was in the hospital she continued to receive treatment for her chronic diastolic heart failure, coronary artery (native vessel) disease with known total chronic occlusion in at least two coronary vessels.

Principal Diagnosis: _____

Secondary Diagnoses: _____

Principal Procedure: _____

Secondary Procedure(s): _____

16

Six months after a house fire in which the patient sustained burns of his right leg, he has developed severe scarring as a result of the third-degree burns. The patient is evaluated in the plastic surgeon's office and scheduled for reconstructive surgery in the near future.

*Note: List all applicable codes **including** the External Cause code.*

First-Listed Diagnosis: _____

Secondary Diagnoses: _____

Chapter 13

Diseases of the Musculoskeletal System and Connective Tissue

Coding Scenarios for *Basic ICD-10-CM/PCS Coding*

The following case studies are organized following the sequence of the chapters in the *ICD-10-CM and ICD-10-PCS* code books. The objective of this book is to provide the student with more detailed clinical information to code, rather than one- or two-line diagnosis and procedure statements. ICD-10-CM diagnosis codes are to be assigned to both the inpatient hospital admission and the outpatient visit case studies. In this book, the ICD-10-PCS procedure codes are to be assigned only to the inpatient hospital admission cases. In actual practice, outpatient cases are assigned CPT/HCPCS codes. The ICD-10-PCS codes are only required for inpatient procedures.

1

A 50-year-old man is treated for severe low back pain and numbness on the left leg over several weeks. The patient thinks the pain is the result of lifting heavy boxes during a recent move to a new residence, but the physician cannot conclude that this was the cause. Diagnostic studies reveal that the patient has a herniated disc. The patient is also found to have osteoarthritis of the spine with radiculopathy. The patient is admitted for a laminotomy and excision of the intervertebral disc at L4-L5 to treat the herniated disc. The patient has an uneventful postoperative recovery and is discharged home to begin rehabilitation therapy in the near future.

Principal Diagnosis: _____

Secondary Diagnoses: _____

Principal Procedure: _____

Secondary Procedure(s): _____

2

An 82-year-old woman had been treated by her family physician for chronic low back pain. One morning upon awakening she could not get out of bed due to severe back pain. She was brought to the emergency department and admitted. X-rays show several severe compression fractures of the lumbar vertebrae as a result of senile osteoporosis. An injection of mixed steroid and local anesthetic agents is administered into the spinal canal to help alleviate her pain from age-related osteoporosis and the pathologic fracture.

Principal Diagnosis: _____

Secondary Diagnoses: _____

Principal Procedure: _____

Secondary Procedure(s): _____

3

This 60-year-old patient is seen again in his primary care physician's office for care of his arthritis. He has generalized degenerative arthritis of the knees, hips, and of the lumbosacral spine. His condition is becoming progressively worse, and different medications have been tried to alleviate the pain and discomfort. Because of his long-standing hypertension, which has not been well-controlled, and angina due to coronary artery disease (with disease in the autologous vein bypass grafts after previous CABG 10 years previously), the patient is not a good candidate for joint replacement surgery. A new arthritis medication is prescribed, and his anti-hypertensive and cardiac medication prescriptions are renewed.

First-Listed Diagnosis: _____

Secondary Diagnoses: _____

4

A 40-year-old woman is admitted to the hospital for chemotherapy for systemic lupus erythematosus (SLE). She is going to receive the next course of intravenous infusion of cyclophosphamide, an effective but highly toxic chemotherapy drug, to treat the SLE. The patient currently has a central venous catheter placed in the superior vena cava in which her chemotherapy treatments are administered. The patient has several complications as a result of SLE, including nephritic syndrome, inflammatory myopathy, anemia of chronic disease, and swan-neck deformities of her fingers. During the hospital stay, the patient receives other medications to manage the complications. Intravenous infusion is started on day 1. She is monitored for toxicity, but none is detected and she is able to go home on day 3.

Principal Diagnosis: _____

Secondary Diagnoses: _____

Principal Procedure: _____

Secondary Procedure(s): _____

5

The patient is a 25-year-old woman who returns to the orthopedic clinic to see her sports medicine physician. She is complaining of gradually increasing pain in her shinbones that used to abate when she resorted to walking instead of running but now is not relieved by such a walking rest. The woman runs several miles 4 days a week. Two weeks ago the physician had ordered x-rays of both lower legs. The results were negative for fractures. Because the patient now complained of pain in her right foot, today the physician ordered the x-rays of the legs to be repeated and an x-ray of the right foot to be performed. The radiologist concluded there was a stress reaction in the right and left lower distal tibias and a stress fracture of the second metatarsal of the right foot. Given the patient's history, physical findings, and radiologic evidence, the physician makes the diagnosis of bilateral stress fractures of the tibias and stress fracture of the right second metatarsal of the foot. The patient is instructed to rest and keep off her feet as much as possible for the next 8 weeks, specifically with no running or other exercising. Based on her complaints of back pain, the physician also describes the patient as having an acute lumbosacral strain. The patient is to return in 4 weeks for repeat x-rays. The physician concluded that her injuries were the result of cumulative trauma from the repetitive impact of running on hard surfaces.

First-Listed Diagnosis: _____

Secondary Diagnoses: _____

6

The patient is admitted to the hospital for debridement of the right fibula bone. After multiple outpatient diagnostic tests are performed, the diagnosis of acute osteomyelitis localized in the right fibula due to a staphylococcal infection is made in this 9-year-old boy. The child began complaining of pain below the right knee and difficulty walking over the past 2 weeks. The patient denied any trauma to the leg but, as an active boy who plays soccer and softball, trauma could not be ruled out, although no evidence of an injury was found on the leg. To prevent bone destruction as well as the possibility of the infection spreading to other bones and joints in the lower leg, the child is admitted for surgery. The procedure is an excisional debridement of the proximal fibula. The child withstands the procedure well and is discharged to his parents for at-home recovery 1 day after surgery.

Principal Diagnosis: _____

Secondary Diagnoses: _____

Principal Procedure: _____

Secondary Procedure(s): _____

7

The patient is a 65-year-old man who had a total knee replacement on the right side 9 years previously. Up until 6 months ago, the patient enjoyed an active retirement, golfing on a daily basis and enjoying walks with his wife around a nearby nature reserve. The patient began to experience pain in the thigh near the knee and in the lower leg on the same side where the joint replacement had occurred. The patient returns to his orthopedic physician with these complaints and x-rays are taken. It appears the prosthetic joint is not in good position. The doctor makes the diagnosis of "aseptic loosening" of the prosthetic joint and recommends a right total knee revision arthroplasty. The patient consents to surgery and is admitted for the procedure. The physician finds he has to replace the femoral, tibial, and patellar components in order to take advantage of the new synthetic substitute metal prosthetic components that were not available when the patient originally had his knee replaced. The previous synthetic joint devices were removed. The new joint replacement devices were cemented in place. The patient also was found to have mild idiopathic gouty arthritis in his knees, which was treated with medications during the hospital stay. The patient is discharged day 5 after surgery to receive physical therapy at home.

Principal Diagnosis: _____

Secondary Diagnoses: _____

Principal Procedure: _____

Secondary Procedure(s): _____

8

The patient comes to the orthopedic surgeon's office complaining of pain, swelling, and tenderness, as well as extreme morning stiffness, in the fingers, hands, wrists, knees, and especially the feet. She also complains of fatigue, anorexia, and unintended weight loss. The patient is a 40-year-old woman who is a partner in a large corporate law firm. Upon physical examination, the physician notes warmth in the joints, especially the knees. The doctor also notes that the patient has simultaneous involvement of the same joints bilaterally. The patient reports that another orthopedic surgeon had told her this condition was simply osteoarthritis, but the patient remains concerned about the other symptoms she has been experiencing. Her grandmother had rheumatoid arthritis, and the patient suspects she has the same disease. The orthopedic surgeon agrees this is a possibility and recommends the patient see a rheumatologist for further investigation. The physician wrote "rule out rheumatoid arthritis" on the progress note he completed for this office visit.

First-Listed Diagnosis: _____

Secondary Diagnoses: _____

9

The patient is a 30-year-old man who comes to the emergency department complaining of joint pain in his shoulder. The patient, who was a state champion wrestler during his college years, reports that his shoulder has dislocated on several occasions since college, when he had several traumatic dislocations of the same shoulder. On this occasion, the patient was lifting a box overhead to place on a shelf in his garage. X-rays were taken to examine the shoulder. The ED physician is unable to reduce the dislocation on the initial attempt. With light intravenous sedation, the physician completes a closed reduction of shoulder dislocation. The physician wrote "chronic recurrent dislocation of right shoulder and traumatic arthritis of the right shoulder" as the final diagnosis on the ED record.

First-Listed Diagnosis: _____

Secondary Diagnoses: _____

10

The patient, a 48-year-old female, was admitted to the hospital for surgical repair of a massive rotator cuff tear of her right shoulder. The patient was known to have hypertension, but it was well controlled and she received medical clearance for surgery. The patient has had pain, weakness, and limited range of motion in her right shoulder, which has been present for several years and has been getting progressively worse. Several years ago she had a fall and injured her right hip but doesn't remember her shoulder being injured at that time. The patient was taken to surgery and placed under general anesthesia. The surgeon found a complete tear of the rotator cuff that appeared nontraumatic and significant tenosynovitis of the shoulder. The surgeon performed a rotator cuff repair, which was accomplished by reattaching the tendon using an arthroscope. A synovectomy of the shoulder was also performed through the arthroscope. The patient was kept overnight in the hospital, received her antihypertensive medication, and was discharged to home on day 2 with a follow-up appointment with the surgeon in 10 days.

Principal Diagnosis: _____

Secondary Diagnoses: _____

Principal Procedure: _____

Secondary Procedure(s): _____

11

The patient is a 56-year-old man with significant hypertensive heart disease who was admitted to the hospital for an arthroscopic partial medial meniscectomy on his right knee. Given his hypertension and heart disease, the cardiologist advised the orthopedic surgeon to admit the patient to the hospital for at least overnight monitoring after the procedure. During a previous orthopedic surgery, this patient had a hypertensive crisis and was placed in the intensive care unit for monitoring. This surgery was performed uneventfully. The patient had an arthroscopic partial medial meniscectomy of the posterior horn of the medial meniscus, right knee. This was determined to be an old tear, likely from a football playing injury. There were no loose bodies in the medial and lateral gutters. The articular cartilage surfaces were in reasonably good condition. The notches of the anterior cruciate and posterior cruciate ligaments were intact. Within the lateral compartment, the meniscus was intact and the articular cartilage surfaces in good condition. At the conclusion of the procedure, all excess fluid was drained, the portal incisions closed with nylon sutures, an injection of Marcaine was administered for pain control, and sterile dressings were applied. The patient was taken to the recovery room and then transferred to a regular bed. He was discharged the following morning with a follow-up appointment with the surgeon in 10 days.

Principal Diagnosis: _____

Secondary Diagnoses: _____

Principal Procedure: _____

Secondary Procedure(s): _____

12

The patient is a 28-year-old female with severe chronic asthmatic bronchitis and a congenital heart condition—ventricular septal defect—that has been monitored for several years. At this time the patient has very painful bunions on both feet that make walking increasingly difficult with the fact she is unable to wear a shoe on her left foot. She has acquired this condition rather quickly over the past couple of years. The patient was referred to a podiatrist for evaluation. After taking the patient's history and performing a physical examination of the patient's lower extremities, the physician concluded the patient had hallux abductovalgus, both feet, worse on the left. The patient consented to an outpatient procedure to be performed one week later, specifically, a McBride bunionectomy with soft-tissue correction. The doctor also included the diagnoses of chronic asthmatic bronchitis and VSD as secondary diagnoses.

First-Listed Diagnosis: _____

Secondary Diagnoses: _____

13

The patient is a 48-year-old woman who was diagnosed with an aggressive form of breast carcinoma in her right breast in the past year and had a radical mastectomy followed by chemotherapy. She has also developed secondary myelofibrosis with therapy-related low grade myelodysplastic syndrome, due to the antineoplastic chemotherapy she has received.

On this occasion, the patient called her physician reporting excruciating low back pain that had developed rapidly over the past two days and was told to go to the emergency department. It was feared the patient had a compression fracture or similar condition due to metastatic bone cancer. The patient was admitted and examined by her attending physician, oncologist, and consulting orthopedic surgeon. Imaging of the spine failed to find any pathology, including no metastatic disease, much to the relief of the patient, family, and physicians. The physicians could not explain the rapid onset of low back pain, which was treated with pain medications. On day 3, the patient reported less back pain and better ambulation and was allowed to go home with her family. Chemotherapy will be performed on schedule in the next two weeks, and the patient continued to receive treatment for her myelofibrosis and myelodysplastic syndrome due to the chemotherapy.

Principal Diagnosis: _____

Secondary Diagnoses: _____

Principal Procedure: _____

Secondary Procedure(s): _____

14

The patient is a 19-year-old female college scholar-athlete who is a scholarship basketball player at the state university. She has had repeated injuries to her knees over the past 7 years while she has played in competitive sports, including basketball, softball, and soccer. Over the past 3 months she had noted a feeling of instability in the right knee, more than usual and with increasing pain over the medial compartment, as a result of these old injuries. The physicians who had treated her over the past year were fairly confident that she had a torn anterior cruciate ligament and suspected possible tears to the medial meniscus and medial collateral ligament. She was admitted to the hospital for reconstructive surgery, with a planned transfer to a sports rehabilitation unit at the university hospital. At surgery, the orthopedic surgeon found a grossly positive Lachman's sign and anterior drawer in neutral, internal, and external rotation. The medial meniscus was torn at the posterior horn in a complex fashion posteriorly. There was no repairable tissue. The medial collateral ligament was torn. The good news was the surfaces of the patellofemoral joint, medial compartment, and lateral compartments were in good condition. The anterior cruciate ligament was completely torn. The posterior cruciate ligament was intact, and the patellar tendons rode laterally in the notch. At the conclusion of the procedure, the knee was stable to Lachman and drawer testing. The procedures performed on the right knee were an arthroscopic reconstruction or repair of the anterior cruciate ligament using nonautologous patellar tendon graft and repair of the medial meniscus and medial collateral ligament, also known as the triad knee repair or O'Donoghue procedure that includes a medial meniscectomy. After 3 days of postoperative recovery, the patient was transferred to the sports rehabilitation unit for a complex rehabilitation program.

Principal Diagnosis: _____

Secondary Diagnoses: _____

Principal Procedure: _____

Secondary Procedure(s): _____

15

Note: Focus on this surgical procedure and not the entire hospital stay to identify musculoskeletal diagnosis and procedure.

HISTORY: This patient is a 65-year-old man who is currently hospitalized under the care of his internal medicine physician for treatment of a duodenal ulcer, gastroesophageal reflux disease (GERD), and an enlarged prostate with urinary retention. His chief complaint, however, is severe pain in his left knee. He is medically stable at this time after treatment by the attending physician and a urologist who performed a prostate exam, and will be ready for discharge soon, pending referral to orthopedics for the chief complaint of severe left knee pain. The pain is limiting his mobility, and he fears falling. He states he has had no particular trauma to the knee but has always felt the left knee to be his "bad knee." The patient wants a knee replacement because his 75-year-old brother had one in the past six months and is back to golfing twice a week. This patient cannot walk the nine holes on the golf course as he was able to do last year. MRI of the left knee showed nonspecific abnormalities and some arthritic changes. The patient consented to an arthroscopic examination of the knee to determine what the abnormalities were, treat the abnormalities, and determine the course of future treatment.

OPERATIVE FINDINGS: An arthroscopic debridement of the left patella was performed. The medial meniscus, lateral meniscus, and anterior cruciate ligament (ACL) were completely normal. Examination of the patellofemoral joints allowed appreciation of the magnitude of the problem with the patella. The entire surface of the patella was involved with chondromalacia with surfaces graded from 3 to mostly 4. He also has a significant degree of prepatellar bursitis of the left knee that likely is also contributing to his pain and stiffness. The pros and cons of a left knee arthroplasty will be discussed with the patient after he recovers from this procedure and determination of pain relief after this debridement is assessed.

DESRIPTION OF PROCEDURE: The patient was provided general endotracheal tube anesthesia and the left lower extremity was prepared and draped in the usual manner for arthroscopic surgery of the left knee. After insufflation of lidocaine and epinephrine, three standard portals, two medial and one lateral, were established in the usual manner. There was difficulty in evaluating the suprapatellar pouch as well as the patellofemoral joint initially because of the extensive chondromalacia and synovial reaction. Prepatellar bursitis was also present. The medial compartment was first able to be evaluated carefully and the medial meniscus was found to be completely normal to observation and to probing, as were the medial femoral condyle and medial tibial plateau. The ACL appeared to be intact. The lateral meniscus and lateral compartment were, in general, completely normal. In order to see the contents of the femoral-tibial joint, some debridement of pedunculated synovial tissue was necessary. On returning to the patellofemoral joint, some debridement of synovial tissues was done as well as some of synovial plica material. At this point, the magnitude of the problem on the patella was evident. Essentially the entire surface of the patella was involved with chondromalacia. There was mostly grade-4 chondromalacia over more of the lateral facet but also on the medial facet with grade-3 chondromalacia. This involved a large portion of the main articular surface of the patella. At the conclusion of this procedure, instrumentation was removed, and sterile dressings applied. The patient was awakened and taken to the recovery room in stable condition.

Principal Diagnosis: _____

Secondary Diagnoses: _____

Principal Procedure: _____

Secondary Procedure(s): _____

16

HISTORY: The patient is a 38-year-old male with a 2-month history of lower back pain radiating down the left leg. The patient reported that he had suffered a work-related injury while acting as a commercial driver and while assisting in the clean-up of the New Orleans hurricane disaster. Because of the severe pain, he was unable to work so he returned home. An MRI of the lumbar spine taken 2 weeks ago shows a large extruded disk herniation on the left side, L5-S1, causing severe nerve impingement. He has failed conservative treatment and is now indicated for nerve root decompression. He reports weakness in the left leg but denies any problems with bowel or bladder control. There is moderate tension in the lower back with flexion to 70 degrees and extension to 10 degrees secondary to lower back pain. He also complains of intermittent pain and numbness in his right hand and fingers that was evaluated during this preoperative episode, and he was diagnosed with right carpal tunnel syndrome, which may be surgically corrected at a later date as an outpatient procedure. His past surgical history is a left knee arthroscopy 12 years ago. He has no medical problems other than his back and the carpal tunnel syndrome in his right upper extremity. His preoperative diagnosis is acute left L5-S1 radiculopathy secondary to large L5-S1 disc herniation. He was admitted to the hospital for surgery.

OPERATIVE FINDINGS: The patient had a L5-S1 laminectomy and discectomy. The nerve root was resting freely at the conclusion of the procedures, and there was no dural injury.

DESCRIPTION OF PROCEDURE: After satisfactory induction of general anesthesia, AV boots were applied to both feet. The patient was turned to the prone position on a Kambin frame. Care was taken to make sure that pressure points were well padded. Once the position of the back was judged to be satisfactory, it was prepped and draped in the usual fashion. Epinephrine 1:500,000 solution was injected into the planned surgical incision site in the right lower back. Sharp dissection was carried down to the level of the fascia. The fascia was incised and subperiosteal dissection was carried out along the spinous processes down to the lamina and facet of each vertebral level. Deep retractors were then used to place a marker and intra-operative fluoroscopy confirmed the L5-S1 level. Once oriented to our level, the laminotomy was begun. The ligamentum flavum was debrided. A partial facetectomy of approximately 10% was carried out on the left side. This allowed identification of the nerve root. Upon retracting the nerve root, we could immediately identify extruded disc fragments. We were able to retrieve a moderate size fragment. Further inspection up behind the body of L5 produced a large extruded fragment. Exploration of the annular defect area identified only a tiny amount of loose material, all of which was retrieved. After multiple inspections, we were satisfied that all of the loose fragments and the disc had been removed. The nerve root was resting freely. Satisfactory hemostasis was achieved. There was no dural injury. A dry piece of Gelfoam was placed over the laminotomy defects. The fascial layer was closed with #1 Vicryl. The subcutaneous layer was closed with 2-0 Vicryl, and the skin was closed with 4-0 Monocryl. The patient was turned to the supine position on the hospital bed and awakened in the operating room. The patient was noted to have intact bilateral lower extremity motor function when asked to move both of his legs, which he could do. The patient was extubated in the operating room and taken to recovery in good condition.

Principal Diagnosis: _____

Secondary Diagnoses: _____

Principal Procedure: _____

Secondary Procedure(s): _____

17

A 46-year-old woman, a former professional athlete, was admitted to the hospital for hip replacement surgery to treat posttraumatic osteoarthritis that involved both hips. Her left hip is considerably worse than her right hip. Otherwise, the patient is in good health. Her past medical history included pneumonia three years ago and a hysterectomy for a fibroid uterus at age 40 years. A successful total left hip replacement was performed using a ceramic-on-ceramic hip replacement bearing surface prosthesis cemented in place. The patient was discharged three days later to receive physical therapy at home. She will be scheduled for the right hip replacement at a later date.

Principal Diagnosis: _____

Secondary Diagnoses: _____

Principal Procedure: _____

Secondary Procedure(s): _____

18

A 65-year-old woman was admitted to the hospital four weeks ago for treatment of a Colles' fracture of the left wrist which she suffered as the result of a fall from an elementary school jungle gym while climbing up it with her grandson. At that time, the patient underwent a closed reduction with application of an external fixator device. The patient is now admitted for an open reduction and bone grafting as part of her traumatic fracture aftercare. The Colles' fracture was considered traumatic and healing routinely: however, she was found to have severe bone loss as a result of senile osteoporosis. The orthopedic surgeon fears the fracture area will collapse at the time the external fixator is removed. She was taken to surgery to remove the external fixator device with an open reduction of the distal radius with bone grafting to the radius performed. Human bone tissue from a bone bank was used. The Colles' fracture site was viewed with no complications noted. The patient was placed in a well-padded secure wrist splint.

Principal Diagnosis: _____

Secondary Diagnoses: _____

Principal Procedure: _____

Secondary Procedure(s): _____

19

A patient comes to the pain clinic for management of chronic neck and shoulder pain that she has suffered since she was the driver in an auto collision with another car in traffic that occurred 10 months previously. The patient has difficulty sleeping due to the pain and has trouble lifting or moving anything with her left shoulder or arm. After taking a complete history and performing a thorough physical examination, the pain management physician diagnoses the condition as "cervicobrachial syndrome, due to auto accident 10 months ago and past whiplash injury."

First-Listed Diagnosis: _____

Secondary Diagnoses: _____

20

The patient is seen in the orthopedic clinic for a complaint of muscle wasting or atrophy of the lower legs. In conducting a thorough history and physical examination, the physician learns that the patient had poliomyelitis 50 years previously. The physician determines the muscle atrophy is a result of her old polio and describes it as postpolio syndrome. The physician recommends a trial of physical therapy in the future to prevent further muscular wasting.

First-Listed Diagnosis: _____

Secondary Diagnoses: _____

21

The patient, an active 60-year-old man, who suffered a fracture of the neck of the left femur in an automobile accident 10 years previously when he was a passenger in a car involved in a collision with a pickup truck, is admitted to the hospital for a left total hip replacement. The patient has suffered progressive disability of his hip joint with severe hip pain on standing, sitting, and lying down. Given the fact the patient has no arthritis in any other joint, it is determined that the arthritis in his left hip is a result of the old fracture or trauma. The patient consents to a total hip replacement with an uncemented ceramic-on-ceramic bearing surface. The patient is discharged home to be followed up by home health nurses and physical therapists.

*Note: List all applicable codes **including** codes from the external causes of morbidity chapter.*

Principal Diagnosis: _____

Secondary Diagnoses: _____

Principal Procedure: _____

Secondary Procedure(s): _____

Chapter 14

Diseases of the Genitourinary System

Coding Scenarios for *Basic ICD-10-CM/PCS Coding*

The following case studies are organized following the sequence of the chapters in the *ICD-10-CM and ICD-10-PCS* code books. The objective of this book is to provide the student with more detailed clinical information to code, rather than one- or two-line diagnosis and procedure statements. ICD-10-CM diagnosis codes are to be assigned to both the inpatient hospital admission and the outpatient visit case studies. In this book, the ICD-10-PCS procedure codes are to be assigned only to the inpatient hospital admission cases. In actual practice, outpatient cases are assigned CPT/HCPCS codes. The ICD-10-PCS codes are only required for inpatient procedures.

1

An 80-year-old female is admitted to the hospital with fever, malaise, and left flank pain. A urinalysis shows bacteria of more than 100,000/mL present in the urine and a subsequent urine culture shows Proteus growth as the cause of the infection. The patient was treated with intravenous antibiotics. Other preexisting conditions of hypertension, arteriosclerotic heart disease (ASHD), previous percutaneous transluminal coronary angioplasty (PTCA) but no history of coronary artery bypass graft (CABG), and long-term chronic obstructive pulmonary disease (COPD) were treated during the hospital stay. The patient also has a history of repeated urinary tract infections (UTI) over the past several years.

Principal Diagnosis: _____

Secondary Diagnoses: _____

Principal Procedure: _____

Secondary Procedure(s): _____

2

A 75-year-old man was admitted to the hospital in acute urinary retention. A transurethral resection of the prostate was performed, and the diagnosis of benign nodular hyperplasia of the prostate was made. The pathologist confirmed the hyperplasia diagnosis and also found microscopic foci of adenocarcinoma of the prostate. The attending physician listed both conditions as discharge diagnoses.

Principal Diagnosis: _____

Secondary Diagnoses: _____

Principal Procedure: _____

Secondary Procedure(s): _____

3

A 52-year-old woman was admitted to the hospital with urinary stress incontinence and is scheduled for surgical repair of a paravaginal cystocele. An open anterior colporrhaphy is performed to repair the cystocele that was causing the incontinence. The patient has mild type 2 diabetes that is also treated during the hospital stay.

Principal Diagnosis: _____

Secondary Diagnoses: _____

Principal Procedure: _____

Secondary Procedure(s): _____

4

An 80-year-old man was brought to the emergency department with complaints of lower abdominal pain and the inability to urinate over the past 24 hours. An indwelling urinary catheter was placed in the patient and he was admitted. After study it was determined that the patient was in subacute to acute renal failure. The acute renal failure was caused by a urinary obstruction. The urologist concluded the urinary obstruction was a result of the patient's benign prostatic hypertrophy. An intravenous pyelogram with low osmolar contrast was performed fluoroscopically and confirmed the physician's diagnoses. The patient was treated with medications and the acute renal failure was resolved. The catheter remained in place for drainage. The patient would require a resection of the prostate but would return for prostate surgery the following week. The patient was discharged home.

Principal Diagnosis: _____

Secondary Diagnoses: _____

Principal Procedure: _____

Secondary Procedure(s): _____

5

A 60-year-old female patient is brought to a small community hospital complaining of flank and back pain, fever with chills, fatigue, and a general ill feeling. The patient was known to have essential hypertension and had a history of renal calculi treated six months ago. The patient was admitted with the diagnosis of possible urinary tract infection. Workup in the hospital showed evidence of acute pyelonephritis. She was treated with intravenous antibiotics, but while in the hospital the patient had a sudden loss of kidney function. A diagnosis was made of acute renal failure complicating the acute pyelonephritis. The physicians were concerned that the patient may need kidney dialysis, but this small community hospital did not have the equipment for dialysis. A urinary catheter was placed in the bladder, and a transfer of the patient to a larger hospital in the same city was quickly accomplished.

Principal Diagnosis: _____

Secondary Diagnoses: _____

Principal Procedure: _____

Secondary Procedure(s): _____

6

The patient is a 21-year-old man who is known to have polycystic kidney disease, which was diagnosed in the past year after he was found to have hypertension. Upon investigating the cause of hypertension in such a young individual, it was discovered he had polycystic kidney disease, an inherited condition. The hypertension was considered secondary to the kidney disease. On this occasion, the patient was admitted to the hospital because of worsening kidney function. After study, it was determined the patient had chronic kidney disease, stage III, as a result of the hypertension and polycystic kidney disease. This patient was referred to the university medical center for further management with hopes for better control of kidney function and avoidance of the need for kidney transplant.

Principal Diagnosis: _____

Secondary Diagnoses: _____

Principal Procedure: _____

Secondary Procedure(s): _____

7

The patient is a 46-year-old woman, gravida 3, para 3, admitted to the hospital for a scheduled vaginal hysterectomy and bilateral salpingo-oophorectomy. The patient has an extensive gynecologic history and was most recently seen for dysmenorrhea and dyspareunia. She stated she was having prolonged, heavy menses with disturbing premenstrual syndrome that was lasting 3–4 days before the onset of the menses. Six months ago, an outpatient laparoscopy was performed and extensive endometriosis of the uterus, ovaries, tubes, and pelvic peritoneum was found. Lysis of adhesions and ablation of the endometriosis was attempted but due to the extensive nature of the disease, it was known the procedure would not be entirely successful. In addition, the patient has been diagnosed and treated for genital herpes on one occasion, molluscum contagiosum, diagnosed by vulvar biopsy, and cervical dysplasia described as mild to moderate that was investigated with 11 different biopsies. All subsequent pap smears have been normal. Despite continued treatment, the patient still suffers from chronic pelvic pain, dysmenorrhea, and dyspareunia. After discussing her treatment options, the patient consented to a vaginal hysterectomy and bilateral salpingo-oophorectomy to treat the extensive endometriosis of the various sites previously described. The surgery was accomplished without difficulty, and the patient was able to go home on day 3. An additional diagnosis was added to the record when the pathology report was reviewed by the surgeon. The pathologist's report confirmed the endometriosis as well as a small lesion of the cervix that was found to be carcinoma in situ of the cervix.

Principal Diagnosis: _____

Secondary Diagnoses: _____

Principal Procedure: _____

Secondary Procedure(s): _____

8

The patient is a 25-year-old woman who is seen in the office today for a follow-up visit for a possible urinary tract infection. Last week the patient was in the office and had complained of pain and burning on urination, frequent urges to urinate, pressure in the lower abdomen, and foul-smelling urine. A urinalysis done last week showed a large number of white blood cells, and a urine culture was collected and sent to the laboratory. The culture confirmed the growth of more than 100,000 E. coli organisms. The diagnosis for this visit is more specifically acute cystitis due to E. coli organism. The patient has had frequent urinary tract infections in the past, and she is being referred to a urologist for further investigation and possible cystoscopy.

First-Listed Diagnosis: _____

Secondary Diagnoses: _____

9

A 45-year-old male patient is sent to the hospital outpatient radiology department with a physician's order for an intravenous pyelogram. Documented on the physician's order is the reason for the x-ray as "renal colic, possible kidney stone." The test is performed, and the diagnosis dictated by the physician on the IVP report is "renal colic due to bilateral nephrolithiasis with staghorn calculi." Following hospital and official coding guidelines, the hospital coder is able to use the radiologist's diagnosis as the reason for the outpatient test.

First-Listed Diagnosis: _____

Secondary Diagnoses: _____

10

The 38-year-old male patient is being admitted for the following procedure: transurethral ureteroscopic lithotripsy using high-energy shock waves. The patient is known to have several large bilateral ureteral stones, and other attempts to remove them have been unsuccessful. The bilateral lithotripsy procedure is performed without complications and the surgeon is satisfied that the ureteral stones were removed.

Principal Diagnosis: _____

Secondary Diagnoses: _____

Principal Procedure: _____

Secondary Procedure(s): _____

11

The patient is a 75-year-old man who was admitted to the hospital for severe weakness and falling multiple times at home over the past several days. The urinalysis performed in the Emergency Department showed evidence of a urinary tract infection, and for this reason he was admitted. The patient was also dehydrated. The patient also has bladder neck carcinoma, which has been an aggressive type treated by chemotherapy. He has bilateral nephrostomy tubes in place. There was some suspicion that there might be an obstruction in one of the nephrostomy tubes, but that was not found to be true. The patient also has coronary artery disease and is status post CABG with venous grafts. He has type 2 diabetes and hypercholesterolemia. The patient was seen in consultation by urology, oncology, and cardiology with his current and chronic conditions evaluated and treated with numerous medications, both intravenous and oral. The patient regained considerable strength and was able to return home with follow-up appointments made with four physicians.

Principal Diagnosis: _____

Secondary Diagnoses: _____

Principal Procedure: _____

Secondary Procedure(s): _____

12

The patient is a 45-year-old woman, gravida 2, para 2, who was electively admitted for a total abdominal hysterectomy and bilateral salpingo-oophorectomy primarily for her menometrorrhagia and severe dysmenorrhea with heavy flow and cramping. She also has uterine fibroids with the uterus being 15–16 weeks of gestation size. On the day of admission, a total abdominal hysterectomy, removal of cervix, and bilateral salpingo-oophorectomy was performed. She was found to have massive intraperitoneal adhesions that took an extended period of time to lyse. In the process of removing the adhesions, a small laceration was made in the small bowel. It was quickly repaired. During surgery she had profuse bleeding tendencies, apparently because of the continuous ingestion of ibuprofen she was taking for the pelvic pain she experienced. Bleeding tendencies are known to be an adverse effect of ibuprofen; the physician was not aware of the amount she was taking. After surgery, the patient experienced several complications. First, she was diagnosed with acute blood-loss anemia. She lost about 1,500 mL of blood during surgery, according to the anesthesiologist. She had hypoxemia, which might be attributed to her current smoking of half of a pack of cigarettes per day, even though she tried to quit prior to surgery but was unsuccessful. She developed atelectasis and fever, both postoperative complications. Finally, during the postoperative management of her conditions, she complained of back pain and was found to have hydronephrosis, which may have been caused by the surgery, as so much packing was placed around the ureters to try to protect them. The urologist performed a cystoscopy, retrograde pyelogram with low osmolar contrast, and inserted a stent into her right ureter for drainage. Within hours, the patient's problems reverted. She became afebrile, the back pain and atelectasis disappeared. She was able to be discharged home on day 4 postop and has an appointment to see the surgeon in her office in two weeks.

Principal Diagnosis: _____

Secondary Diagnoses: _____

Principal Procedure: _____

Secondary Procedure(s): _____

13

A 46-year-old female was admitted to the hospital through the emergency room feeling tired, weak, and stating that she had not been feeling well for the past 3 days. She also stated she had diarrhea alternating with vomiting off and on for the past week. Laboratory tests were performed including an electrolyte panel, BUN, and creatinine, all of which were abnormal. The impression written by the doctor on the history and physical examination report was "dehydration with suspected acute renal failure," and intravenous hydration was started. The patient was monitored closely by the nursing staff, including the documentation of fluid intake and output. The patient did not have diarrhea or vomiting. Laboratory tests including the BUN and creatinine were repeated over the next 48 hours. Given the patient's general healthy history and the other tests performed, there was no underlying chronic kidney condition. No reason for the patient's diarrhea and vomiting that occurred prior to admission was found. No dialysis was required, as the patient's normal kidney function returned as the patient was rehydrated. The physician concluded the patient's condition was acute renal failure due to dehydration.

Principal Diagnosis: _____

Secondary Diagnoses: _____

Principal Procedure: _____

Secondary Procedure(s): _____

14

The patient is a 68-year-old female who had a hysterectomy 22 years ago and had a cystocele repair 8 years ago. Now the patient has very significant urinary stress incontinence for the past 2 years and is admitted at this time for surgical treatment. She had failed conservative management with medications that had provided no improvement of her stress incontinence.

The patient required inpatient recovery and monitoring because of her oxygen dependence due to severe COPD. The day of admission the patient was taken to surgery for a suprapubic sling operation. The procedure is a suspension of the urethra using the levator muscle to reposition the bladder neck to restore support to the bladder and urethra. The patient was able to be released from the hospital late in the afternoon of the day after surgery, with no complications from the anesthesia and her lung function returned to her baseline status. Home health care services were ordered for the patient, and a follow-up appointment in the urologist office was scheduled for 7 days after surgery.

Principal Diagnosis: _____

Secondary Diagnoses: _____

Principal Procedure: _____

Secondary Procedure(s): _____

15

The patient is a 26-year-old female who is gravida 4, para 3, AB 1 with two past cesarean deliveries and one normal spontaneous vaginal delivery. She had one voluntary interruption of pregnancy at 10 weeks prior to the birth of her children. The patient states she does not want any more children and cannot tolerate oral contraceptives because of the side effects of nausea and vomiting. She also complains of irregular menstrual and intermenstrual uterine bleeding with two periods a month that last between 5 and 7 days. The patient is given the facts about the proposed procedures, the alternatives, risks, complications, and possible failure rate. Nevertheless, the patient consents to the surgery to be performed on an outpatient basis at the hospital. The procedures performed are a dilation and curettage with a diagnostic laparoscopy with bilateral tubal Falope ring application. The pre- and postoperative diagnoses are the same: dysfunctional uterine bleeding and desire for elective sterilization.

First-Listed Diagnosis: _____

Secondary Diagnoses: _____

16

HISTORY: The patient is a 38-year-old woman who gave birth 10 weeks ago. This past week she developed abdominal pain and symptoms of a urinary tract infection (UTI), and was admitted to the hospital. She was found to have a left ureteral stone, and small bilateral renal stones, as well as bilateral hydronephrosis and UTI. It was recommended that the left collecting system be stented because of the hydronephrosis and the infection. Once the infection has been adequately treated, she will undergo ESWL of the ureteral stone at a later date.

OPERATIVE FINDINGS: The urethra is normal. The bladder is smooth and without stone or tumor. Orifices are in normal location bilaterally. Right retrograde pyelogram showed no evidence of persistent filling defect; however, there is dilation of the collecting system and very mild hydronephrosis on the right side. One the left side, there was a 1-cm stone over the left ureterovesical junction with ureteral dilatation both distal and proximal to this, but especially proximal, and also left hydronephrosis. No other obvious stones were identified.

DESCRIPTION OF PROCEDURE: The patient was taken to the operating area where she underwent IV sedation without problems. Following successful anesthesia, she was placed in the dorsal lithotomy position and prepped and draped in the sterile fashion. A #21 French cystoscopy with lens was introduced into the bladder and thorough inspection of the bladder and urethra was carried out. Following examination, bilateral retrograde pyelograms were obtained and reviewed. Next, under fluoroscopic control, a .035 guidewire was placed up to the left orifice into the renal pelvis. Over this, a 24 cm × 6 F double-J stent was passed without problems, so that the proximal end curled in the left renal pelvis, and the distal end curled in the bladder. The bladder was then evaluated and the cystoscope was withdrawn. The patient was awakened and transported to the recovery room in good condition, tolerating the procedure well. She will be kept on a course of Ampicillin 500 mg 4 times a day for the next week and will then return at that time for ESWL of her left ureteral stone at a later date.

Principal Diagnosis: _____

Secondary Diagnoses: _____

Principal Procedure: _____

Secondary Procedure(s): _____

17

A 75-year-old male was admitted to the hospital because of refractory temperature elevation, documented as "probable urinary sepsis" that did not respond to outpatient antibiotics. He became more acutely ill the day before admission. He lives alone but was coherent enough to call a neighbor to ask for help. His fever was 104.5°F at home the day of admission. He had been on Ciprofloxacin for approximately 12 hours prior to admission with no change in his fever. He has a history of urinary tract infections (UTI) and was hospitalized six months ago for life-threatening septic shock. He is known to have an enlarged prostate without lower urinary tract symptoms. His only other medical problem is chronic atrial fibrillation, which has been under treatment for several years with an anticoagulant medication that was continued in the hospital. A consultation with a urologist resulted in a nonsurgical workup. After appropriate cultures were drawn, he was started on IV antibiotics and vigorous IV hydration. His blood cultures were returned as negative. His urine culture demonstrated large amounts of a mixed growth that was suggestive of a possible contaminant. This was not unexpected, with the source of his infection considered to be his prostate. He responded dramatically to the IV antibiotics, but it took several days before he became close to afebrile. After four days in the hospital he was well enough to be taken off all IV support and was transferred to a skilled (swing) bed for two more days of observation on oral antibiotics to be sure it is safe to discharge him to home care. His discharge diagnoses were urinary sepsis/UTI due to chronic prostatitis with possible acute prostatitis, BPH, and atrial fibrillation. The physician was queried regarding the diagnosis "urinary sepsis/UTI" and responded to clarify that the diagnosis was "urinary tract infection."

Principal Diagnosis: _____

Secondary Diagnoses: _____

Principal Procedure: _____

Secondary Procedure(s): _____

Chapter 15

Pregnancy, Childbirth, and the Puerperium

Coding Scenarios for *Basic ICD-10-CM/PCS Coding*

The following case studies are organized following the sequence of the chapters in the *ICD-10-CM and ICD-10-PCS* code books. The objective of this book is to provide the student with more detailed clinical information to code, rather than one- or two-line diagnosis and procedure statements. ICD-10-CM diagnosis codes are to be assigned to both the inpatient hospital admission and the outpatient visit case studies. In this book, the ICD-10-PCS procedure codes are to be assigned only to the inpatient hospital admission cases. In actual practice, outpatient cases are assigned CPT/HCPCS codes. The ICD-10-PCS codes are only required for inpatient procedures.

1

A 35-year-old woman at 22 weeks of pregnancy underwent a 1-hour glucose screening test that was found to be abnormal, with a blood sugar level reported to be over 200 mg/dL. The patient was sent to the outpatient laboratory for a 3-hour glucose tolerance test. The reason for the laboratory test was documented on the order as "rule out gestational diabetes; abnormal glucose tolerance on screening during pregnancy."

First-Listed Diagnosis: _____

Secondary Diagnoses: _____

2

The patient is a 26-year-old female, gravida 2, para 1, in her 10th week of pregnancy. While at work, she developed severe cramping and vaginal bleeding. Coworkers brought her to the hospital emergency department, and she was admitted to the hospital. After examination, the physician described her condition as an "inevitable abortion." When the physician was asked to further define her condition, she stated that an inevitable abortion meant the cervix was dilated and fetal and placental material probably had already passed from the patient's body. According to the physician, another description of this condition was an incomplete early spontaneous abortion. During this pregnancy the patient had been treated for transient hypertension of pregnancy, for which she was monitored during this hospital stay. She was taken to the operating room where a dilation and curettage was performed to remove the products of conception in order to treat the abortion. There were no complications from the procedure.

Principal Diagnosis: _____

Secondary Diagnoses: _____

Principal Procedure: _____

Secondary Procedure(s): _____

3

A 34-year-old female is admitted in active labor during week 39 of pregnancy. She had a previous cesarean section 2 years ago as a result of fetal distress and cephalopelvic disproportion (CPD). No fetal distress was found during this admission, but it was determined that the patient still had CPD; therefore, a repeat low cervical cesarean section had to be performed. A healthy 8 lb, 10 oz female was safely delivered.

Principal Diagnosis: _____

Secondary Diagnoses: _____

Principal Procedure: _____

Secondary Procedure(s): _____

4

A 45-year-old woman, gravida 1, para 0, was admitted in labor to the hospital obstetrical department. Unexpectedly but happily, this woman found herself pregnant after 15 years of marriage. She had been under the care of a physician who specialized in high-risk pregnancies. Because of her age, the woman was thought to be at higher risk for complications, but her pregnancy was uneventful. The physician described her as an "elderly primigravida, full term 38 week pregnancy." She had a manually assisted vaginal delivery of a healthy 7 lb, 5 oz girl. Mother and baby were able to leave the hospital on day 2 after delivery.

Principal Diagnosis: _____

Secondary Diagnoses: _____

Principal Procedure: _____

Secondary Procedure(s): _____

5

The patient is a 30-year-old woman, gravida 3, para 2, in week 40 of pregnancy. The patient is admitted for "induction of labor at term." There is no other reason documented by the physician as the reason for labor induction. The patient was not in labor at the time of admission. The induction is performed by artificial rupture of membranes. Labor proceeds normally, and the woman delivers a healthy male infant vaginally without complications. The mother and baby were able to be discharged on the hospital day 2.

Principal Diagnosis: _____

Secondary Diagnoses: _____

Principal Procedure: _____

Secondary Procedure(s): _____

6

The obstetrics patient at 15 weeks gestation (second trimester) is seen for her regular antepartum visit. The woman has confessed to using cocaine both prior to and during her current pregnancy. A drug screen performed during this visit is positive for cocaine. She feels she is unable to quit using the drug on her own, but wishes to become drug-free for the safety of her baby and herself. The patient has consented to admission later today to a specialized antepartum unit at a nearby hospital for drug detoxification and cocaine dependence treatment. The patient will be seen again in the OB clinic in 1 month for continued antepartum care. The patient is also being treated for a urinary tract infection during the pregnancy.

First-Listed Diagnosis: _____

Secondary Diagnoses: _____

7

The patient is seen in her OB physician's office 2 weeks after a normal vaginal delivery that produced a healthy full-term female infant. The patient has been breast feeding the infant, but over the past 2 days had developed redness, pain, and swelling of her right breast. Upon examination there appears to be a hard lump in the right breast, and the diagnosis of a postpartum purulent breast abscess is made. The patient is given a prescription for an antibiotic and advised she may take an anti-inflammatory drug to reduce the pain and inflammation. She is also advised to discontinue breast feeding until the infection resolves. The patient will return to the office within 7 days for a reevaluation.

First-Listed Diagnosis: _____

Secondary Diagnoses: _____

8

The patient is admitted to the hospital 6 weeks after delivering a healthy female infant following a full-term pregnancy with the admitting diagnosis of acute cholecystitis with chole-lithiasis. The patient was known to have gallstones prior to her pregnancy and had symptoms of the disease recur during the pregnancy and become more serious during the immediate postpartum period. A laparoscopic cholecystectomy is performed without complications. Pathologic examination confirmed the admitting diagnosis. The patient is able to go home 1 day after the surgery.

Principal Diagnosis: _____

Secondary Diagnoses: _____

Principal Procedure: _____

Secondary Procedure(s): _____

9

The patient is admitted to the hospital with excessive vaginal bleeding 2 days following an elective abortion at an outpatient surgical facility. The patient is immediately taken to surgery for a dilatation and curettage. The pathology report describes the tissue removed as "retained products of conception." The previous elective abortion was not completed as expected. At the time of the procedure it was determined the patient had anemia due to the acute blood loss and it was treated. The physician's final diagnosis is "delayed hemorrhage following elective abortion, now completed, anemia of pregnancy due to acute blood loss." The patient is able to be discharged the next day.

Principal Diagnosis: _____

Secondary Diagnoses: _____

Principal Procedure: _____

Secondary Procedure(s): _____

10

A pregnant woman is admitted to the hospital during week 12 of her pregnancy. The patient had called her physician describing vague symptoms, and the physician ordered a complete obstetrical ultrasound. The fetus is seen in utero, but no fetal heart tones are detected and further examination confirms the fetus is dead. The physician describes the condition in one progress note as an inevitable abortion and in another progress note as a missed abortion. No medical or obstetrical complication can be found to explain the loss of the pregnancy. A D&C is performed to complete the missed abortion. The mother receives grief counseling and is able to be discharged 1 day after the procedure.

Principal Diagnosis: _____

Secondary Diagnoses: _____

Principal Procedure: _____

Secondary Procedure(s): _____

11

The patient was admitted from home on May 31 with vaginal bleeding. This is the patient's third admission to labor and delivery during this pregnancy. The patient is 33 years old, gravida 1, para 0, with an estimated date of confinement of July 9. She has twin gestation (two placentae and two amniotic sacs) and complete placenta previa. Because of this last episode of bleeding, it was decided to keep her at bed rest in labor and delivery at the hospital so that, should any further excessive bleeding occur, she would be available for emergency cesarean delivery if necessary. The intent was to keep her until she reached 36 weeks gestation as recommended by the perinatologist in consultation. On June 10 she had bright red bleeding from the vagina. There were contractions of preterm labor noted. Because she was one day short of 36 weeks gestation, it was decided to go forward with a primary low cervical cesarean delivery for the complete placenta previa with hemorrhage. She delivered a 4 pound, 9 ounce viable female with Apgars of 8 and 9 at 16:01 p.m. She delivered a 4 pound, 15 ounce viable male with Apgars of 7 and 9 at 16:02 p.m. Intraoperative blood loss was approximately 1 liter. She was anemic due to acute blood loss prior to surgery. She had a good recovery from the surgery and her hemoglobin stabilized at 8.2 gm. She was discharged home to follow up in the office in 2 weeks for an incision check. Her twin infants remained in the premature nursery for further treatment.

Principal Diagnosis: _____

Secondary Diagnoses: _____

Principal Procedure: _____

Secondary Procedure(s): _____

12

The patient was admitted to the hospital from the obstetrician's office at 38 and 3/7 weeks gestation. She came to the office today complaining of not feeling well and noticing a lack of fetal movement over the past day or two. She had been in the office 3 days ago and the baby was reactive. The biophysical profile in the office today was 6/8 with no breathing movement. The nonstress test was reactive. The patient also has severe iron deficiency anemia of pregnancy and gestational hypertension complicating her pregnancy. She desires a tubal ligation during this delivery for her grand multiparity. She is 38 years old and gravida 6, para 3, AB 2 with an estimated date of delivery of June 30. She has had two previous cesarean deliveries, one in 1995 and one in 2005. Her oldest child was delivered vaginally in 1993. Because of the decreased fetal movement, a repeat low cervical cesarean delivery was performed on June 19,

2008. A bilateral tubal ligation was also performed by ligation and crushing. Delivered at 4:55 p.m. was a 6 pound, 2 ounce live female infant with Apgar scores of 7 and 8. The patient had an uneventful recovery from the delivery, was continued on her medications for anemia and gestational hypertension, and asked to return to the office in 2 weeks. Mother and daughter were discharged home together on post-op day 3.

Principal Diagnosis: _____

Secondary Diagnoses: _____

Principal Procedure: _____

Secondary Procedure(s): _____

13

The patient is a 23-year-old female, gravida 2, para 1, AB 0, who was admitted to the hospital in the early morning hours reporting she had sporadic contractions for the past 24 hours. She is 38 and 1/7 weeks gestation. At 2:45 a.m. she had an artificial rupture of membrane, her cervix was 4-5 cm dilated and 90% effaced. She had some variable fetal heart rate decelerations on the external fetal monitor. She was pushing with some of her contractions, and the fetal distress appeared to worsen. Presentation was vertex, and station was minus 1 for most of the morning. The fetal head came down to about zero station. However, since the fetal distress did not abate, a long discussion was held with the patient and her mother about a change in the management of her anticipated delivery. The doctor recommended a cesarean delivery for the intrauterine pregnancy be performed because of the fetal distress caused by fetal heart rate decelerations, and the patient consented to it. A low cervical cesarean section was performed at 10 a.m. under spinal anesthesia. A viable male infant with spontaneous respiration and cry was delivered. The cord was doubly clamped and cut, and the infant was placed in the warmer and examined by the pediatrician. The mother's placenta was removed, uterine cavity cleaned, and the uterine incision closed in two layers. Careful inspection of the uterus, fallopian tubes, and ovaries did not reveal any unusual findings or bleeding. The peritoneum was closed vertically, and the fascia was closed. Subcutaneous tissue was closed with plain silk, and the skin was closed with subcuticular sutures followed by staples. The patient received Pitocin and a gram of Ancef, per protocol. The patient's estimated blood loss was about 500 cc with no surgical complications. Postoperatively the patient complained of the typical abdominal discomfort from the incision. The patient was known to have microcytic anemia during her pregnancy, and the anemia was present at the time of delivery and at discharge as well. The anemia continued to be treated. The patient was discharged with her newborn son on day 3 with a follow-up appointment in the obstetrician's office in 10 days.

Principal Diagnosis: _____

Secondary Diagnoses: _____

Principal Procedure: _____

Secondary Procedure(s): _____

14

The 45-year-old female was admitted to the hospital in premature labor at 36 and 4/7th weeks gestation with 5 cm dilation. The patient is gravida 6, para 5 with five daughters at home ranging in age from 8 to 18 years. This was a "surprise" pregnancy to this elderly multigravida patient and her husband. Two antepartum ultrasounds predicted the birth of a male infant, which has brought considerable excitement to the family. The patient's labor was augmented with Pitocin drip, and she was placed on an external fetal monitor. The patient has a known cystocele that was monitored during the pregnancy and will probably require surgical treatment in the near future. After a short period of labor, the patient had a manually assisted delivery of a healthy male infant at 4 lb 2 oz with Apgar scores of 8 and 9 at one and five minutes. When the patient was visited by the delivering physician in her room later the same day, the patient asked if it was "too late" for tubal ligation, as she and her husband concluded their family was complete and she desired permanent sterilization. The next day the patient was taken to the operating room for a postpartum endoscopic tubal ligation by division and ligation, which was completed uneventfully. The patient was discharged home on day 3, but the male infant remained in the nursery for observation and weight gain. Discharge instructions and a follow-up appointment with her obstetrician were given to the patient.

Principal Diagnosis: _____

Secondary Diagnoses: _____

Principal Procedure: _____

Secondary Procedure(s): _____

15

HISTORY: The patient is a 28-year-old, gravida 2, para 1, with complete/total placenta previa with four bleeding episodes was admitted to the hospital. She has a previous cesarean section for her first child. The patient has received steroids and has consented for a repeat preterm cesarean delivery because of the placenta previa and the threat-to-life hemorrhage that could occur again as the pregnancy continued or during a vaginal delivery. The patient is aware that a hysterectomy may need to be performed if the placenta cannot be removed but will be avoided if at all possible. The patient also is known to have the baby in a double footling breech presentation and had gestational hypertension during this pregnancy. Labor was not allowed to occur in this patient. The patient is a 32 5/7 week gestation.

FINDINGS:
1. Complete placenta previa
2. Viable male infant in double footling breech presentation. Weight 5 pounds even. Apgar scores were 6 at one minute, 8 at five minutes, and 9 at ten minutes. The uterus did not have to be removed. There were normal-appearing tubes and ovaries. Of note: the pathologist reported on examination of the placenta that mild-to-moderate amnionitis was present in this mid third-trimester placenta.

DESCRIPTION OF PROCEDURE: The patient was taken to the operating room, where a spinal anesthesia was found to be adequate. She was then prepped and draped in the normal, sterile fashion in the dorsal supine position with a left-ward tilt. A Pfannenstiel skin incision was made with the scalpel and carried through to the underlying layer of the fascia. The fascia was incised in the midline, and the incision extended laterally with the use of Mayo scissors. The superior aspect of the fascial incision was then grasped with the Kocher clamps, and the underlying rectus muscles were dissected with the Mayo scissors. Attention was then turned to the inferior aspect of this incision, which in a similar fashion was grasped with the pickups and entered, and the underlying rectus muscles were dissected with the Mayo scissors. The rectus muscle was spread in the midline, and the peritoneum was entered bluntly. The peritoneum was extended superiorly and inferiorly, with good visualization of the bladder, using the Metzenbaum scissors. The bladder blade was placed and the vesico-uterine peritoneum was identified, tented up, and entered sharply with the Metzenbaum scissors. A bladder flap was then created digitally, and the bladder blade was replaced. The uterine incision was made about a centimeter and a half higher than usual due to the placenta previa, and the incision was widened with blunt force. At this time we were able to reach past the placenta previa and were able to grab both feet. At this point, the bag seemed to rupture. The infant was delivered in double footling breech with the typical breech maneuvers. The head delivered atraumatically. The nose and mouth were bulb suctioned. The cord was doubly clamped and cut. The infant was handed off to the waiting pediatrician. Cord gases and blood were obtained. The placenta was removed. The uterus was exteriorized and cleared of all clots and debris. The uterine incision was then repaired with a 0 Vicryl in a running, locked fashion, and a second layer of the same was used to ensure excellent hemostasis. The uterus was then replaced into the abdomen and the gutters were irrigated and cleared of all clots and debris. The peritoneum was repaired with a 2-0 Vicryl. The 0 Vicryl was then used to reapproximate the rectus muscle in the midline. The fascia was repaired with a 0 Vicryl in a running fashion. The subcutaneous layer was then closed with plain 2-0 silk on a GI needle. The skin was closed with staples. The sponge, lap, and needle counts were correct times two. The patient had been given a gram of Ancef at cord clamp. The patient was taken to the recovery room in stable condition.

Principal Diagnosis: _____

Secondary Diagnoses: _____

Principal Procedure: _____

Secondary Procedure(s): _____

Chapter 16

Certain Conditions Originating in the Perinatal Period

Coding Scenarios for *Basic ICD-10-CM/PCS Coding*

The following case studies are organized following the sequence of the chapters in the *ICD-10-CM and ICD-10-PCS* code books. The objective of this book is to provide the student with more detailed clinical information to code, rather than one- or two-line diagnosis and procedure statements. ICD-10-CM diagnosis codes are to be assigned to both the inpatient hospital admission and the outpatient visit case studies. In this book, the ICD-10-PCS procedure codes are to be assigned only to the inpatient hospital admission cases. In actual practice, outpatient cases are assigned CPT/HCPCS codes. The ICD-10-PCS codes are only required for inpatient procedures.

1

A premature female infant was transferred for admission to the high risk neonatal intensive care unit at the university hospital from a smaller hospital for treatment at the age of 5 hours. The infant weighed 975 grams as the result of a pregnancy that last 29 weeks and 5 days. The patient was also treated for neonatal respiratory distress syndrome and spent 10 weeks in the hospital before being discharged to home with pediatric home care services provided.

Principal Diagnosis: _____

Secondary Diagnoses: _____

Principal Procedure: _____

Secondary Procedure(s): _____

2

A 2-day-old full-term male infant was transferred for admission to the high risk neonatal intensive care unit at the university hospital from a smaller hospital for treatment of sepsis due to streptococcus, group B. The physicians concluded that the infant acquired the infection during or shortly after birth from organisms colonizing the maternal genital tract. The mother was found to be a carrier of group B streptococci. The infant had the typical symptoms of neonatal sepsis: respiratory distress, lethargy and hypotension. Cultures from the infant confirmed group B streptococci found in the blood. The infant was treated with intravenous antibiotics. No complications such as meningitis developed, and the infant was able to be discharged 16 days later and will be followed by pediatric home care.

Principal Diagnosis: _____

Secondary Diagnoses: _____

Principal Procedure: _____

Secondary Procedure(s): _____

3

An 8-day-old male infant was brought by his mother to his pediatrician's office for his first well baby exam. The mother told the physician she was concerned about the malodorous discharge from his umbilical stump that she had been cleaning several times a day. Upon examination, the physician found periumbilical erythema and tenderness as well as discharge from the umbilical stump but no hemorrhage from the site. The baby did not have a fever or other signs of systemic infection. The physician prescribed liquid antibiotics to be started the same day and arranged for an appointment with an infectious disease specialist the next day to confirm the antibiotic was appropriate. A culture was taken from the umbilical drainage. The physician's final diagnosis for the office visit was neonatal omphalitis.

First-Listed Diagnosis: _____

Secondary Diagnoses: _____

4

A 2-day-old infant is transferred for admission to the larger community hospital for evaluation and treatment from a small rural hospital where he was born. The baby's mother has type 1 diabetes mellitus. The infant was large at birth (more than 10 pounds) and exhibited hypoglycemia, transient tachypnea, and possibly other endocrine disorders that are characteristic of a syndrome of infants born to diabetic mothers. The baby required special surveillance because, as an "infant of a diabetic mother," he was at increased risk for a variety of complications and congenital defects. The baby was also observed for suspected sepsis or other infectious process because of the mother's sepsis. Fortunately, no major problems were found. The infant was discharged to his parents 3 days after admission to be followed closely by a pediatric specialist.

Principal Diagnosis: _____

Secondary Diagnoses: _____

Principal Procedure: _____

Secondary Procedure(s): _____

5

A 2-day-old baby girl was transferred for admission to the Children's Hospital after being noted to be hypoxemic soon after birth. She was a full-term infant from an uneventful pregnancy. A transthoracic contrast echocardiogram of the pediatric heart done on admission did not reveal any major cardiac defects. However, there was right-to-left shunting suggestive of pulmonary hypertension. The doctors were concerned about her episodes of significant hypoxemia. During the morning of day 2 the baby required significantly increased inotropic medication support to maintain her hemodynamics. Given the lability as well as the increase in inotropes, it was felt that she would benefit from ECMO support. Neurologically, some movements had been noted earlier today and the liver function and renal function tests were within normal range suggesting that there was no significant end-organ injury related to the hypoxia. The baby was taken to the operating room and sedated with fentanyl, Versed, and vecuronium. A transverse skin incision was made 2 cm above the medial aspect of the clavicle and extended down through the subcutaneous tissues and platysma. The internal jugular vein and the carotid artery were identified. Two Ethibond ties were passed proximal and distal around each of the vessels. Intravenous heparin of 50 units/kg was administered. The distal carotid artery was ligated and the proximal carotid cannulated with a 10-French Biomedicus arterial cannula. A longitudinal venotomy was performed and a 12-French Biomedicus cannula was inserted into the superior vena cava while a 12-French polystan cannula was introduced cephalad and both were secured to the vessel with a 2-0 tie. The ECMO circuit was brought into the field and tubing divided. The arterial cannula was connected to the arterial end of the circuit taking care to avoid air entry and the venous cannulae were connected to the venous end of the circuit. ECMO flows were initiated. The patient tolerated the procedure, and no complications were encountered. The sternocleidomastoid was reapproximated with a 3-0 Vicryl suture and skin was closed with multiple interrupted 3-0 nylon sutures. Dressings were applied in standard fashion. The doctors provided a final diagnosis of persistent fetal circulation or primary pulmonary hypertension of newborn. The continuous extracorporeal membrane oxygenation was successful in treating the patient's symptoms of hypoxemia due to the pulmonary hypertension.

Principal Diagnosis: _____

Secondary Diagnoses: _____

Principal Procedure: _____

Secondary Procedure(s): _____

6

A 12-hour-old infant was transferred for admission to the university hospital neonatal intensive care unit for respiratory problems after being born at a community hospital by vaginal delivery to a woman who had just completed her 39th week of pregnancy. The infant was exhibiting respiratory symptoms consistent with aspiration of meconium at the time of the delivery. The infant had low Apgar scores of 5 and 6 with tachypnea and cyanosis. Within 1 day, the infant's chest x-ray demonstrated patchy infiltrates. The neonatologist diagnosed the infant as having meconium aspiration pneumonia with no signs of pulmonary hypertension as a consequence of the pneumonia. The physician also described the infant as "small for dates," weighing 2,200 grams.

Principal Diagnosis: _____

Secondary Diagnoses: _____

Principal Procedure: _____

Secondary Procedure(s): _____

7

The patient is an infant who was transferred for admission to the university hospital neonatal intensive care unit after being born at a community hospital by vaginal delivery to a woman who had just completed her 38th week of pregnancy. The mother of the infant was addicted to prescription narcotics for back pain from a car accident but had switched to prescription methadone during her pregnancy. The infant admitted to the neonatal ICU in narcotic withdrawal after being born addicted to the methadone the mother was taking during her pregnancy. The baby was attached to cardiac and oxygen monitors and exhibited symptoms of drug withdrawal with difficulty sleeping, long periods of crying, diarrhea, and trouble with feeding. A slow process of weaning was started with the baby receiving small doses of methadone to wean her off the drugs. Over time, the baby had fewer symptoms of withdrawal and was gaining weight and sleeping for longer periods of time. On discharge, the physician described the infant as "small for dates," weighing 2,400 grams and infant of an addicted mother suffering withdrawal. The baby and her mother will be followed by a pediatric home care team.

Principal Diagnosis: _____

Secondary Diagnoses: _____

Principal Procedure: _____

Secondary Procedure(s): _____

8

A seven-day-old infant was brought by her parents to the University Hospital's outpatient high-risk pediatric clinic for her first post-hospital discharge examination. The physician examined the patient and was most concerned about the child's fetal growth retardation. The physician was pleased to see the child had gained weight since leaving the hospital. The physician described the child's condition as premature infant with fetal growth retardation, 36 week 3 day gestation, with a birth weight of 1,600 grams. The parents will bring the child back to the clinic in three weeks.

First-Listed Diagnosis: _____

Secondary Diagnoses _____

9

A 25-day-old infant is brought to the university hospital's high-risk pediatric clinic by her foster mother for evaluation of her status as a "crack baby." The child's mother was dependent on cocaine, and the baby had a positive drug screen for cocaine at birth and exhibited several symptoms. The baby continues to exhibit transitory tachypnea of newborn. The physician orders a continuation of pediatric home health services to monitor the child's respiratory status and the effect of the noxious substance (cocaine) on the baby. The reason for the clinic visit documented by the physician is crack baby with continued transitory tachypnea. The baby will be brought back to the clinic in 2 weeks.

First-Listed Diagnosis: _____

Secondary Diagnoses: _____

10

The parents of a 10-day-old baby bring the newborn to the pediatrician's office to evaluate her feeding problems. The child vomits after bottle feedings. When the baby was born, the umbilical cord was found loosely wrapped around the newborn's neck. It was quickly removed by the obstetrician, and the baby was observed for respiratory and other difficulties. Feeding problems were evident while the baby was in the hospital, and the pediatricians considered the nuchal cord problem as the cause. The physician recommends a change in baby formula and different feeding bottles. The physician also orders pediatric home health services to assist the parents in the child's care at home. A follow-up appointment is scheduled to return to the office in 2 weeks. The physician's diagnosis is feeding problems in an infant born with nuchal cord around his neck.

First-Listed Diagnosis: _____

Secondary Diagnoses: _____

11

This male infant was born today at 32-3/7th weeks premature weighing 1,920 grams by a repeat cesarean delivery. The baby had Apgar scores of 8 and 9. He had bag-mask inhalation for 30 seconds. His oxygen saturation was then 99 on room air. The baby was admitted to the premature nursery and placed on monitors. He was observed for a suspected infection but found to have none. Otherwise his physical exam showed no abnormalities other than Light-for-Dates, and he remained in the nursery after his mother's discharge for additional monitoring and weight gain. He was discharged at day 10 to be followed by pediatric home care nurses. No circumcision was performed.

Principal Diagnosis: _____

Secondary Diagnoses: _____

Principal Procedure: _____

Secondary Procedure(s): _____

12

This female infant was born to a 17-year-old mother, gravida 1, para 0, by spontaneous vaginal delivery with vertex presentation. She was born at 38 4/7 weeks gestation and small for gestational age, weighing 2,035 grams (4 pounds, 4 ounces). Her Apgar scores were 6 and 9. The baby required bag-mask inhalation for 2 minutes and 30 seconds and was admitted to the neonatal intensive care nursery for continuing monitoring and treatment. Initially the baby had transient tachypnea that became respiratory distress, and metabolic acidosis. She had hypermagnesemia, as her mother received magnesium therapy. She also had neonatal hyperbilirubinemia of prematurity. She was observed for possible sepsis, but none was found. The intravenous antibiotics were discontinued after 2 days. The baby's physical examination on discharge was within normal limits for a premature infant as her condition improved with laboratory data showing more normal findings. She was discharged at age 5 days to be followed by pediatric home care nurses with an appointment in the physician's office 2 days after discharge.

Principal Diagnosis: _____

Secondary Diagnoses: _____

Principal Procedure: _____

Secondary Procedure(s): _____

13

The mother of a 7-day-old baby brought the newborn to the pediatrician's office for her first post-hospital discharge evaluation. Upon examination, the physician noted bilateral conjunctivitis with mild erythema and scant mucoid discharge. A culture was taken from both eyes. Given the fact that the mother was diagnosed and treated for a chlamydial infection at the time of delivery the pediatrician decided the infant had a mild form of neonatal chlamydial conjunctivitis. The baby was prescribed to receive a 14-day course of oral erythromycin. A follow-up appointment is scheduled to return to the office in 2 weeks.

First-Listed Diagnosis: _____

Secondary Diagnoses: _____

14

A full-term male infant was born at Community Hospital to a mother who acquired a severe case of herpes simplex virus (HSV) during her pregnancy. At the age of one day old, the infant was transferred for admission to University Hospital's special care unit to "rule out HSV visceral and/or central nervous system (CNS) infection." The infant was diagnosed with congenital HSV but did not develop a visceral or CNS specific infection. The infant was treated with intravenous acyclovir for 10 days. An additional diagnosis of small-for-dates was made for the infant, who weighed 2,040 grams with a gestational age of 38 1/7th weeks. The infant was discharged to his mother's care with neonatal home nursing services to follow the infant's care at home.

Code for the infant at University Hospital only.

Principal Diagnosis: _____

Secondary Diagnoses: _____

Principal Procedure: _____

Secondary Procedure(s): _____

15

A preterm male infant was born at Community Hospital at 33 and 5/7th weeks to a primi-gravida 30-year-old female. The infant was having respiratory difficulties and was transferred within hours for admission to University Hospital to care for his prematurity and to rule out respiratory distress syndrome. While in the neonatal intensive care unit, the infant's respiratory symptoms abated. A thorough evaluation of the infant included laboratory and imaging studies. One unexpected diagnosis established through the imaging studies was the diagnosis of spina bifida occulta, the mildest form of spina bifida. Only through imaging examinations could the physician see an opening in the vertebrae of the spinal column, with no apparent damage to the spinal cord, which is the definition of spina bifida occulta. The infant remained in the hospital for 4 weeks gaining weight and maturing. The infant was discharged with the final diagnoses of preterm infant, 33 5/7th weeks gestation, birthweight of 1,600 grams with spina bifida occulta. The infant was discharged to the care of his parents with neonatal home nursing services to follow the infant's care at home. An appointment was made for the parents to return with the infant to see a pediatric neurologist in 4 weeks.

Code for the infant at University Hospital only.

Principal Diagnosis: _____

Secondary Diagnoses: _____

Principal Procedure: _____

Secondary Procedure(s): _____

Chapter 17

Congenital Malformations, Deformations, and Chromosomal Abnormalities

Coding Scenarios for *Basic ICD-10-CM/PCS Coding*

The following case studies are organized following the sequence of the chapters in the *ICD-10-CM and ICD-10-PCS* code books. The objective of this book is to provide the student with more detailed clinical information to code, rather than one- or two-line diagnosis and procedure statements. ICD-10-CM diagnosis codes are to be assigned to both the inpatient hospital admission and the outpatient visit case studies. In this book, the ICD-10-PCS procedure codes are to be assigned only to the inpatient hospital admission cases. In actual practice, outpatient cases are assigned CPT/HCPCS codes. The ICD-10-PCS codes are only required for inpatient procedures.

1

A 6-month-old infant, born with a congenital anomaly of the inner ear with impairment of hearing, is admitted for surgery to treat his mixed hearing loss. The patient is taken to surgery to place bilateral single channel cochlear prosthesis (hearing) implants via an open approach. He quickly recovers from the procedure and anesthesia and is discharged home.

Principal Diagnosis: _____

Secondary Diagnoses: _____

Principal Procedure: _____

Secondary Procedure(s): _____

2

A 3-month-old infant was born with a biliary atresia. The patient has severe obstructive jaundice due to the congenital condition. The patient was admitted and the diagnosis is confirmed by surgical exploration with an operative cholangiography done under fluoroscopic guidance with low osmolar contrast (this included views of the gallbladder and bile ducts). The biliary atresia is treated with an open roux-en-Y cholecystojejunostomy of the gallbladder.

Principal Diagnosis: _____

Secondary Diagnoses: _____

Principal Procedure: _____

Secondary Procedure(s): _____

3

A 2-month-old female infant, who has been in critical condition and in the NICU since being transferred to this hospital for admission one day after her birth, is brought to the operating room for excisional repair of the coarctation of the thoracic aorta with end-to-end anastomosis done with the pump oxygenator.

Principal Diagnosis: _____

Secondary Diagnoses: _____

Principal Procedure: _____

Secondary Procedure(s): _____

4

The mother of an 8-day-old infant brought the child to the pediatrician's office for the first well infant check-up. During the physical examination, the femoral head is felt to displace with a jerk, which is repeated as the femur slides back into the acetabulum upon release of the displacing force. The pediatrician is certain the baby has what is called a congenital dislocatable right hip. The mother is requested to bring the baby back to the office in 3 days. The mother is advised that the condition is likely to resolve within a week or two after birth. If the condition is still present at the next visit, the child will be referred to a pediatric orthopedic physician.

First-Listed Diagnosis: _____

Secondary Diagnoses: _____

5

The patient is admitted to the children's hospital for open heart surgery to repair her congenital heart defects. The patient is a 7-year-old girl who was born with Tetralogy of Fallot that was corrected by surgical repair at age 2 years. She has been seen by the pediatric cardiologist every 6 months since that surgery, aware of the fact that further surgery would be necessary later in childhood. Since birth, it has also been known that she suffers from the following diagnoses as listed on her discharge summary: "Stenosis of the pulmonary valve with right ventricular outflow obstruction causing pulmonary insufficiency and stenosis of the left pulmonary artery; status post previous cardiac surgery; surgically repaired congenital heart defects 5 years ago." The corrective surgery for these congenital conditions is "right ventricular outflow reconstruction with replacement of pulmonary valve with homograft; left pulmonary artery reconstruction to hilum with patch arterioplasty; right pulmonary artery stenosis arterioplasty." The surgery is performed under cardiopulmonary bypass and an intraoperative transesophageal echocardiogram of the pediatric heart with no contrast is performed.

Principal Diagnosis: _____

Secondary Diagnoses: _____

Principal Procedure: _____

Secondary Procedure(s): _____

6

A two-week-old male infant is brought to the University Medical Center pediatric gastroenterology clinic upon the request of the child's pediatrician based on findings of a recent well-baby exam. The infant was full-term when born and fed well after birth but then experienced occasional regurgitation of feedings. Several days later, the vomiting became more frequent and projectile containing the previous feedings. Shortly after the vomiting, the baby is ready to feed again. Imaging studies confirm the suspected diagnosis of congenital hypertrophic pyloric stenosis. The parents were instructed on the type of feedings to provide. A follow-up appointment is made for 1 week later. The parents were advised to return with the infant to the emergency department of the University Medical Center if the vomiting occurs more frequently. The possible need for surgery, specifically a pyloromyotomy, was discussed with the parents but will be reconsidered at the next visit.

First-Listed Diagnosis: _____

Secondary Diagnoses: _____

7

The patient is an 18-month-old boy who was born with a complete bilateral cleft lip and palate deformity. He is seen in the University Hospital's outpatient pediatric clinic. The child has had reconstruction surgery to correct the congenital defect. The child continues to have feeding difficulties. While he is free of infection now, he has had a few ear infections. Both the feeding and ear problems are attributed to the cleft lip and palate that appears to be incompletely repaired. The physician recommended to the parents that one more surgery should be performed to improve the symmetry of the palate and lip and alleviate the feeding problems and ear infections. However, it is possible that the child will need ear tubes placed in the future because of the chronic ear infections. A revision of the cleft palate and advancement flap graft is scheduled for the next month.

First-Listed Diagnosis: _____

Secondary Diagnoses: _____

8

After admission to the hospital, the patient is a 21-day-old male who is brought to the operating room and general anesthesia induced. The child had been previously diagnosed with Hirschsprung's disease by a rectal biopsy that showed no ganglion cells. A left lower quadrant oblique incision was made and dissection continued with electrocautery until the peritoneal cavity was entered. A stool-filled sigmoid colon was identified and delivered into the wound. A small biopsy was taken from the sigmoid portion of the bowel and sent for frozen section. This was returned normal with normal numbers of ganglion cells. The colon was then tacked to the fascia and peritoneum using interrupted 4-0 silk suture. A #12 red-rubber catheter was placed through the mesentery of the colon and looped upon itself and sutured with 2-0 silk suture. The colostomy of the sigmoid colon was then opened using electrocautery and both the limbs were found to be widely patent through the fascia. The colostomy was brought to the cutaneous level and a colostomy bag was applied. The sponge, needle, and instrument counts were reported to be correct at the conclusion of the procedure. The child was awakened and taken to the recovery room in satisfactory condition.

Principal Diagnosis: _____

Secondary Diagnoses: _____

Principal Procedure: _____

Secondary Procedure(s): _____

9

A seven-day-old male infant was examined by a pediatric ophthalmologist in the doctor's office. The child had been recently discharged from the hospital after birth. He was the product of a full-term gestation whose mother had an uneventful prenatal period. Based on physical findings and testing the male infant was diagnosed with Trisomy 13. In order to rule out a retinoblastoma, the infant was referred for this examination. The external examination of the lids was normal. There was haziness overlying the limbus superiorly in both eyes, consistent with an anterior embryotoxon. The pupils dilated readily. The lens were clear. The vitreous was clear. Examination of the fundus revealed normal-appearing disks and macular blood vessels with no evidence of any lesion. The consultant wrote the diagnoses on the report returned to the primary pediatrician as "Bilateral anterior embryotoxon, otherwise normal examination with no evidence of retinoblastoma in this newborn infant with Trisomy 13."

First-Listed Diagnosis: _____

Secondary Diagnoses: _____

10

A 1-day-old male infant with a prenatal history of hypoplastic left heart syndrome with ventricular septal defect was transferred for admission to the Mid Size Community Hospital from a rural regional hospital for evaluation and management. Noninvasive cardiac testing confirmed the congenital cardiac conditions. The patient was also found to have E. coli sepsis and was ordered to receive 7 days of intravenous antibiotics. The pediatric cardiovascular surgeon came to the hospital for a consultation and to meet with the parents to discuss performing a cardiac catheterization and a possible Hybrid Stage I procedure with median sternotomy and bilateral pulmonary artery banding versus a Norwood procedure. The parents agreed with the proposed Hybrid Stage I procedure, and the infant was transferred on day 3 to the University Medical Center for the surgical procedure.

Code for the baby at Mid Size Community Hospital.

Principal Diagnosis: _____

Secondary Diagnoses: _____

Principal Procedure: _____

Secondary Procedure(s): _____

11

The patient is a 3-week-old female infant who is brought to the pediatrician's office because the mother has observed the patient to appear to be arching her head and neck in an effort to breathe, especially after the child has been sucking on a bottle. The physician examined the baby and was unable to pass a small tube through the right nares to the pharynx, but the left nares was completely open. The physician ordered an immediate CT scan of the nasopharynx to determine if there was bony or membranous occlusion that was producing the complete obstruction of the posterior nares owing to choanal atresia. The doctor's diagnosis was choanal atresia, left side.

First-Listed Diagnosis: _____

Secondary Diagnoses: _____

12

The patient is 2-year-old male who was brought to the pediatrician's office by his parents for a routine well-baby check. During the physical examination, the physician noted the child had an undescended testicle on the right side. No other abnormalities or conditions were found. The parents were given a referral to take the child to a pediatric urologist within the next two weeks to determine the appropriate medical or surgical intervention needed to treat the unilateral cryptorchism.

First-Listed Diagnosis: _____

Secondary Diagnoses: _____

13

A 32-year-old female patient returns to her obstetrician-gynecologist's office to review the findings of her recent transvaginal uterine ultrasound. The patient has been married for 3 years and has not become pregnant as desired. The doctor informs the patient that the ultrasound examination showed that she had a bicornuate uterus, which is sometimes described as a heart-shaped uterus because of the distinct shape of the uterus when viewed externally, for example, on an ultrasound. The doctor also explained this is a congenital condition that occurs when the uterine fundus fails to fuse. The patient's condition is a partial bicornuate uterus with an evidenced cleft in the uterine dome. Given the fact that patients with this type of Mullerian abnormality often have a kidney abnormality as well, the patient was given an order to return to the radiology department for a renal ultrasound. The physician's review of the literature about this condition found that reproductive function is generally good in patients with partial bicornuate uteri, but the patient will be referred to a reproductive endocrinologist if she does not become pregnant within the next 6 months. The patient will return to this physician's office in 2 weeks to discuss the results of the renal ultrasound if an abnormality is found.

First-Listed Diagnosis: _____

Secondary Diagnoses: _____

14

A 3-day-old female infant was transferred for admission to the city's Children's Hospital because of noisy breathing or stridor. The doctors who ordered the transfer were concerned about the child having partial respiratory tract obstruction or partial occlusion in the airway. After imaging studies, the pediatrician concluded the infant had laryngomalacia, but not a severe form. The patient's stridor lessened when the patient was placed in the prone position with head extension. The doctors informed the parents that stridor usually resolves in most infants within 2 to 3 months as the child grows. The parents were requested to bring the infant back to the pediatric pulmonary disease clinic in one month. If the stridor had not improved at that time, it was expected that the parents will be asked to consent to an endoscopic exam of the infant's upper respiratory tract. The discharge diagnosis was infantile stridor due to laryngomalacia.

Principal Diagnosis: _____

Secondary Diagnoses: _____

Principal Procedure: _____

Secondary Procedure(s): _____

15

The parents of a one-year-male brought the child to the pediatric urologist's office for re-evaluation of his coronal or balanic hypospadias. The condition was diagnosed at the time of birth. The doctor reminded the parents that this urethral anomaly is the most common urethral anomaly that occurs in one out of 300 births. The child's congenital condition is not particularly severe, as his urethra is functional and the child does not have undescended testicles that often accompany hypospadias. Originally the urologist had advised the surgical plastic repair of the hypospadias be completed prior to school age. However, the parents were requesting the surgery to be completed sooner. The parents and physician agreed to wait until the child was at least 18 months old before surgery is scheduled.

First-Listed Diagnosis: _____

Secondary Diagnoses: _____

Chapter 18

Symptoms, Signs, and Abnormal Clinical and Laboratory Findings, Not Elsewhere Classified

Coding Scenarios for *Basic ICD-10-CM/PCS Coding*

The following case studies are organized following the sequence of the chapters in the *ICD-10-CM and ICD-10-PCS* code books. The objective of this book is to provide the student with more detailed clinical information to code, rather than one- or two-line diagnosis and procedure statements. ICD-10-CM diagnosis codes are to be assigned to both the inpatient hospital admission and the outpatient visit case studies. In this book, the ICD-10-PCS procedure codes are to be assigned only to the inpatient hospital admission cases. In actual practice, outpatient cases are assigned CPT/HCPCS codes. The ICD-10-PCS codes are only required for inpatient procedures.

1

A 50-year-old man is an inpatient who is scheduled for a colonoscopy. The reason for the colonoscopy is stated as "change in bowel habits, family history of colon cancer, and possible colonic polyp." A colonoscopy is performed. At the conclusion of the colonoscopy, the physician documents the final diagnosis as (1) change in bowel habits, unexplained, (2) normal colon examination.

Principal Diagnosis: _____

Secondary Diagnoses: _____

Principal Procedure: _____

Secondary Procedure(s): _____

2

A 59-year-old woman is referred by her primary care physician to the hospital outpatient radiology department with an order for a CT scan of the abdomen. The patient has been complaining of generalized abdominal pain, fatigue, and nausea but no vomiting over the past several weeks. Previous x-rays taken were abnormal. The doctor's diagnosis on the order is "abnormal radiology findings of GI tract, require further definition by CT exam, generalized abdominal pain, fatigue, nausea, rule out abdominal malignancy."

First-Listed Diagnosis: _____

Secondary Diagnoses: _____

3

A patient is admitted for a bronchoscopy with a transbronchial lung biopsy to determine the etiology of a lung mass found on recent x-ray and CT studies. The patient had been complaining of a cough and chest pressure over the past several weeks. The patient is taken to the outpatient endoscopy suite. Following administration of conscious sedation, the fiberoptic bronchoscopy is performed. During the process to obtain the transbronchial biopsy, the patient experiences a prolonged episode of bradycardia, and the physician terminates the procedure before the biopsy is obtained. The procedure will be rescheduled after the cardiologist evaluates the patient.

Principal Diagnosis: _____

Secondary Diagnoses: _____

Principal Procedure: _____

Secondary Procedure(s): _____

4

A 50-year-old man is admitted through the emergency department (ED) with a complaint of chest pain. The EKG and laboratory tests done in the ED are inconclusive, but an acute myocardial infarction is ruled out. During the hospital stay, the cardiovascular workup could not disprove the existence of coronary artery disease. Results of a thallium cardiac stress test were mildly abnormal. The patient did not want to have a cardiac catheterization study performed. Gastrointestinal studies, including an EGD, found some abnormalities including evidence of gastroesophageal reflux disease. Given the conflicting information, the physician concludes the patient had "atypical chest pain due to either angina or GERD." The patient is requested to visit both a cardiologist and gastroenterologist for additional testing.

Principal Diagnosis: _____

Secondary Diagnoses: _____

Principal Procedure: _____

Secondary Procedure(s): _____

5

A 38-year-old woman comes to her physician's office for the results of recent diagnostic studies. The woman had several complaints including numbness of her legs, difficulty in walking, lack of coordination, and trembling in her hands. The symptoms are not present all the time but have occurred more frequently over the past couple of weeks. The patient had also been examined by a neurologist. The patient was told the MRI and neurologic tests, as well as the conclusion of the neurologist, consider her condition to be consistent with multiple sclerosis (MS). When the patient asked whether the doctor was certain that she had MS, he said he was not 100% certain and made arrangements for her to be examined by physicians in a neurology group that specializes in treating patient with MS.

First-Listed Diagnosis: _____

Secondary Diagnoses: _____

6

A 52-year-old woman with known fibrocystic disease of the right breast has an appointment for a diagnostic mammogram at the hospital outpatient department. A screening mammogram done 3 days previously was abnormal with a suspicious lesion noted in the upper quadrant of the left breast. Findings of fibrocystic disease of the right breast were noted again. The diagnostic mammogram is performed and interpreted by the radiologist. The patient's physician meets with the radiologist to review the findings. The patient's physician agrees with the radiologist's findings of "microcalcifications of breast tissue, left breast" and advises the patient of the benign findings. The status of the fibrocystic disease of the right breast had not changed since last year's mammogram. The patient will have a follow-up diagnostic mammogram in 6 months.

First-Listed Diagnosis: _____

Secondary Diagnoses: _____

7

A 30-year-old woman has a repeat visit in her gynecologist's office to review the results of a recent abnormal Pap smear. Over the past year, the woman had experienced genital warts that appear and disappear on the external areas of her genitals. During the last visit, the gynecologist had performed a colposcopy and a Pap smear. Cells were scraped from the cervix and sent for cytologic and DNA testing. The patient is advised today that the conclusion of the test is "DNA positive for cervical high-risk human papillomavirus (HPV)." The patient consents to a cervical biopsy, which is scheduled for the following week. The patient's genital warts on her external genitalia today were examined and appear to be decreasing.

First-Listed Diagnosis: _____

Secondary Diagnoses: _____

8

A mother brought her 7-week-old infant to the pediatrician's office for intermittent diarrhea. The physician examines the infant and takes a comprehensive history, including the baby's food history and eating pattern. The physician considers the possibility that the baby is allergic to the infant formula being fed to the patient, which includes milk products. The physician recommends certain laboratory tests be performed and includes the following diagnosis on the order for the tests "Failure to thrive, diarrhea, possible milk allergy."

First-Listed Diagnosis: _____

Secondary Diagnoses: _____

9

Family members bring a 19-year-old man to the hospital emergency department. The patient had stated he had a severe headache, fever, and nausea and vomiting. A thorough physical examination is performed, including a spinal tap. The physician arranges for the transfer of the patient to a larger hospital with the diagnosis of "Rule out meningitis." All records and test results are transferred with the patient. In addition to the physical complaints stated by the patient, the physician adds the diagnosis of meningismus.

First-Listed Diagnosis: _____

Secondary Diagnoses: _____

10

A 56-year-old woman is admitted through the emergency department complaining of right upper quadrant abdominal pain. In addition, the patient says she is having nausea and had vomited several times at home. The patient is admitted with the diagnosis of possible cholecystitis. Several tests are performed, and all results are normal, except those of an ultrasound of the abdomen. It is also discovered that the patient has elevated blood pressure readings, but a diagnosis of hypertension is not made. The physician stated "no conclusive diagnosis found." When asked for more documentation concerning the patient diagnosis, the physician stated that the only conclusive findings were the patient's initial complaints, her elevated blood pressure readings, and the abnormal ultrasound of the GI abdominal area. The patient is discharged for outpatient management.

Principal Diagnosis: _____

Secondary Diagnoses: _____

Principal Procedure: _____

Secondary Procedure(s): _____

11

The patient is a 66-year-old woman who was admitted to the hospital after being seen in her physician's office with the complaint of difficulty in swallowing, first solid food and now difficulty with swallowing liquids. She was found to be dehydrated and was admitted. A gastroenterology consult was obtained, and the physician recommended an esophagogastro-duodenoscopy to rule out esophageal stricture or obstruction. The patient became very anxious during the start of the EGD, and it was postponed. After discussion with the patient and the primary care physician, the gastroenterologist recommended the procedure be performed under general anesthesia, which was accomplished. The EGD was performed, and no obstruction, stricture, or other disease was found in the esophagus, in the stomach, or small bowel, which was also examined. After being reassured that there was no disease or cancer present in her upper GI tract, the patient appeared very relieved. That evening she was able to eat a soft diet meal and drink liquids. The primary care physician listed the final diagnoses as dysphagia, cause unknown; anxiety disorder; and dehydration.

Principal Diagnosis: _____

Secondary Diagnoses: _____

Principal Procedure: _____

Secondary Procedure(s): _____

12

The patient is a 15-year-old female who has experienced a fever of 102 with chills overnight and was brought to the Emergency Department by her mother at 5 AM. Laboratory tests, including a complete blood count and urinalysis, were performed with normal results produced. The patient also complained of body aches, weakness, and fatigue. The patient's family physician was contacted and advised the patient be discharged home and come to his office the same afternoon if she did not feel better. The Emergency Department physician wrote the final diagnosis as "fever with chills, possible viral syndrome."

First-Listed Diagnosis: _____

Secondary Diagnoses: _____

13

The patient is a 45-year-old man who was referred by his primary care physician to the cardiologist in his office "to diagnosis and treat for possible cardiac disease." Three days earlier the patient had an abnormal test stress study that was done for preventive health purposes. The patient did not have any complaints typical of cardiac disease. When the nurse in the cardiologist's office was taking the patient's history and recording the vital signs, she noted the patient's blood pressure to be 138/88. The patient admitted to being somewhat "stressed-out" by being there, so the nurse waited 10 minutes and took the blood pressure again. This time the blood pressure values were 138/84. After the cardiologist reviewed the patient's history with him and completed the physical examination, the physician personally took the patient's blood pressure and found it to be 136/86. The physician explained to the patient that it was possible that he had hypertension, but he would not make the diagnosis during the first patient visit. The patient was prescribed a mild diuretic and given a follow-up appointment to return in 2 weeks. The doctor completed his progress note about the visit with the impressions of (1) abnormal cardiovascular stress test, (2) elevated blood pressure readings, and (3) rule out hypertension.

First-Listed Diagnosis: _____

Secondary Diagnoses: _____

14

A 58-year-old woman requested a same-day appointment with her primary care physician because of recurrent jaw and shoulder pain that had occurred over the past 2 days and was increasing in intensity. The physician examined the patient and had the nurse perform an immediate electrocardiogram (EKG) on the patient. The physician recognized these symptoms as a possible acute myocardial infarction (AMI). When the physician noted the EKG was markedly abnormal, he had the staff call for an ambulance immediately and transferred the patient to the nearest hospital's emergency room. The diagnoses recorded by the physician on the progress note for the visit was jaw and shoulder pain, rule out AMI.

First-Listed Diagnosis: _____

Secondary Diagnoses: _____

15

The parents of a seven-week-old female infant returned to the pediatrician's office for a follow-up visit to examine the baby, who had been previously diagnosed with "colic." Laboratory work performed during the last visit was reported with normal values. The parents stated there had not been much change in the baby since their last appointment, 2 weeks ago. The infant was inconsolable 3 or 4 times a week with symptoms that lasted 4–5 hours, from the late afternoon through the evening hours. Some of the physician's recommended calming techniques worked, such as the "football hold," placing the baby face down along the length of the father's arm, as well as putting the baby in the car seat and driving around for several hours, but other efforts failed. The breast-feeding mother had eliminated recommended items from her diet, including caffeine, chocolate, and gas-producing foods. The pediatrician encouraged the parents that he had seen many babies like their baby and fortunately most of the babies did not experience as much colic after the age of 12–14 weeks. The parents made note of additional calming techniques recommended by the physician and his nurse. The physician's examination of the infant during this visit found an otherwise healthy infant. A follow-up appointment was made for 3 weeks later. The final diagnosis recorded for the visit was full-term female infant with colic.

First-Listed Diagnosis: _____

Secondary Diagnoses: _____

16

The patient is a 25-year-old male Army veteran of the Iraq war, He was in a vehicle that was damaged by an improvised explosive device that did not hit the vehicle directly. However, the four soldiers inside the vehicle had minor injuries. This patient recalls hitting his head on the side door of the vehicle when it crashed but otherwise was uninjured with no loss of consciousness. Since the soldier has been discharged, his family at home describe him as exhibiting irritability and impulsiveness behaviors that are uncharacteristic of him. Today's visit at the Veterans Administration Outpatient Center is to review test results to explain his behavior change which the patient also notices but cannot explain. Given the circumstances, the physician concludes the patient has "Late effect symptoms (irritability, impulsiveness) of diffuse traumatic brain injury." The patient was referred to a specialized treatment center that focuses on patients with traumatic brain injury.

First-Listed Diagnosis: _____

Secondary Diagnoses: _____

Chapter 19A

Injuries, Effects of Foreign Body, Burns and Corrosions, and Frostbite

Coding Scenarios for *Basic ICD-10-CM/PCS Coding*

The following case studies are organized following the sequence of the chapters in the *ICD-10-CM and ICD-10-PCS* code books. The objective of this book is to provide the student with more detailed clinical information to code, rather than one- or two-line diagnosis and procedure statements. ICD-10-CM diagnosis codes are to be assigned to both the inpatient hospital admission and the outpatient visit case studies. In this book, the ICD-10-PCS procedure codes are to be assigned only to the inpatient hospital admission cases. In actual practice, outpatient cases are assigned CPT/HCPCS codes. The ICD-10-PCS codes are only required for inpatient procedures.

1

A 16-year-old boy is brought to the emergency department with second- and third-degree burns of the chest wall and first- and second-degree burns of the upper arms, above the elbows. The total body surface burn is 25 percent with 9 percent being third-degree. The patient is transferred to the burn unit at the city's university hospital.

*Note: List all applicable codes **excluding** the External Cause codes.*

First-Listed Diagnosis: _____

Secondary Diagnoses: _____

2

The patient, a 22-year-old man, was brought to the emergency department by friends after being involved in a fight. The patient complains of severe jaw pain, and his face appears asymmetric with the left side of his face appearing out of alignment. The physician obtains x-rays of the man's facial bones and jaw and is advised by the radiologist that a dislocation of the left side of the mandible exists. One 3.0 cm laceration across the metacarpal area of the right hand required skin suturing, which was done in the emergency department. The patient is admitted to the hospital. The next morning the patient is taken to surgery for a closed reduction of the dislocation of the mandible. The patient is discharged the next day with a follow-up appointment scheduled with the surgeon in 10 days.

*Note: List all applicable codes **excluding** the External Cause codes.*

Principal Diagnosis: _____

Secondary Diagnoses: _____

Principal Procedure: _____

Secondary Procedure(s): _____

3

A 42-year-old man was in an auto accident that involved the collision of his vehicle into the expressway median divider. He was brought to emergency department complaining of leg and foot pain. X-rays showed a displaced left distal or lower femur fracture and a displaced fracture of the neck of the talus (tarsal) bone of the left foot. He was admitted to the hospital and taken to the operating room for an immediate open reduction with internal fixation for both fractures.

*Note: List all applicable codes **excluding** the External Cause codes.*

Principal Diagnosis: _____

Secondary Diagnoses: _____

Principal Procedure: _____

Secondary Procedure(s): _____

4

The patient is a semiprofessional baseball player who is a pitcher. He is seen in the orthopedic sports medicine physician's office because of a painful right shoulder. The patient felt a pain in his right shoulder while pitching during a game within the past three days. After the game, he felt more severe muscular pain in the shoulder and was unable to use his arm. The physician suspects a severe injury to the biceps tendon and muscles of the shoulder. The patient consents to exploratory surgery and shoulder repair if indicated. The patient is admitted to the hospital for the surgery. During the open procedure, the physician examines the superior labrum that attaches the biceps tendon to the bones of the shoulder. The physician finds the superior labrum is torn from front to back. An immediate repair or arthroplasty of the shoulder is done to repair the labrum or glenoid ligament and reattach it to the bones of the shoulder joint. The physician describes the injury as a SLAP, or superior glenoid labrum lesion. (This procedure is a repair of the shoulder glenoid ligament also known as the labrum). The physician advises the patient-athlete that the injury is fairly common among athletes who use their upper extremities in strenuous activities. Physical therapy and athletic training will be the next plan of care for the patient so that he may return to playing baseball.

*Note: List all applicable codes **excluding** the External Cause codes.*

Principal Diagnosis: _____

Secondary Diagnoses: _____

Principal Procedure: _____

Secondary Procedure(s): _____

5

The patient is a 19-year-old man who is brought to the emergency department (ED) by fire department ambulance, which was called by neighbors to the scene of a street fight. Apparently the patient was beaten by rival gang members. The patient was unconscious when found by the paramedics. The ED physician performs a comprehensive physical examination, and the patient is taken for an MRI of the brain. The patient regains consciousness within 40 minutes of arriving in the ED, less than an hour after being found by the paramedics. The MRI is negative for fractures or internal bleeding. The patient is admitted to the ICU for monitoring. The physician describes the injury as a closed head injury with loss of consciousness of less than 1 hour. The patient also has multiple lacerations on the face, including his cheek, forehead, upper lip, and jaw. There are abrasions on both his hands as well as multiple contusions on the abdominal wall and both the knees and lower legs. The skin lacerations are suture repaired in the ICU after the patient is stabilized. The patient is transferred out of the ICU within 48 hours with no signs of permanent neurologic injury. He is discharged home 7 days after his injury occurred.

*Note: List all applicable codes **excluding** the External Cause codes.*

Principal Diagnosis: _____

Secondary Diagnoses: _____

Principal Procedure: _____

Secondary Procedure(s): _____

6

The patient is a 25-year-old man brought to the emergency department (ED) after being shot in the abdomen during a drive-by shooting. The trauma team assembled in the ED, and it was quickly determined that the gunshot wound of the epigastric area of the abdomen was complicated by injury to the abdominal aorta, with the retained bullets in the peritoneal cavity. The trauma surgeons attempt to control the bleeding and prepare the patient for surgery to repair the aorta, but there is a complete transection of the abdominal aorta, and the patient expires prior to being admitted and taken to surgery.

*Note: List all applicable codes **excluding** the External Cause codes.*

First-Listed Diagnosis: _____

Secondary Diagnoses: _____

7

The patient is a 44-year-old woman who works as a road construction flag holder. The patient was directing traffic on an expressway where road resurfacing was being performed. A truck came too close to the worker and its tires rolled over her left foot. The patient is brought to the nearest hospital's emergency department, where the physician on duty immediately examines the patient and x-rays are performed. The physician describes the patient's trauma as a crush injury of the foot with open fracture. The radiologist's impression documented on the radiology report describes the injury as open fracture of the first metatarsal of the foot. The orthopedic surgeon on call comes to the hospital, and the patient is admitted and taken to surgery for an open reduction and internal fixation of the first metatarsal bone with a fasciotomy. The patient remains in the hospital 3 days before being discharged to home health services follow-up care, with an appointment to see the orthopedic surgeon in 7 days.

*Note: List all applicable codes **excluding** the External Cause codes.*

Principal Diagnosis: _____

Secondary Diagnoses: _____

Principal Procedure: _____

Secondary Procedure(s): _____

8

The patient is a 50-year-old man brought to the emergency department (ED) by fire department ambulance that was called to a restaurant in which the patient was eating dinner with friends. The patient was eating steak when he felt something stick in his chest. He could not dislodge it, and was becoming rather panicky because of the intense epigastric pain. He was still able to breathe unassisted and able to speak. The emergency department physician examines the patient and immediately calls the gastroenterologist for what the ED physician describes as "Steakhouse Syndrome." The patient is examined by the gastroenterologist who suspects that food is lodged in the patient's esophagus. The patient is taken immediately to the gastroenterology procedure suite, and an upper GI endoscopy is performed. The physician finds several large pieces of poorly chewed meat at the level of the lower esophagogastric junction. The physician is able to remove some of the obstruction, but smaller pieces of meat had already passed into the stomach. The physician also documents that reflux esophagitis is present. The physician is able to examine the upper GI tract, including the stomach, and no injury to the mucosa is found. Prior to the procedure, the patient was admitted to the hospital for overnight monitoring and discharged the next morning.

*Note: List all applicable codes **excluding** the External Cause codes.*

Principal Diagnosis: _____

Secondary Diagnoses: _____

Principal Procedure: _____

Secondary Procedure(s): _____

9

The patient is a 15-year-old girl who is brought to the emergency department by ambulance from a motor vehicle accident where she was thrown from the car. After a complete history and physical examination, multiple radiologic studies are obtained. The trauma physician determines the patient has an unstable burst fracture of the L2 and L3 vertebrae, but there is no evidence of spinal cord injury. With the parents' consent, the patient is admitted and taken to surgery for repair of her injury. The physician performs an open reduction of the L2-L3 fracture. He also performs a posterior spinal fusion of L2-L3 with an interbody fusion device by posterior approach and posterior column. The procedure also includes L2-L3 interspinous process wiring. Bone is harvested from the right posterior iliac crest for bone grafting. The primary closure includes a L1-L2 laminotomy. The patient tolerates the surgical procedure and is taken to the surgical ICU. Fifteen days later the patient is transferred to an acute rehabilitation facility for ongoing therapy and recovery.

*Note: List all applicable codes **excluding** the External Cause codes.*

Principal Diagnosis: _____

Secondary Diagnoses: _____

Principal Procedure: _____

Secondary Procedure(s): _____

10

The patient is a 40-year-old man brought to the emergency department by fire department ambulance after falling off a ladder at home while doing home repairs. Apparently, in an attempt to catch himself, his left hand and wrist broke a window, and he was cut severely by the broken glass. The ED physician examines the patient and orders x-rays of the fingers, hand, and wrist. No fractures are seen. Based on the physical examination, the physician concludes that there is a major injury to the ulnar nerve and also an injury to the tendon in addition to the laceration of the wrist. The physician repairs the laceration loosely and makes arrangements for the patient to be transferred to another hospital in the city where a hand surgeon waits to examine him and possibly take him to surgery for definitive repair. The patient is transferred by private ambulance to the nearby hospital.

Note: List all applicable codes ***excluding*** *the External Cause codes.*

First-Listed Diagnosis: _____

Secondary Diagnoses: _____

11

The patient is a 20-year-old man who sustained a drunken fall through a plate-glass window and was cut by the broken glass. He was brought to the Level I trauma emergency department at a local hospital. On examination the patient had a large penetrating wound to the right thoracoabdominal region. The patient had no memory of the event and could not describe how it happened. According to friends, he had been told to leave the nightclub/bar. They saw him leave alone and agreed he was "drunk." The fall through the glass of a store occurred about a half a block down on the same street. The patient was hemodynamically stable in the ER, but the CT scan revealed several retained objects in the right upper quadrant that had violated the liver, as well as possible violation of the right kidney. The patient was admitted and taken by the trauma surgeons to the operating room for an exploratory laparotomy. The injuries found during the procedure were a major laceration through and through of the liver, a laceration of the jejunum, and a hematoma of the right kidney. Exploratory laparotomy was performed with repair of the liver laceration, repair of the jejunum laceration, examination of the right kidney, and removal of 3 fragments of leaded glass from the abdominal wall and fascia. Examination of the colon revealed no injuries. A #10 JP drain was placed into the abdomen at the operative site, for postoperative drainage. The fascia, subcutaneous tissue, and skin edges were closed with sutures and staples. The patient was taken to the recovery area in stable condition. In addition to the injuries described with the operative findings, the patient was treated for acute alcoholic poisoning and multiple small skin lacerations (that did not need repair) of the right shoulder and right lower leg. After an extended hospital stay that included physical therapy, antibiotic and postoperative treatment, wound care management, and substance abuse preventative counseling, the patient was discharged home.

Note: List all applicable codes ***excluding*** *the External Cause codes.*

Principal Diagnosis: _____

Secondary Diagnoses: _____

Principal Procedure: _____

Secondary Procedure(s): _____

12

Fire department ambulance and paramedics brought a 14-year-old boy to the Level I trauma emergency room after he was shot in the head by a drive-by shooter while standing with some friends on a neighbor's porch. The entrance was into the right posterior parietal area of the skull, and the bullet was lodged in the occipital area. The inlet gunshot wound was hemorrhaging. The injury traumatized a major portion of the brain. When the patient arrived at the hospital, he was deeply comatose with cerebrate rigidity. His pupils were fixed and dilated with severe respiratory compromise. He was intubated and placed on a ventilator and admitted to the pediatric ICU. After discussing his condition with his parents, consent was obtained and the patient was taken to surgery, even though everyone understood the patient was in extremely critical condition. The following procedures were performed: decompressive craniotomy of the right parietal bone, duraplasty, and insertion of an intracranial pressure (ICP) monitor. The objectives of the procedure were to drain blood from beneath the skull bone and to repair the dura. Massive injuries to the brain were found as a result of the gunshot wound: comminuted skull fractures of the parietal bone, cerebral contusion, subdural hemorrhaging, diffuse cerebral edema, and herniation of the brainstem. The patient never regained consciousness. It became evident that the patient could not recover from these injuries, and the family consented to organ donation of his lungs, liver, kidneys, skin, and other tissue. The family did not consent to donating his heart. A flexible fiberoptic bronchoscopy was performed to examine the lung to determine the suitability for donation, and no injuries or inflammation was found. The patient was pronounced dead approximately 50 hours after the original injury.

*Note: List all applicable codes **excluding** the External Cause codes.*

Principal Diagnosis: _____

Secondary Diagnoses: _____

Principal Procedure: _____

Secondary Procedure(s): _____

13

The patient is a 21-year-old male who was found by a passing police car sitting on the side of a city street with a bleeding face and dazed appearance. A fire department ambulance brought the patient to the emergency room. The patient claimed to have no memory of what happened or chose not to tell the healthcare providers the circumstances that caused his injury. He did remember being on the street, walking home from a friend's house. Alcohol and drug screens were negative, but the patient was extremely quiet and sleepy. He did not complain of the amount of pain the physicians would have expected in a patient with the injuries found, which were bilateral mandibular angle fractures, laceration of the skin of the jaw, and a fractured tooth. The patient was admitted and taken to surgery the following morning and given IV antibiotics to prevent infection. The procedures performed were an open reduction and internal fixation of the mandibular fractures, a repair of the jaw laceration, and forceps extraction of one fractured tooth of the lower jaw. The patient had no complications during or after the procedure. The preoperative urinalysis and subsequent urine culture showed a urinary tract infection, which was treated. X-rays of his skull and neck showed no fractures or injuries. The patient also had abrasions on the right hand that were cleaned and bandaged. At the time of discharge, the patient still claimed to have no memory of what happened to him but otherwise appeared to be alert, cooperative, and thinking clearly. City police interviewed the patient during the hospital stay to investigate a possible crime but were unable to gain any information and found no witnesses to the event. He was discharged to the care of his older sister, with whom he lives, and follow-up appointments were given, primarily for care of his fractured mandible.

Note: List all applicable codes *excluding* the External Cause codes.

Principal Diagnosis: _____

Secondary Diagnoses: _____

Principal Procedure: _____

Secondary Procedure(s): _____

14

The patient is a 30-year-old man brought to the emergency department by his mother after being injured in an argument with a male neighbor two days ago. The patient fell down his front steps at this home trying to grab the neighbor, who had come to the patient's home complaining of loud music. The patient complained of pain and significant swelling of his right leg, near his knee, which had been replaced two years ago. Neither the patient nor the mother could tell the doctor the reason for the knee replacement other than it "collapsed" and had to be replaced. The patient also has had hemophilia A disease since birth and was diagnosed as HIV positive 10 years ago. He is asymptomatic related to his HIV status and has had no infections or consequences of it. X-ray of the leg showed a right tibia fracture at the upper or proximal end. Because of his hemophilia, the fact the patient had a replaced joint near the site of the fracture, and the potential complications of an open reduction type treatment, the patient was admitted to the hospital. The leg was splinted and elevated for 48 hours until the swelling was under control. He was taken to the operating room on day 3, and a closed reduction, closely monitored under imaging, was performed, and an excellent reduction was achieved. A cast was applied. He complained of severe pain from the time of admission, and this was managed fairly well with injectable and oral analgesic medications. He was also given intravenously via a peripheral vein a total of 3,000 units of Factor VIII on a daily basis for the hemophilia status. The patient and his mother were instructed that the patient was to use the wheelchair they had at home to get around and not to put any weight on the right leg. Home healthcare services were ordered, and a medical car was arranged to take the patient home and get him into the house. A follow-up appointment with his orthopedic surgeon for fracture care was given to the patient, and he was encouraged to contact his hematologist at University Hospital as soon as possible. Copies of his record were given to the patient.

Note: List all applicable codes *excluding* the External Cause codes.

Principal Diagnosis: _____

Secondary Diagnoses: _____

Principal Procedure: _____

Secondary Procedure(s): _____

15

The patient is an 80-year-old female who fell out of bed and injured her left ankle. Examination in the emergency room revealed pain, swelling, and deformity around the left ankle. The patient denied any other pain or injury. She was admitted to the orthopedic floor and seen promptly by an orthopedic surgeon and her attending physician. X-rays were taken that showed a trimalleolar fracture of the left ankle with displacement. The patient had a significant past medical history with a previous cerebrovascular accident (CVA) last year in this right-handed woman. The left hemiplegia was due to an old cerebral infarction of the distribution of the right middle cerebral artery. She had vigorous physical therapy following this and had been doing well with ambulation and self care since that time. She is also has type 2 diabetes of long standing and ischemic heart disease that continues under treatment. While she was in the hospital she continued to receive her oral diabetic medication. An EKG show inferior lateral ischemia that was not a new finding. The day after admission, the orthopedic surgeon performed a closed reduction and casting of the left ankle. X-rays taken following the reduction revealed alignment to be in good position. The patient tolerated the procedure well and had no intra- or postoperative complications. A slight urinary tract infection was noted, and an antibiotic was prescribed. The patient was discharged home with home health services ordered.

*Note: List all applicable codes **excluding** the External Cause codes.*

Principal Diagnosis: _____

Secondary Diagnoses: _____

Principal Procedure: _____

Secondary Procedure(s): _____

16

HISTORY: The patient is an 11-year-old boy who was riding his bicycle in front of his home, hit a bump in the pavement, and fell off his bicycle. Because of severe wrist pain, he was taken to the emergency department, where X-rays confirmed displaced right distal radius Salter-Harris type I fracture and right distal Salter-Harris type I ulna fracture. The patient was seen by an orthopedic surgeon, who advised admission and a closed reduction of the fractures that was agreed to by the patient and his parents.

OPERATIVE FINDINGS: The right wrist has a deformity with some expected level of swelling. His fingers are moving, and he is neurovascularly intact. The skin is intact. Contralateral wrist is nontender. Fingertips are pink with good capillary refill. Lower extremities are nontender. X-ray films have been reviewed, which reveal fractures of both the distal radius and distal ulna with 100% displacement.

DESCRIPTION OF PROCEDURE: The patient was taken to the operating room and placed supine on the table with all of his extremities adequately padded. The patient was given laryngeal mask anesthesia. A closed reduction was performed. The fractures were found to reduce. Fluoroscopy was used to view the fractures in multiplanar views. Given the nature of the fracture pattern, it was deemed appropriate to pin the radius to increase stability. Two K-wires were then placed percutaneously under direct fluoroscopic guidance across the fracture site. The growth plate was avoided. The fracture and pins were then visualized in multiplanar fluoroscopy, and the fracture and pins were noted to be in good position. The pins were bent and cut. Final films were obtained. Sterile dressings followed by a sugar tong type of splint were then applied. The patient tolerated the procedure well, was awakened in the operating room, and was taken to recovery. There were no complications of this procedure.

*Note: List all applicable codes **excluding** the External Cause codes.*

Principal Diagnosis: _____

Secondary Diagnoses: _____

Principal Procedure: _____

Secondary Procedure(s): _____

17

HISTORY: The patient is a 79-year-old retired woman from Iowa, in general good health, brought to the emergency department (ED) with the complaint of acute pain in her right hip. The patient is on bus trip vacation with a senior citizen's group, with the destination Nashville, Tennessee and the Grand Ole Opry. After the group stopped at a restaurant en route, she fell off a curb in the parking lot while walking back to the bus. She was able to be helped up and got back on the bus and rode on to their hotel in Nashville. Someone got a wheelchair from the hotel, and she was able to be pushed around, including to the show at the Opry's Ryman Auditorium. After the show, she told her companion that she thought she should go to the emergency room because the hip was hurting more than earlier in the day. Radiographs in the ED revealed a subcapital impacted right hip fracture. Emergent orthopedic consultation was obtained, and the patient was admitted. The patient's physician in Iowa was contacted, and he provided her medical history including the type of medication she received for her essential hypertension, which was her only medical problem. The day after admission, the patient was taken to the operating room, where a 3-pin fixation utilizing cannulated screws to the right hip was performed without difficulty. A day after surgery, physical therapy was started and by discharge on day 3, the patient was able to ambulate with a walker. Her son and daughter came to Nashville with a rented motor home to transport the patient back to Iowa. Access to the patient's electronic health record was provided to her physician in Iowa for continuation of care.

DESCRIPTION OF PROCEDURE: The patient was taken to the operating room, placed in the supine position on the fracture table for an open internal fixation. Once adequate anesthesia was obtained, the right hip girdle was sterilely prepped and draped. The hip was well aligned, and no traction was required. Image intensification was brought into appropriate position, and the AP and lateral projections were obtained. This showed the fracture to be well reduced on its own. A 3-cm incision was then made just distal to the greater trochanter and carried down to the level of the subcutaneous tissues. Small bleeders were cauterized along the way. Great care was taken to ensure that no harm came to any significant neurovascular structures. The iliotibial band was identified, incised in line with its fibers, and gently retracted. Access was gained to the lateral femoral cortex. A guide pin was placed without difficulty into the femoral head and neck. AP and lateral projections revealed adequate guide pin placement. Then an appropriately sized 16-mm thread 7.0 cannulated screw was placed over the guide pin. Image intensification revealed adequate screw placement. Two additional screws were then passed in a parallel fashion into the inferior and posterior portion of the femoral head and neck. Once the 3-pin fixation was completed, AP and lateral projections revealed adequate fracture stabilization and hardware placement. The wound was irrigated with copious amounts of normal saline solution. The iliotibial band was reapproximated with 0-Vicryl suture in an interrupted fashion. Subcutaneous tissues were closed with 2-0 Vicryl sutures, the skin was closed with clips, and a sterile dressing was applied. The patient was taken to the recovery room by the anesthesiologist and nursing staff in stable condition.

*Note: List all applicable codes **excluding** the External Cause codes.*

Principal Diagnosis: _____

Secondary Diagnoses: _____

Principal Procedure: _____

Secondary Procedure(s): _____

18

The patient is a 50-year-old woman who was previously treated by closed reduction and external fixation of a fracture of her right tibia, distal medial malleolus, which she suffered as the result of a fall down stairs. During follow-up care, it becomes evident that the fracture is not healing. X-rays demonstrate a nonunion of the distal tibia. The patient is admitted for surgical repair of the nonunion. The surgery performed is an open reduction of the tibia with bone grafting. Bone for the grafting is harvested from the patient's left iliac crest. The distal medial malleolus tibial bone, at the site of the non-union, is osteotomized and repositioned. The harvested bone graft is packed into the fracture site to replace the missing bone, and three screws are inserted to secure the area. The patient is discharged the day after surgery for recovery at home.

*Note: List all applicable codes **excluding** the External Cause codes.*

Principal Diagnosis: _____

Secondary Diagnoses: _____

Principal Procedure: _____

Secondary Procedure(s): _____

19

The patient fell out of a chair at the nursing home and was previously treated by closed reduction with external fixation for a fracture on the surgical neck of the right humerus. There was a malunion of the fracture in the 80-year-old female patient and she was admitted for an open reduction of the humerus with bone grafting. During the surgical procedure, the orthopedic surgeon harvested bone from the patient's left iliac crest. The humeral fracture site was opened and the area of malunion was osteotomized, cleaned, and repositioned. Internal fixation was accomplished with screws and the harvested bone was packed into the fracture site to replace the missing bone segment. The patient recovered from the procedure uneventfully and was discharged on the second hospital day. Other chronic conditions treated in the hospital were arteriosclerotic heart disease, chronic renal insufficiency, and type 2 diabetes mellitus. The patient was given an appointment to see the orthopedic surgeon in his office in 5 days and was going to be followed by home health nurses for postoperative care.

*Note: List all applicable codes **excluding** the External Cause codes.*

Principal Diagnosis: _____

Secondary Diagnoses: _____

Principal Procedure: _____

Secondary Procedure(s): _____

Chapter 19B

Poisoning by Adverse Effect, Underdosing, Toxic Effects of Substances, Other Effects of External Causes, Certain Early Complications of Trauma, and Complications of Surgical and Medical Care

Coding Scenarios for *Basic ICD-10-CM/PCS Coding*

The following case studies are organized following the sequence of the chapters in the *ICD-10-CM and ICD-10-PCS* code books. The objective of this book is to provide the student with more detailed clinical information to code, rather than one- or two-line diagnosis and procedure statements. ICD-10-CM diagnosis codes are to be assigned to both the inpatient hospital admission and the outpatient visit case studies. In this book, the ICD-10-PCS procedure codes are to be assigned only to the inpatient hospital admission cases. In actual practice, outpatient cases are assigned CPT/HCPCS codes. The ICD-10-PCS codes are only required for inpatient procedures.

1

A 25-year-old woman was found unresponsive in her apartment by her roommate and brought to the hospital by fire department ambulance paramedics. She had recently been treated for depression, and her roommate found the patient's prescription bottle of antidepressant medication empty. The patient's other prescription bottle of Lorazepam was also empty. The emergency department (ED) staff talked to the patient's psychiatrist and confirmed these medications had been prescribed for depression. An empty bottle of vodka was found in the bedroom near the patient's body. The ED examination and toxicology studies confirm a drug overdose of these two medications and alcohol. Another friend received a suicide e-mail note from the patient the same afternoon. While the patient was receiving treatment in the ED, she suffered a cardiopulmonary arrest and died. Physician documented poisoning in a suicide attempt with antidepressant, Lorazepam, and vodka.

First-Listed Diagnosis: _____

Secondary Diagnoses: _____

2

A patient with congestive heart failure and 6 weeks status post acute MI had been prescribed and was correctly taking Lanoxin (digoxin). She began to experience nausea and vomiting with extreme fatigue. She was admitted to the hospital. Blood drug levels are taken and it is determined the patient is experiencing a side effect of the medication. A different medication is prescribed for her heart disease to avoid these symptoms. The patient's cardiac conditions are evaluated and found to be stable.

Principal Diagnosis: _____

Secondary Diagnoses: _____

Principal Procedure: _____

Secondary Procedure(s): _____

3

The patient had surgery 1 week previously for acute appendicitis with a peritoneal abscess. She is admitted now for fever, pain, and redness at the operative site. There is evidence of cellulitis of the operative wound, and cultures of the abdominal wall wound drainage confirm Staphylococcus aureus, methicillin resistant, as the cause. She receives intravenous (IV) antibiotics for the infection and also receives treatment for type 2 diabetes mellitus. The physician's diagnoses on discharge were: status postappendectomy with wound infection, MRSA (methicillin resistant staphylococcus aureus); diabetes type 2.

Principal Diagnosis: _____

Secondary Diagnoses: _____

Principal Procedure: _____

Secondary Procedure(s): _____

4

An 80-year-old man was brought to the emergency department (ED) by his family with the chief complaint of "nose bleed." The patient is taking Coumadin under prescription by his internist for atrial fibrillation. The patient is also known to have congestive heart failure. The patient said his nose began bleeding about 2 hours ago and he was unable to stop the bleeding with other methods he had used in the past. He reported that he had these nose bleeds before today. However, today the bleeding is more pronounced and could not be stopped at home. In the ED, the physician is able to control the bleeding somewhat but recognized that an ENT physician should be called in for consultation. The patient's laboratory work revealed anemia and an EKG showed the existing atrial fibrillation. Because of his various conditions, his internist admitted him to the hospital. He was seen by the ENT physician, who was able to stop the bleeding with an anterior and posterior packing. The packing was removed on day 2, and the epistaxis had stopped. Repeated laboratory work confirmed the doctor's diagnosis of "chronic blood loss anemia." The patient continued to receive medications for the atrial fibrillation and congestive heart failure, and new medications were started to treat the anemia. The patient's Coumadin was continued, but the dosage was lowered. In the physician's discharge progress note, he wrote "Epistaxis due to Coumadin therapy with resulting chronic blood loss anemia in a patient with atrial fibrillation and congestive heart failure."

Principal Diagnosis: _____

Secondary Diagnoses: _____

Principal Procedure: _____

Secondary Procedure(s): _____

5

A 12-year-old girl is brought to the primary care physician's office by her mother. The mother states that she had taken the child to the Urgent Care Center 5 days previously because the child had acute otitis media. The Urgent Care doctor had prescribed azithromycin. The child's condition did not improve, and, in fact, she developed red spots and itchiness on her arms and chest. The primary care physician examines the patient and concludes that the child has an allergy to the medication. The acute otitis media is still present as the medication seemed to have no effect on the infection. The physician tells the mother to discontinue the azithromycin medication and a new prescription is given. On the encounter form the physician writes "Pruritic drug allergy and acute otitis media."

First-Listed Diagnosis: _____

Secondary Diagnoses: _____

6

The patient, a 35-year-old man, is brought to the emergency department (ED) by friends who report that the patient has chest pain. Upon questioning, the patient admitted to being a cocaine addict and to having used cocaine several times over the past 24 hours. The patient stated "maybe I overdosed," as he experienced chest pain on a previous occasion when he used more cocaine than he normally used. The patient is placed on telemetry in the ED and is later admitted to a telemetry bed on a nursing unit. Further cardiovascular testing finds no evidence of an acute myocardial infarction or respiratory disease. However, it is determined that the patient has hypertension that had never been treated. The physician determines that this event is a cocaine overdose that occurred with the consequence of chest pain. The patient is also treated for hypertension and is strongly advised to continue the antihypertensive medications and to seek help to overcome the cocaine addiction, as the two conditions have serious consequences on his long-term health. A referral is given to the local community mental health center, which offers a drug counseling service. The patient agrees and is discharged accompanied by his brother.

Principal Diagnosis: _____

Secondary Diagnoses: _____

Principal Procedure: _____

Secondary Procedure(s): _____

7

The patient is a 67-year-old man who comes to his cardiologist's office with complaints of pain and warmth around the pacemaker generator pocket in his left upper chest wall. The physician examines the patient and determines the patient has cellulitis of the chest wall due to an infected pacemaker pocket and needs to have the pacemaker generator moved to a different location of the chest wall to allow the infected pocket to heal. The patient has a history of a MRSA infection being treated in the past. The type of infection that appears present at this time will be investigated to check for a recurrence. The physician makes arrangements for the patient to have outpatient surgery the next day.

First-Listed Diagnosis: _____

Secondary Diagnoses: _____

8

The family practice physician examines a 56-year-old male established patient who comes to the office with his wife. The patient states that he has felt dizzy and lightheaded over the past three days. The patient is on medications for hypertension and states he has been taking all as prescribed. The physician and the physician's nurse take the patient's blood pressure and find it to be 100/70 mm Hg, which is much lower than the patient's pressure as normally recorded. The patient had been taking antihypertensive medications of irbesartan (Avapro) and metoprolol (Toprol) with a low-dose diuretic. The physician is unable to determine which medication was the cause but is certain the patient's symptoms of vertigo and light-headedness are the side effects of the antihypertensive medications. New prescriptions are issued for adjusted dosages of the medications, and the patient is advised to go to the emergency department and call this physician if the symptoms get worse over the next 24 hours.

First-Listed Diagnosis: _____

Secondary Diagnoses: _____

9

The patient is a 25-year-old woman who was prescribed Ciprofloxacin by her family physician for an E. coli urinary tract infection and advised to take one 250-mg tablet every 12 hours for 10 days. Because she was leaving on a vacation cruise on Saturday, the patient doubled up the dosages and for the past 3 days had taken two 250-mg tablets every 12 hours. Over the past 24 hours, the patient had diarrhea severe enough for her to come to the emergency department (ED). A urinalysis shows bacteria still present to support the diagnosis of UTI. The physician recognizes these symptoms as not only side effects of the medication but, in this patient's situation, an accidental overdose of Ciprofloxacin, as she had not followed the physician's directions in the amount of the medication she was to take. The ED physician advises her to continue taking the medication as prescribed without alterations.

First-Listed Diagnosis: _____

Secondary Diagnoses: _____

10

The patient had surgery 2 weeks previously for insertion of a central venous vascular catheter for infusion to treat colon carcinoma. The patient is admitted to the hospital extremely ill with the admitting diagnosis of "sepsis." The patient's signs and symptoms include elevated temperature, rapid heart rate and respirations, and elevated white blood cell count. After study, the physician determines that the patient has sepsis due to the vascular catheter that apparently is the source of the infection. The physician and consultants further describe the patient's condition as systemic inflammatory response syndrome or sepsis in a patient with an infection. Blood cultures show evidence of methicillin susceptible staphylococcal aureus (MSSA) organisms as the cause of the septicemia or bloodstream infection. Intravenous antibiotic medications and other therapy are given for the infection and the carcinoma. The partially implantable venous access device is removed by incision. The patient recovers and is discharged home in 10 days to be followed in the oncology clinic in 1 week.

Principal Diagnosis: _____

Secondary Diagnoses: _____

Principal Procedure: _____

Secondary Procedure(s): _____

11

The patient is an 80-year-old man with multiple medical problems: Parkinson's disease, glaucoma, total blindness in right eye and low vision in left eye, old MI 6 months ago, recent abnormal cardiac stress test, status post right total knee replacement, and primary osteoarthrosis, generalized. On this occasion he is admitted to the hospital for a planned revision of his right total knee arthroplasty. The patient has been evaluated by cardiology and cleared for surgery. He had been seen by the orthopedic surgeon several weeks ago and scheduled for this revision arthroplasty. About 10–12 years ago the patient had a total knee replacement on the right side for osteoarthritis. He developed increasing pain in his knee, and the orthopedic evaluation found aseptic loosening of the tibial component of his knee. The patient was taken to surgery on the day of admission and had a revision right knee arthroplasty of the tibial component. The surgeon found femoral and patellar components of the previous knee replacement to be stable and in good working order. The tibial component was found to be grossly loose and was able to be removed with little effort. The tibial tray had divided completely from the cement mantle. The orthopedic surgeon proceeded to replace the tibial component only. The patient recovered well from surgery without complications and was transferred to a skilled unit facility for rehabilitation and to increase his ability to perform activities of daily living independently. All of his medical conditions were monitored and treated while he was in the hospital for this surgery.

Principal Diagnosis: _____

Secondary Diagnoses: _____

Principal Procedure: _____

Secondary Procedure(s): _____

12

One year ago this 40-year-old female received a left kidney transplant from an unrelated donor to treat her end-stage renal disease. The doctors were notified by the transplant network that the donor was diagnosed with low grade lymphoma, and the transplant patient was tested for any evidence of the lymphoma in the donated kidney. Unfortunately the transplanted kidney was proven by biopsy to have non-Hodgkin's lymphoma. The patient was admitted to the hospital. A nephrectomy was performed to remove the transplanted kidney. The patient received one session of hemodialysis for the end-stage kidney disease still present. The patient had an uneventful recovery and was discharged home with home health services.

Principal Diagnosis: _____

Secondary Diagnoses: _____

Principal Procedure: _____

Secondary Procedure(s): _____

13

The patient is a 24-year-old male who received an orthotopic liver transplant 2 months ago to treat his primary biliary cirrhosis. The patient was admitted at this time after a transplant clinic visit on the same day because of a generalized macular rash on his chest. The patient also complained of diarrhea and an enlarging abdomen that the doctors identified as ascites. A skin biopsy of the chest was performed and revealed a significant number of donor lymphocytes due to acute graft-versus-host (GVH) disease. The doctors informed the patient that his acute GVH disease is a complication of his liver transplant but can be treated with medications such as corticosteroids, immunosuppressants, antibiotics, and immunoglobulins. The patient remained in the hospital for 5 days and started on a medication regimen with relief of his diarrhea and lessening of the symptoms of the ascites and the rash. The patient was discharged home with home health services and an appointment with the transplant clinic in 2 weeks.

Principal Diagnosis: _____

Secondary Diagnoses: _____

Principal Procedure: _____

Secondary Procedure(s): _____

14

The patient is a 7-year-old male who was brought to the emergency department by his mother because of a suspected allergic reaction. The patient was experiencing wheezing, urticaria, and itching and tingling on his lips and in his mouth. The patient was at a party at school and ate cookies that contained small bits of peanuts, unknown to him at the time. The mother states he has a known allergy to peanuts and has had reactions in the past when exposed to peanuts, even without eating them. The physician described the patient's condition as a relatively mild anaphylactic reaction to food (peanuts), and the patient received an injection of epinephrine. He was observed in the emergency room for another 3 hours and had a complete resolution of his symptoms.

First-Listed Diagnosis: _____

Secondary Diagnoses: _____

15

A 30-year-old man was brought to the emergency department by a fire department ambulance that was called by police to a building where suspected drug sales and use were occurring. The patient was found unresponsive on the floor in the apartment where other individuals were arrested for solicitation and illegal possession of narcotics, including cocaine and heroin. The patient was later identified by his sister and known to be a chronic drug addict. Upon arrival to the emergency department, the patient was found to be in acute respiratory failure. He required immediate intubation and was placed on continuous mechanical ventilation and admitted to ICU. The drug toxicology screening test later returned the finding of a high level of cocaine, known to be a central nervous system stimulant. The patient's respiratory function continued to worsen. He developed acute renal failure and became unresponsive to treatment. The patient expired within 72 hours of admission. The physician's final diagnosis was "Acute respiratory failure as a result of an accidental cocaine overdose, cocaine dependency with intoxication delirium, acute renal failure."

Principal Diagnosis: _____

Secondary Diagnoses: _____

Principal Procedure: _____

Secondary Procedure(s): _____

16

The patient is a 60-year-old woman who came to the emergency room with a variety of complaints, including diarrhea, swelling of her face, especially around her eyes, weakness, and fatigue. Given the variety of her complaints and her extensive medical history, the patient was admitted to the hospital. The emergency department physician was most concerned with her facial swelling, and documented facial swelling as the admitting diagnosis.

The patient is known to have multiple primary and secondary malignancies for which she is currently receiving outpatient chemotherapy and radiation therapy. She has primary carcinoma of the right kidney with metastasis to the intra-abdominal lymph nodes, primary non-small-cell carcinoma of the lung, left upper lobe, with metastasis to the anterior mediastinum, and a past history of carcinoma of the anal canal which was cured surgically. She is also under treatment for hyperthyroidism. She has had diarrhea for two days and was found to be severely dehydrated. She has been at home receiving antibiotic therapy through a peripherally inserted central catheter (PICC), placed prior to this admission, for a staph aureus septicemia infection from an implanted chemotherapy port that was removed. The antibiotic treatment via the PICC was continued this admission. She has significant swelling of her face and neck with prominent periorbital swelling. Upon further investigation, it was thought that she had angioneurotic edema, as a result of an allergic reaction, possibly to one or more of the medications she was taking, or possibly as a result of a food allergy. The patient also presented with cellulitis of the face and orbital areas. She received her ongoing antibiotic therapy for the septicemia, additional antibiotic therapy for the facial cellulitis, which did not involve the orbits themselves, intravenous therapy for her dehydration, and medications for the diarrhea and hyperthyroidism. She was seen by oncology to assess the progression of her renal and pulmonary malignancies and metastases. The patient was relieved of some of her distressing symptoms and allowed to go home to continue receiving antibiotic therapy through her PICC. She was discharged with home health care services.

There were three final diagnoses that appeared to meet the definition of principal diagnosis: angioneurotic edema, cellulitis of the face, and dehydration. The attending physician was queried for assistance with the determination of the principal diagnosis, and together with the coder, determined that the main circumstance of the admission and most extensive therapy was directed at diagnosing and treating the angioneurotic edema.

Principal Diagnosis: _____

Secondary Diagnoses: _____

Principal Procedure: _____

Secondary Procedure(s): _____

17

The patient is a 53-year-old male with end-stage renal disease and chronic glomerulonephritis. He has been dialyzed through an arteriovenous (AV) fistula (radial artery to cephalic vein) in his left arm for two years, most recently two days ago. His end-stage renal disease is the result of his long-standing hypertension. When he went for his dialysis treatment this morning it was noted that the access was clotted, and he was taken to an emergency department for direct admission for inpatient care. Because of his urgent need for dialysis, a central venous (Quinton) catheter was placed percutaneously in the left internal jugular vein, and dialysis was accomplished on the day of admission. He was placed on antibiotics and taken to surgery on day two for an open thrombectomy of the right AV fistula. The clot was located in the cephalic vein. The AV fistula did not have to be revised. The patient had no complications from the procedure or during his six-day hospital stay. The Quinton catheter that was used for his dialysis access while in the hospital was left in place for the doctor at the renal dialysis center to evaluate at his next dialysis appointment in order to determine whether it can be removed, and when the AV fistula will be available for access for dialysis. His discharge diagnoses were written by the physician as (1) end-stage renal disease, (2) chronic glomerulonephritis, (3) hypertension, (4) clotted obstructive AV fistula. The procedures performed were dialysis, insertion of the left internal jugular vein catheter, and arteriotomy of the right AV fistula with thrombectomy.

Principal Diagnosis: _____

Secondary Diagnoses: _____

Principal Procedure: _____

Secondary Procedure(s): _____

Chapter 20

External Causes of Morbidity

Coding Scenarios for *Basic ICD-10-CM/PCS Coding*

Note: Assign only External Cause of Morbidity codes (V01–Y99) for the following scenarios.

Reminders from the ICD-10-CM guidelines for external cause codes:

- An external cause code may be used with any code in the range of A00.0–T88.9, Z00–Z99, classification that is a health condition due to an external cause. Though they are most applicable to injuries, they are also valid for use with such things as infections or diseases due to an external cause, and other health conditions, such as a heart attack that occurs during strenuous physical activity.

- Assign the external cause code, with the appropriate 7th character (initial encounter, subsequent encounter, or sequela) for each encounter for which the injury or condition is being treated.

- An external cause code can never be a principal or first-listed diagnosis.

- No external cause code from Chapter 20 is needed if the external cause and intent are included in a code from another chapter, for example, poisoning codes.

- When applicable, place of occurrence, activity, and external cause status codes are sequenced after the main external cause code(s). Regardless of the number of external cause codes assigned, there should be only one place of occurrence code, one activity code, and one external cause status code assigned to an encounter.

- A place of occurrence code is used only once, at the initial encounter for treatment. Do not use place of occurrence code Y92.9, Place of occurrence of the external cause, unspecified place or not applicable, if the place is not stated or is not applicable.

- An activity code is used only once, at the initial encounter for treatment. The activity codes are not applicable to poisonings, adverse effects, misadventures, or sequela. Do not assign Y93.9, Activity codes, unspecified activity, if the activity is not stated.

- An external cause status code is used only once, at the initial encounter for treatment. A code from category Y99, External cause status, indicates the work status of the person at the time the event occurred. The external cause status codes are not applicable to poisonings, adverse effects, misadventures, or late effects. Do not assign code Y99.9, unspecified external cause statue, if the status is not stated.

INSTRUCTIONS: For this chapter's exercises, consider all the scenarios in questions 1 through 20 as "Initial Encounters." Code ONLY the external cause codes for each scenario.

1. Injury in a fight between spectators at a football game, location was a sports stadium. Patient is a student and was a spectator at the sports event.

   External cause code(s): _____

2. Self-inflicted gunshot wound using a handgun, stated to be intentional; location was his garage at home, a single family house. Patient is an unemployed worker.

   External cause code(s): _____

3. Driver injured in a car accident involving a collision with another car on a highway. Patient is an employed driver for a delivery company.

   External cause code(s): _____

4. Patient is a construction worker who fell off scaffolding at a building construction site. Patient is an employed construction worker.

   External cause code(s): _____

5. Homeowner fell off a ladder in his yard while washing exterior windows at his home, a single family house. Patient is an unemployed homeowner.

   External cause code(s): _____

6. Patient was the driver of a motor vehicle that struck a bridge abutment on a highway. Patient is a student driving his vehicle while talking on a handheld cellular phone.

   External cause code(s): _____

7. Patient was a passenger on a commercial (fixed wing) airplane flight who was injured when the plane experienced a forced hard landing at the city public airport. Patient was flying to a vacation destination.

   External cause code(s): _____

8. Patient was a vacationer who stepped on broken glass in the sand while walking on the beach at the oceanside resort. Patient was on vacation and walking on the beach.

   External cause code(s): _____

9. Child was injured when he dove into the swimming pool at the next-door neighbor's home, a single family residence, and struck the side of the pool with his leg. Patient was a student and diving off a springboard platform.

   External cause code(s): _____

10. Patient was brought to the emergency department with wounds suffered in a drive-by gang shooting using a handgun, which appeared to be a homicide attempt. Shooting occurred on a local residential street. Patient was riding a bike and is a high school student.

    External cause code(s): _____

11. A hospital patient fell out of bed and injured his hip while in the hospital. Patient was a retired individual in the hospital.

    External cause code(s): _____

12. A patient was assaulted by an acquaintance and was stabbed in the abdomen with a knife during the argument, which occurred in a parking lot. Patient was an unemployed worker.

    External cause code(s): _____

13. The patient has a closed head injury as result of a tree falling on him in the front yard of his home, a single family residence, during a tornado. Patient was off work on vacation at home.

    External cause code(s): _____

14. The child was scalded with hot tap water while in the bath in his mother's apartment bathroom. This was confirmed as child abuse. The abuser was the boyfriend of the child's mother, and the incident occurred in the home. Patient was a student.

    External cause code(s): _____

15. The patient was overcome by heat exhaustion while working near a blast furnace in a steel mill. Patient was an employed steel worker in the mill.

    External cause code(s): _____

16. The patient was working as a paid landscaper and injured his back by straining to lift excessively heavy stones being placed for a decorative border around the entrance to a city park.

    External cause code(s): _____

17. A teenager was brought to the emergency room with an injured right wrist that was the result of the patient running and falling off his skateboard. The accident occurred in a parking lot. The patient was a student in high school.

    External cause code(s): _____

18. A 30-year-old man was brought to the emergency room complaining of back and neck pain from a fall that occurred after he collided with another player while playing basketball at the local outdoor basketball court. The patient was spending leisure time playing basketball.

    External cause code(s): _____

19. A 50-year-old man was brought to the emergency room and diagnosed with a right hip fracture that was a result of a fall off his skis while snow skiing downhill on a mountain at a local ski resort. Patient was on vacation at the ski resort.

    External cause code(s): _____

20. A child was struck by a car and dragged several feet when he ran across the residential street in front of his home. He sustained head injuries and multiple fractures and was admitted to the trauma intensive care unit at the hospital after being brought to the emergency department by fire ambulance. Patient was a student who was running across the street.

    External cause code(s): _____

Chapter 21

Factors Influencing Health Status and Contact with Health Services

Coding Scenarios for *Basic ICD-10-CM/PCS Coding*

The following case studies are organized following the sequence of the chapters in the *ICD-10-CM and ICD-10-PCS* code books. The objective of this book is to provide the student with more detailed clinical information to code, rather than one- or two-line diagnosis and procedure statements. ICD-10-CM diagnosis codes are to be assigned to both the inpatient hospital admission and the outpatient visit case studies. In this book, the ICD-10-PCS procedure codes are to be assigned only to the inpatient hospital admission cases. In actual practice, outpatient cases are assigned CPT/HCPCS codes. The ICD-10-PCS codes are only required for inpatient procedures.

1

A 27-completed-week gestation infant is delivered by cesarean section. The baby weighs 945 grams. The baby's lungs are immature, and she subsequently develops respiratory distress syndrome, requiring a long inpatient stay in the neonatal intensive care unit. The baby eventually is able to go home with her family. The physician's diagnosis is "liveborn infant, delivered by cesarean section, extreme immaturity with a birthweight of 945 grams at 27 weeks of gestation, with resulting respiratory distress syndrome."

Principal Diagnosis: _____

Secondary Diagnoses: _____

Principal Procedure: _____

Secondary Procedure(s): _____

2

While an inpatient in the hospital for atrial fibrillation, the 60-year-old male patient is scheduled for a cystoscopy. This is a follow-up examination because the patient has a history of bladder carcinoma that was resected 7 years previously. At that time, the patient received chemotherapy but has not been treated for the cancer for nearly 6 years. He has had yearly cystoscopic examinations, and no recurrence of the bladder cancer has been found. The cystoscopy of the bladder is performed by the urologist who documents as the postoperative diagnosis "history of transitional cell carcinoma of the bladder with no recurrence found, follow-up examination, mild benign prostatic hypertrophy evaluated."

Principal Diagnosis: _____

Secondary Diagnoses: _____

Principal Procedure: _____

Secondary Procedure(s): _____

3

While the 35-year-old patient, gravida 6, para 6, is in the hospital for newly diagnosed uncontrolled hypertension, she requests a tubal ligation/sterilization to be performed by her OB-GYN physician as she does not want to have more children. The procedure is scheduled after her hypertension is controlled. The physician performs the following procedure with the following diagnosis: laparoscopic tubal ligation using Falope rings, admission for desired sterilization and multiparity.

Principal Diagnosis: _____

Secondary Diagnoses: _____

Principal Procedure: _____

Secondary Procedure(s): _____

4

A full-term, 38-week gestation, infant is born by vaginal birth in the hospital to a 35-year-old woman who develops gestational diabetes during the pregnancy. The mother required close monitoring during the pregnancy because of rather severe fluctuations in blood glucose level. The infant, weighing 8 lb, 5 oz, appears normal and healthy. However, because of the mother's gestational diabetes, the infant is kept as an inpatient in the hospital 2 days longer than usual to observe for possible metabolic disorders as a result of his mother's condition. No symptoms are exhibited by the infant, and the results of diagnostic studies performed are negative. The pediatrician writes the discharge diagnosis as normal, full-term infant, observed for possible effects of mother's gestational diabetes, no disease found.

Principal Diagnosis: _____

Secondary Diagnoses: _____

Principal Procedure: _____

Secondary Procedure(s): _____

5

A 75-year-old retired nun has a total hip replacement for localized osteoarthritis of the right hip. After surgery, she experiences significant difficulty in ambulating, along with gait abnormalities. Physical therapists treat the patient while she is in the hospital, but on day 6, she is discharged to home to be followed up by home health services.

The patient is seen three times a week by a nurse and physical therapists. The patient receives an anticoagulant drug to prevent clots. This requires the nurse to draw blood for a PT/PTT laboratory test weekly. Physical therapists treat the patient for her gait abnormality and difficulty in walking as part of her aftercare following the hip joint replacement. Physical therapy performed includes gait training and strengthening exercises to increase the patient's mobility.

Code for the home health services received:

First-Listed Diagnosis: _____

Secondary Diagnoses : _____

6

A premature twin infant with a liveborn mate is admitted to the special care nursery after the cesarean delivery during which he was delivered. The infant is treated for his prematurity and low birth weight as well as neonatal jaundice associated with the preterm delivery. The infant receives phototherapy to skin over multiple days for the jaundice and is discharged to his parents after 1 month in the hospital. The pediatrician's discharge diagnoses were premature twin infant, result of a 34-week pregnancy, with a birthweight of 1,800 grams, with newborn jaundice of prematurity.

Principal Diagnosis: _____

Secondary Diagnoses: _____

Principal Procedure: _____

Secondary Procedure(s): _____

7

The fire ambulance brings a family to the hospital emergency department (ED) after a serious car accident when their car was in a collision with another car on the interstate highway. The father and mother were seriously injured and are admitted to the hospital with multiple fractures and head trauma. During the accident, the 10-month-old baby was secured in a rear-facing child seat in the backseat. The ED physicians examine the baby carefully and request several x-rays to be performed. All x-rays are negative, but the physicians are still particularly concerned about the infant given the serious nature of the accident. They decide to admit the baby to the hospital for monitoring and further testing for undetected injuries. After day 2, no injuries can be found in the infant, and he is discharged to the care of his maternal grandparents.

Note: Assign codes only for the infant.

Principal Diagnosis: _____

Secondary Diagnoses: _____

Principal Procedure: _____

Secondary Procedure(s): _____

8

The patient is a 32-year-old woman who is 24 weeks pregnant. She is being followed up by her physician as a high-risk pregnancy because of her history of having a hydatidiform mole 10 years previously. The patient is considered to have a history of infertility as the patient has not been pregnant since she was treated for the hydatidiform mole with surgical evacuation. The physician orders ongoing laboratory testing for monitoring of the current pregnancy, and no problems have been detected. The patient will return for her next prenatal visit at 27 weeks.

First-Listed Diagnosis: _____

Secondary Diagnoses: _____

9

The first visit of the day for this pediatrician is a 2-week-old infant who was born by vaginal delivery to a woman during the 39th week of pregnancy. All laboratory tests done in the hospital were normal and the baby was discharged with her mother on day 2. The mother reports that the infant has been nursing well and has generally been a delight. The pediatrician examines the infant and does not find any problems or abnormalities at the age of 14 days. The mother is counseled regarding infant care, nursing, and the recommended infant vaccinations to be performed during the follow-up visits.

First-Listed Diagnosis: _____

Secondary Diagnoses: _____

10

The patient admitted to the hospital is a 28-year-old woman who is a third-grade school teacher. She is donating her left kidney for a young boy in her class who has polycystic kidney disease and is in need of a kidney transplant. The donor has a history of an allergy to latex, so she was protected from any exposure to latex supplies during her hospital stay. This allergy did not prevent her from being a donor. The teacher's surgery, a unilateral open nephrectomy, is performed uneventfully, and she is discharged to her home to recover.

Principal Diagnosis: _____

Secondary Diagnoses: _____

Principal Procedure: _____

Secondary Procedure(s): _____

11

The patient was seen in the physician's office for change of the dressings on both hands. The patient is a construction worker who was injured on the job 7 days ago. He was handling a rope used to pull up a heavy metal structure when the rope began to run through his gloved hands. He tried to stop the rope and states that his gloves actually caught fire. He developed pain to both of his hands. He was brought to the Emergency Department of the hospital near the construction site. The ER physician applied cool dressings to the hands and removed some avulsed skin from several fingers. During this office visit, the patient's dressings were changed with Silvadene applied to the fingers. The wounds did not appear infected. The reason for the visit documented by the physician was "Change of dressings to protect the healing deep abrasions on both hands."

First-Listed Diagnosis: _____

Secondary Diagnoses : _____

12

The patient was seen in his primary care physician's office for routine fracture healing. The patient suffered traumatic fractures of his pelvis that occurred 4 weeks ago. The patient was walking across a street when he was hit by a car, knocked down, and the car ran over his pelvis. The fractures did not require surgical treatment. After the hospital stay, the patient was transferred to an acute rehabilitation facility, and he improved dramatically over the past 4 weeks. He was discharged from the rehabilitation facility 2 days ago and will begin outpatient physical therapy tomorrow. During this office visit, his fracture was evaluated. The physician also reviewed and signed the physical therapy plan of treatment and orders for the patient to continue to receive fracture aftercare.

First-Listed Diagnosis: _____

Secondary Diagnoses: _____

13

The patient, a 70-year-old man, was seen in his cardiologist's office for a report of the echocardiogram that was performed on the patient within the past week. The man had the mitral valve in his heart replaced about 20 years ago and has had some vague symptoms that led the doctor to order the echocardiogram. Based on the physical examination and the report of the echocardiogram, the cardiologist concluded the heart valve was near the end of its life and needed to be replaced. The doctor informed the patient that this was an expected event, that valves do not last forever, and that the need to replace it did not mean the valve was defective or causing a complication. To prevent the patient from experiencing serious problems by delaying the inevitable replacement, the doctor arranged for the patient to be admitted to the hospital the same evening, with consultation with the cardiothoracic surgeon immediately. Two days later the patient had the mitral valve replaced with a new synthetic prosthetic valve by thoracotomy and had an uneventful recovery.

Principal Diagnosis: _____

Secondary Diagnoses: _____

Principal Procedure: _____

Secondary Procedure(s): _____

14

The patient is a 17-year-old high school senior who was in his chemistry laboratory when another student spilled a non-medicinal chemical during a lab assignment. Other students in the classroom complained of nausea and shortness of breath. This patient had no symptoms or complaints. The student was examined by the Emergency Department physician and found to be well. The diagnosis written by the doctor on the record was "Well adolescent, exposed to non-medicinal chemical, no injury or disease found."

First-Listed Diagnosis: _____

Secondary Diagnoses: _____

15

A five-month-old female was brought by her mother to the pediatrician's office for her scheduled "Synagis" shot. Synagis is a medication given prophylactically to high-risk infants to protect them from acquiring the respiratory syncytial virus (RSV) and avoid an acute respiratory illness. The doctor's progress note for the visit concludes with his impression of "Ex-30 week premature infant here for Synagis injection, subcutaneous, completed."

First-Listed Diagnosis : _____

Secondary Diagnoses: _____

16

The patient is a 35-year-old female who is admitted for prophylactic robotic-assisted laparoscopic total abdominal hysterectomy (TAH) and bilateral laparoscopic salpingo-oophorectomy (BSO). She is having this elective removal of her uterus, tubes, and ovaries because she has a strong history of ovarian cancer in her family, including her grandmother, aunt, sister, and cousin. She has three healthy children. The surgery was performed without complications, and the patient had an uneventful postoperative period. After surgery, the gynecologic oncologist who performed the surgery informed the patient that a tiny area of malignancy, Stage 1 ovarian carcinoma, was found in the right ovary. The patient was discharged for recovery at home with the assistance of a home health agency and will return to her oncologist's office in two weeks to discuss further treatment.

Principal Diagnosis: _____

Secondary Diagnoses: _____

Principal Procedure: _____

Secondary Procedure(s): _____

Answer Key for Coding Scenarios

Chapter 1

Certain Infectious and Parasitic Diseases

1. **First-Listed Diagnosis:** **A56.09** Cervicitis, chlamydial. This combination code includes in its description the diagnosis cervicitis and the causative infectious agent, chlamydia.

   Secondary Diagnoses: None indicated by the documentation provided

2. **Principal Diagnosis:** **B20** HIV; Disease, Human immunodeficiency virus; or Human immunodeficiency virus

   Secondary Diagnoses: **B59** Pneumonia, pneumocystis. (As a manifestation of HIV disease, the code for this diagnosis is listed following code B20.)
   B37.0 Candidiasis, oralis also listed as a secondary code, whether present on admission or not present on admission, because this disease is a manifestation of HIV disease.

   Principal Procedure: None indicated by the documentation provided

   Secondary Procedure(s): None indicated by the documentation provided

3. **First-Listed Diagnosis:** **B18.1** Hepatitis, viral, chronic, Type B
   Secondary Diagnoses: **K74.60** Cirrhosis of liver. The suspected liver failure is not coded because conditions documented as suspected are not coded for outpatient encounters.
   F11.21 Addiction, heroin, see Dependence, Drug, Opoid, in remission.

4. **Principal Diagnosis:** **A41.51** Sepsis, Escherichia coli [E. coli].

   Secondary Diagnoses: **R65.20** Sepsis, severe;
   J96.00 Failure, respiratory, acute. Code R65.20 is sequenced following the code for the underlying infection, sepsis. Additional codes for any acute organ dysfunction are sequenced next, for example, J96.00.

Principal Procedure:

Character	Code	Explanation
Section	5	Extracorporeal Assistance & Performance
Physiological System	A	Physiological Systems
Root Operation	1	Performance
Body Part	9	Respiratory
Duration	4	24–96 Consecutive Hours
Function	5	Ventilation
Qualifier	Z	No Qualifier

INDEX: Mechanical ventilation see Performance, Respiratory

Note: Mechanical ventilation is coded to the extracorporeal assistance and performance section. Insertion of the endotracheal tube as part of a mechanical ventilation procedure is not coded as a separate device insertion procedure, because it is merely the interface between the patient and the equipment used to perform the procedure, rather than an end in itself. On the other hand, insertion of an endotracheal tube in order to maintain an airway in patients who are unconscious or unable to breathe on their own is the central objective of the procedure. Therefore, insertion of an endotracheal tube as an end in itself is coded to the root operation INSERTION and the device ENDOTRACHEAL AIRWAY. Refer to Appendix C in the *ICD-10-PCS Reference Manual*—page C.8–9

Secondary Procedure(s): None indicated by the documentation provided

5. **First-Listed Diagnosis:** **A46** Erysipelas. See the main Index term Erysipelas, or the main Index term Cellulitis, subterm erysipelatous.

   Secondary Diagnoses: None indicated by the documentation provided

6. **First-Listed Diagnosis:** **B26.9** Parotitis, infectious see Mumps

   Secondary Diagnoses: None indicated by the documentation provided

7. **First-Listed Diagnosis:** **A54.01** Urethritis, gonococcal or Cystitis, gonococcal. This combination code includes all components of the diagnosis

   Secondary Diagnoses: None indicated by the documentation provided

8. **First-Listed Diagnosis:** **A15.0** Tuberculosis, lung—see Tuberculosis, pulmonary

   Secondary Diagnoses: **I10** Hypertension (essential);
   I25.10 Disease, artery, coronary;
   Z98.61 Status, angioplasty, coronary artery.
   No mention was made of implants (stents) or grafts.

9. **First-Listed Diagnosis:** **G14** Postpolio syndrome

   Secondary Diagnoses: None indicated by the documentation provided.
   Code B91, sequela of poliomyelitis, is not used as a specific diagnosis is provided, postpolio syndrome, and the Excludes1 note present at B91 and G14 indicate these codes may not be assigned together.

10. **Principal Diagnosis:** **A87.0** Meningitis, coxsackie virus

    Secondary Diagnoses: None indicated by the documentation provided

    Principal Procedure:

Character	Code	Explanation
Section	0	Medical and Surgical
Body System	0	Central Nervous System
Root Operation	9	Drainage
Body Part	U	Spinal Canal
Approach	3	Percutaneous
Device	Z	No Device
Qualifier	Z	No Qualifier

INDEX: Puncture, lumbar see Drainage, spinal canal

Secondary Procedure(s): None indicated by the documentation provided

11. **Principal Diagnosis:** **A41.59** Sepsis, gram negative (organism). An additional code for severe sepsis or associated acute organ dysfunction is not assigned because neither was documented. See the Index, main term Sepsis, subterm Gram-negative. There is no subterm for Klebsiella.

    Secondary Diagnoses: **N39.0** Infection, Urinary tract. Follow the instruction note to use an additional code to identify infectious agent. Assign B96.1 Infection, Klebsiella pneumoniae [K. pneumoniae] as the cause of diseases classified elsewhere;
    E87.1 Hyponatremia;
    E87.6 Hypokalemia;
    C77.3 Neoplasm, malignant, Secondary axilla and upper limb lymph nodes;
    Z85.3 History, personal malignant neoplasm (of) breast.

    Principal Procedure: None indicated by the documentation provided

    Secondary Procedure(s): None indicated by the documentation provided

12. **First-Listed Diagnosis:** **B01.2** Chickenpox—see Varicella with pneumonia

    Secondary Diagnoses: **E86.0** Dehydration;
    H65.191 Otitis media, nonsuppurative acute (right ear)

13. **First-Listed Diagnosis:** **B60.13** Keratoconjunctivitis, Acanthamoeba

    Secondary Diagnoses: None indicated by the documentation provided

14. **First-Listed Diagnosis:**   **B18.2** Hepatitis, "C" Chronic

     Secondary Diagnoses: **K75.4** Hepatitis, Autoimmune

15. **First-Listed Diagnosis:**   **A02.0** Poisoning, food, due to salmonella, with, gastroenteritis

     Secondary Diagnoses: **E86.0** Dehydration

16. **First-Listed Diagnosis:**   **A69.23** Arthritis due to or associated with, Lyme disease

     Secondary Diagnoses: **B94.8** Sequela, infectious disease, specified

Chapter 2

Neoplasms

1. **Principal Diagnosis:**   **C34.01** Neoplasm, bronchus main, malignant, primary

     Secondary Diagnoses: **C79.51** Neoplasm, bone, malignant, secondary;
          J43.9 Emphysema;
          Z87.891 History, Personal, nicotine dependence

Principal Procedure:

Character	Code	Explanation
Section	0	Medical and Surgical
Body System	B	Respiratory System
Root Operation	B	Excision
Body Part	3	Main Bronchus, Right
Approach	8	Via Natural or Artificial Opening Endoscopic
Device	Z	No Device
Qualifier	X	Diagnostic

INDEX: Biopsy, see excision, bronchus, with qualifier diagnostic, bronchus, main, right

Secondary Procedure(s): None indicated by the documentation provided

2. **Principal Diagnosis:**   **Z51.11** Encounter, chemotherapy for neoplasm

     Secondary Diagnoses: **C94.20** Leukemia, acute myeloid M7. The patient is receiving chemotherapy because the leukemia is not in remission.

Principal Procedure:

Character	Code	Explanation
Section	3	Administration
Physiological System	E	Physiological Systems and Anatomical Regions
Root Operation	0	Introduction
Body System	4	Central Vein

Approach	3	Percutaneous
Substance	0	Antineoplastic
Qualifier	5	Other Antineoplastic

INDEX: Chemotherapy, infusion for cancer, see Introduction of substance in, vein, central, antineoplastic

Secondary Procedure(s): None indicated by the documentation provided

3. **Principal Diagnosis:**   **E87.1** Dehydration, hypotonic

    Secondary Diagnoses: **C18.7** Neoplasm, sigmoid colon, Malignant, primary;
    C78.7 Neoplasm, liver and intrahepatic bile duct, malignant, secondary;
    Z51.5 Palliative care;
    Z66 DNR (do not resuscitate)

    Principal Procedure: None indicated by the documentation provided

    Secondary Procedure(s):   None indicated by the documentation provided

4. **Principal Diagnosis:**   **C25.0** Neoplasm, pancreas, head, malignant, primary. A diagnosis documented as "probable" is coded as though it were confirmed. This code is listed as the principal diagnosis because it was determined, after study, that the carcinoma of the pancreas was the underlying etiology of the patient's symptoms.

    Secondary Diagnoses: **I12.9** Hypertension, kidney, stage 1 through stage 4 chronic kidney disease;
    N18.4 Disease, kidney, Chronic stage 4 (severe);
    E86.0 Dehydration;
    G89.3 Pain, due to malignancy

    Principal Procedure: None indicated by documentation provided

    Secondary Procedure(s):   None indicated by documentation provided

5. **First-Listed Diagnosis:**   **D06.9** Neoplasm, cervix, CA-in situ

    Secondary Diagnoses: None indicated by the documentation provided

6. **First-Listed Diagnosis:**   **C43.62** Melanoma (Malignant), skin, upper arm or shoulder

    Secondary Diagnoses: None indicated by the documentation provided

7. **First-Listed Diagnosis:**   **C43.39** Melanoma (Malignant), skin, forehead. Although there was no more malignant tissue found, because treatment was directed at the site of the melanoma, the code for malignant melanoma is assigned.

    Secondary Diagnoses: **Z80.8** History, Family malignant neoplasm of other organs or systems;
    Z77.123 Contact, radiation, naturally occurring

8. **Principal Diagnosis:**   **N13.39** Hydronephrosis, specified type NEC. The subterm obstruction does not apply here because the obstruction was not due to a calculus or stricture, but caused by the metastasis.

    Secondary Diagnoses: **C79.19** Neoplasm, ureter, malignant, secondary;
    C16.2 Neoplasm, stomach, malignant, primary;
    C78.6 Neoplasm, peritoneum, malignant, secondary;
    R18.0 Ascites, Malignant (Sequence following the code for the secondary malignancy of the peritoneum.)

Principal Procedure:

Character	Code	Explanation
Section	0	Medical and Surgical
Body System	T	Urinary System
Root Operation	9	Drainage
Body Part	0	Kidney, Right
Approach	3	Percutaneous
Device	0	Drainage device
Qualifier	Z	No Qualifier

INDEX: Nephrostomy, see Drainage, urinary system or kidney

Secondary Procedure(s):

Character	Code	Explanation
Section	0	Medical and Surgical
Body System	W	Anatomical Regions, General
Root Operation	9	Drainage
Body Part	G	Peritoneal Cavity
Approach	3	Percutaneous
Device	Z	No Device
Qualifier	X	Diagnostic

INDEX: Paracentesis, peritoneal cavity, see Drainage, peritoneal cavity

9. **First-Listed Diagnosis:**   **C79.51** Neoplasm, bone, malignant, secondary. This is the site where treatment was directed during this encounter.

    Secondary Diagnoses: **C79.31** Neoplasm brain, malignant, secondary;
                                        C50.912 Neoplasm, breast, left, female, malignant, primary

10. **Principal Diagnosis:**   **C7a.020** Tumor, carcinoid, malignant, appendix. Do not use the Neoplasm Table when assigning codes for carcinoid tumors.

     Secondary Diagnoses: **E34.0** Syndrome, Carcinoid

Principal Procedure:

Character	Code	Explanation
Section	0	Medical and Surgical
Body System	D	Gastrointestinal System
Root Operation	T	Resection
Body Part	J	Appendix
Approach	4	Percutaneous Endoscopic
Device	Z	No Device
Qualifier	Z	No Qualifier

INDEX: Appendectomy, see Resection, appendix

Secondary Procedure(s): None indicated by the documentation provided

11. **Principal Diagnosis:** **C18.4** Neoplasm, intestine, large, colon, transverse, malignant, primary. When the admission is for management of anemia and anemia is the only treatment, the guideline states the code for the malignancy is sequenced first.

   Secondary Diagnoses: **D63.0** Anemia in neoplastic disease

Principal Procedure:

Character	Code	Explanation
Section	3	Administration
Body System	0	Circulatory
Root Operation	2	Transfusion
Body Part	3	Peripheral Vein
Approach	3	Percutaneous
Substance	N	Red Blood Cells
Qualifier	1	Nonautologous

INDEX: Transfusion, vein, peripheral, blood, red cells

Secondary Procedure(s): None indicated by the documentation provided

12. **Principal Diagnosis:** **D61.2** Anemia, aplastic, due to radiation.
   Note: The aplastic anemia is sequenced as the principal diagnosis because guidelines direct users to assign the anemia associated with an adverse effect of radiation; the anemia code is sequenced first followed by the appropriate neoplasm code and code Y84.2 for radiotherapy as the cause of an abnormal reaction.

   Secondary Diagnoses: **C62.12** Seminoma, specified site—see Neoplasm, testis, left, malignant, primary;
   Y84.2 (External cause) Reaction, abnormal, to medical procedures—see Complication, radiological

Principal Procedure:

Character	Code	Explanation
Section	3	Administration
Body System	0	Circulatory
Root Operation	2	Transfusion
Body Part	3	Peripheral
Approach	3	Percutaneous
Substance	H	Whole Blood
Qualifier	0	Nonautologous

INDEX: Transfusion, peripheral vein, blood, whole

Secondary Procedure(s): None indicated by the documentation provided

13. **Principal Diagnosis:** **C71.3** Glioblastoma, giant cell, specified site—Neoplasm, brain, parietal lobe, malignant, primary

   Secondary Diagnoses: **C78.01** Neoplasm, lung, right, secondary, malignant;
   F17.210 Dependence, drug, Nicotine, cigarettes;
   R73.09 Prediabetes

Principal Procedure:

Character	Code	Explanation
Section	0	Medical and Surgical
Body System	0	Central Nervous System
Root Operation	B	Excision
Body Part	7	Cerebral Hemisphere
Approach	3	Percutaneous
Device	Z	No Device
Qualifier	X	Diagnostic

INDEX: Biopsy, see Excision with qualifier diagnostic, Use Appendix C Body Part Key to search for parietal lobe and find parietal lobe see cerebral hemisphere

Secondary Procedure(s):

Character	Code	Explanation
Section	0	Medical and Surgical
Body System	B	Respiratory System
Root Operation	B	Excision
Body Part	K	Lung, Right

Approach	8	Via Natural or Artificial Opening Endoscopic
Device	Z	No Device
Qualifier	X	Diagnostic

INDEX: Bronchoscopy with biopsy, see Excision lung right

14. **Principal Diagnosis:**   **C54.1** Neoplasm, endometrium, malignant, primary

    Secondary Diagnoses: **E89.0** Hypothyroidism, Postprocedural;
    Z85.850 History, Personal malignant neoplasm of thyroid;
    Z90.79 Absence, fallopian tubes, (acquired);
    Z90.722 Absence, ovary (acquired), bilateral;
    I10, Hypertension;
    F41.9, Disorder, anxiety;
    E11.9, Diabetes, type 2

Principal Procedure:

Character	Code	Explanation
Section	0	Medical Surgical
Body System	U	Female Reproductive System
Root Operation	T	Resection
Body Part	9	Uterus
Approach	0	Open
Device	Z	No Device
Qualifier	Z	No Qualifier

INDEX: Hysterectomy, see Resection, Uterus,

Secondary Procedure(s):

Character	Code	Explanation
Section	0	Medical Surgical
Body System	U	Female Reproductive System
Root Operation	T	Resection
Body Part	C	Cervix
Approach	0	Open
Device	Z	No Device
Qualifier	Z	No Qualifier

INDEX: Resection, cervix; Additional code required for cervix as it is a separate body part that is removed with the uterus.

15. **First-Listed Diagnosis:** **C50.912** Neoplasm, breast, malignant, primary (left). This is still under treatment.

    Secondary Diagnoses: **Z17.0** Status, estrogen receptor, positive (See Tabular, there was error in 2011 Index.)

16. **Principal Diagnosis:** **C54.1** Neoplasm, endometrium, malignant, primary

    Secondary Diagnoses: **N83.1** Cyst, Corpus luteum;
    E11.9 Diabetes, type 2;
    Z79.4 Long term (current) use of insulin. See the instruction note pertaining to code category E11 Type 2 diabetes mellitus to "Use additional code to identify any insulin use."

Principal Procedure:

Character	Code	Explanation
Section	0	Medical Surgical
Body System	U	Female Reproductive System
Root Operation	T	Resection
Body Part	9	Uterus
Approach	0	Open
Device	Z	No Device
Qualifier	Z	No Qualifier

INDEX: Hysterectomy, Resection, Uterus

Secondary Procedure(s):

Character	Code	Explanation
Section	0	Medical Surgical
Body System	U	Female Reproductive System
Root Operation	T	Resection
Body Part	C	Cervix
Approach	0	Open
Device	Z	No Device
Qualifier	Z	No Qualifier

INDEX: Resection, cervix; additional code required for cervix as it is a separate body part that is removed in a hysterectomy

Secondary Procedure(s):

Character	Code	Explanation
Section	0	Medical Surgical
Body System	U	Female Reproductive System
Root Operation	T	Resection
Body Part	2	Ovaries, bilateral
Approach	0	Open
Device	Z	No Device
Qualifier	Z	No Qualifier

INDEX: Resection of bilateral ovaries

Secondary Procedure(s):

Character	Code	Explanation
Section	0	Medical Surgical
Body System	U	Female Reproductive System
Root Operation	T	Resection
Body Part	7	Fallopian tubes, bilateral
Approach	0	Open
Device	Z	No Device
Qualifier	Z	No Qualifier

INDEX: Resection of bilateral fallopian tubes

17. **Principal Diagnosis:** **C50.211** Neoplasm, breast, upper-inner quadrant malignant, primary
    Secondary Diagnoses: **Z80.3** History, Family malignant neoplasm of breast
    Principal Procedure:

Character	Code	Explanation
Section	0	Medical and Surgical
Body System	H	Skin and Breast
Root Operation	B	Excision
Body Part	T	Breast, Right
Approach	0	Open
Device	Z	No Device
Qualifier	Z	No Qualifier

INDEX: Excision, breast, right for lumpectomy

Secondary Procedure(s): None indicated by the documentation provided

18. **Principal Diagnosis:** **C19** Neoplasm, rectosigmoid, malignant, primary

    Secondary Diagnoses: **I25.118** Arteriosclerosis, coronary, native, with angina specified NEC (stable angina);
E78.0, Hypercholesterolemia;
Z95.5 Status, angioplasty, coronary artery with implant;
Z87.891 History personal nicotine dependence

Principal Procedure:

Character	Code	Explanation
Section	0	Medical and Surgical
Body System	D	Gastrointestinal System
Root Operation	T	Resection
Body Part	N	Sigmoid Colon
Approach	0	Open
Device	Z	No Device
Qualifier	Z	No Qualifier

INDEX: Resection, colon, sigmoid

Secondary Procedure(s): None indicated by the documentation provided

Chapter 3

Diseases of Blood and Blood-forming Organs and Certain Disorders Involving the Immune Mechanism

1. **Principal Diagnosis:** **D57.811** Disease, sickle cell, Hb-SE, with crisis, with acute chest syndrome

    Secondary Diagnoses: None indicated by the documentation provided

    Principal Procedure: None indicated by the documentation provided

    Secondary Procedure(s): None indicated by the documentation provided

2. **Principal Diagnosis:** **C25.0** Neoplasm, pancreas, head, malignant, primary

    Secondary Diagnoses: **D63.0** Anemia in neoplastic disease. See the instruction note "Code first neoplasm (C00–D49)"
Coding guideline I.C.2.c.1: When admission/encounter is for management of an anemia associated with the malignancy, and the treatment is only for anemia, the appropriate code for the malignancy is sequenced as the principal or principal diagnosis followed by the appropriate code for the anemia, such as D63.0, Anemia in neoplastic disease.

Principal Procedure:

Character	Code	Explanation
Section	3	Administration
Physiological System	0	Circulatory
Root Operation	2	Transfusion
Body Part	3	Peripheral Vein
Approach	3	Percutaneous
Substance	N	Red Blood Cells
Qualifier	1	Nonautologous

INDEX: Transfusion, Vein, Peripheral, Blood, Red Cells

Secondary Procedure(s): None indicated by the documentation provided

3. **Principal Diagnosis:** **D50.9** Anemia, Iron deficiency

   Secondary Diagnoses: None indicated by the documentation provided

Principal Procedure:

Character	Code	Explanation
Section	0	Medical and Surgical
Body System	7	Lymphatic and Hemi Systems
Root Operation	D	Extraction
Body Part	R	Bone Marrow, Iliac
Approach	3	Percutaneous
Device	Z	No Device
Qualifier	X	Diagnostic

INDEX: Extraction, bone marrow, iliac.

Note: Aspiration is not the root operation for this case because it does not meet the definition of taking or letting out fluids and/or gases from a body part. Excision is not applicable for bone marrow "biopsy" because the removal of bone marrow does not meet the definition of excision: cutting out a portion of a body part. In this example, bone marrow is extracted or pulled out of the site.

Secondary Procedure(s): None indicated by the documentation provided

4. **First-Listed Diagnosis:** **D53.9** Anemia, Nutritional

   Secondary Diagnoses: **J44.9** Disease, lung/pulmonary, obstructive (chronic);

                                      I25.2 Infarction, myocardium, healed or old

5. **Principal Diagnosis:**   **D59.1** Anemia, hemolytic, autoimmune

    Secondary Diagnoses: **M32.9** Lupus, erythematous, systemic

    Principal Procedure:

Character	Code	Explanation
Section	0	Medical and Surgical
Body System	7	Lymphatic and Hemi Systems
Root Operation	T	Resection
Body Part	P	Spleen
Approach	0	Open
Device	Z	No Device
Qualifier	Z	No Qualifier

INDEX: Splenectomy, see Resection, Lymphatic and Hemi System (Spleen)

Secondary Procedure(s): None indicated by the documentation provided

6. **Principal Diagnosis:**   **K25.4** Ulcer, gastric see stomach, Chronic with hemorrhage

    Secondary Diagnoses: **D62** Anemia, posthemorrhagic, Acute

    Principal Procedure:

Character	Code	Explanation
Section	0	Medical and Surgical
Body System	D	Gastrointestinal System
Root Operation	J	Inspection
Body Part	0	Upper Intestinal Tract
Approach	8	Via Natural or Artificial Opening Endoscopic
Device	Z	No Device
Qualifier	Z	No Qualifier

INDEX: Esophagogastroduodenoscopy

Secondary Procedure(s): None indicated by the documentation provided

7. **First-Listed Diagnosis:**   **K29.40** Gastritis, atrophic (Chronic) (without bleeding)

    Secondary Diagnoses: **D51.0** Anemia, pernicious;
    D80.1 Agammaglobulinemia

8. **Principal Diagnosis:**   **D61.1** Anemia, aplastic, drug-induced or due to drugs.

       See coding guideline I.C.2.c.2: When the admission/encounter is for management of an anemia associated with an adverse effect of the administration of chemotherapy or immunotherapy and the only treatment is for the anemia, the anemia code is sequenced first followed by the appropriate codes for the neoplasm and the adverse effect (such as T45.1x5, Adverse effect of antineoplastic and immunosuppressive drugs).

Secondary Diagnoses: **T45.1x5A** Table of Drugs and Chemicals, antineoplastic, (Adverse effect of antineoplastic and immunosuppressive drugs), initial encounter;
C56.2 Neoplasm, ovary, malignant, primary, and assign 4th character "2" to denote left side

Principal Procedure: None indicated by the documentation provided

Secondary Procedure(s):   None indicated by the documentation provided

9. **Principal Diagnosis:**   **D66** Hemophilia, A

    Secondary Diagnoses: **M36.2**, Arthritis in hemophilia NEC

    Principal Procedure:

Character	Code	Explanation
Section	6	Extracorporeal Therapies
Physiological Systems	A	Physiological Systems
Root Operation	5	Pheresis
Body System	5	Circulatory
Duration	0	Single
Qualifier	Z	No Qualifier
Qualifier	3	Plasma

INDEX: Plasmapheresis, therapeutic

Secondary Procedure(s):   None indicated by the documentation provided

10. **Principal Diagnosis:**   **D69.3** Purpura, thrombocytopenic, Idiopathic

    Secondary Diagnoses: None indicated by the documentation provided

    Principal Procedure:

Character	Code	Explanation
Section	0	Medical and Surgical
Body System	7	Lymphatic and Hemi Systems
Root Operation	B	Excision
Body Part	P	Spleen
Approach	4	Percutaneous Endoscopic
Device	Z	No Device
Qualifier	Z	No Qualifier

INDEX: Excision, Spleen

Secondary Procedure(s):   None indicated by the documentation provided

11. **Principal Diagnosis:**   **L89.153** Ulcer, pressure, sacral, stage 3

     Secondary Diagnoses: **R15.9**, Incontinence, feces;

L89.212 Ulcer, Pressure ulcer stage 2, hip. Assign 6th character 2 to denote right hip;

D62 Anemia, posthemorrhagic, acute;

E11.9 Diabetes, type 2;

I10 Hypertension;

M47.26, Osteoarthritis, spine, see Spondylosis, with radiculopathy, lumbar region (Chronic back pain not coded due to Excludes1 note with R52 and M54)

Principal Procedure:

Character	Code	Explanation
Section	0	Medical and Surgical
Body System	D	Gastrointestinal System
Root Operation	1	Bypass
Body Part	M	Descending Colon
Approach	0	Open
Device	Z	No Device
Qualifier	4	Cutaneous

INDEX: Colostomy, see Bypass, Gastrointestinal System

Secondary Procedure(s):

Character	Code	Explanation
Section	3	Administration
Physiological System	0	Circulatory
Root Operation	2	Transfusion
Body Part	3	Peripheral Vein
Approach	3	Percutaneous
Substance	N	Red Blood Cells
Qualifier	1	Nonautologous

INDEX: Transfusion, Vein, Peripheral, Blood, Red Cells

12. **First-Listed Diagnosis:**   **D61.2** Anemia, aplastic, due to, radiation

     Secondary Diagnoses: **C50.911** Neoplasm, breast, malignant, primary. Assign 6th character 1 to denote right breast;

C79.51 Neoplasm, bone, malignant, secondary;

Y84.2 Radiation complication or abnormal reaction to radiotherapy, without mention of misadventure at the time of the procedure. (See guideline I.C.2.c.2).

13. **First-Listed Diagnosis:**   **N18.6** Disease, renal, End stage

    Secondary Diagnoses: **D63.1** Anemia, in, end-stage renal disease. See the Tabular instruction note to Code first underlying chronic kidney disease (CKD) (N18-);
    Z99.2 Dependence on renal dialysis

14. **Principal Diagnosis:**   **O47.02** False labor before 37 completed weeks of gestation, second trimester

    Secondary Diagnoses: **O99.012**, Pregnancy, complicated by, anemia, 2nd trimester (Includes conditions from D50–D64, which includes the sickle-cell trait code);
    D57.3 Sickle-cell trait

Principal Procedure:

Character	Code	Explanation
Section	B	Imaging
Body System	Y	Fetus and Obstetrical
Root Type	4	Ultrasonography
Body Part	C	Second Trimester, Single Fetus
Contrast	Z	None
Qualifier	Z	None
Qualifier	Z	None

INDEX: Ultrasonography, Fetus, Single, Second Trimester

Secondary Procedure(s): None indicated by the documentation provided

15. **Principal Diagnosis:**   **R55** Syncope

    Secondary Diagnoses: **D56.1** Thalassemia, beta, major (Splenomegaly not coded as it is symptom of the disease.)

Principal Procedure:

Character	Code	Explanation
Section	3	Administration
Physiological System	0	Circulatory
Root Operation	2	Transfusion
Body Part	3	Peripheral Vein
Approach	3	Percutaneous
Substance	N	Red Blood Cells
Qualifier	1	Nonautologous

INDEX: Transfusion, Vein, Peripheral, Blood, Red Cells

Secondary Procedure(s): None indicated by the documentation provided

Chapter 4

Endocrine, Nutritional, and Metabolic Diseases

1. **Principal Diagnosis:** **E10.329** Diabetes mellitus, type 1 with retinopathy, nonproliferative, mild. The term "uncontrolled" is not used for code assignment.

    Secondary Diagnoses: None indicated by the documentation provided
    Note: Although not addressed in the guidelines, Z79.4, long term [current] use of insulin, is not to be assigned with codes from E10 for type 1 diabetes mellitus. Instead the classification provides a use additional note to identify any insulin use in all the diabetes categories with the exception of E10 for type 1 diabetes mellitus. The Z79.4 code would not be assigned with type 1 cases because insulin is required to sustain life.

    Principal Procedure: None indicated by the documentation provided

    Secondary Procedure(s): None indicated by the documentation provided

2. **First-Listed Diagnosis:** **E11.42** Diabetes, type 2 with polyneuropathy

    Secondary Diagnoses: **E11.22**, Diabetes, type 2 with chronic kidney disease;
    N18.2 Disease, Chronic kidney, stage 2 (mild).
    Note that either code could be first-listed as both are diabetic diseases.

3. **Principal Diagnosis:** **T85.614A**, Complication, insulin pump, Mechanical, breakdown for initial encounter

    Secondary Diagnoses: **T38.3x6A** Table of Drugs and Chemical, insulin, Underdosing, initial encounter;
    E10.10 Diabetes, type 1 with ketoacidosis

    Principal Procedure: None indicated by the documentation provided

    Secondary Procedure(s): None indicated by the documentation provided

4. **First-Listed Diagnosis:** **E11.9** Diabetes mellitus (If the type of diabetes mellitus is not specified, the default is type 2 according to guideline C.4.a.2.)

    Secondary Diagnoses: **Z79.4** Long-term (current) use of insulin

5. **First-Listed Diagnosis:** **E21.0** Hyperparathyroidism, Primary. This is the condition treated during this encounter.

    Secondary Diagnoses: **D35.1** Adenoma (see also Neoplasm, benign, by site), Neoplasm, parathyroid, benign

6. **First-Listed Diagnosis:** **E05.90** Hyperthyroidism

    Secondary Diagnoses: **R00.2** Palpitations

7. **Principal Diagnosis:** **E10.9** Diabetes type 1. No complications were documented for this encounter.

    Secondary Diagnoses: None indicated by the documentation provided

    Principal Procedure:

Character	Code	Explanation
Section	0	Medical and Surgical
Body System	J	Subcutaneous Tissue and Fascia

Root Operation	H	Insertion
Body Part	8	Subcutaneous Tissue and Fascia, Trunk
Approach	0	Open
Device	V	Infusion Pump
Qualifier	Z	No Qualifier

INDEX: Infusion Device, insertion of device in abdomen

Secondary Procedure(s):

Character	Code	Explanation
Section	3	Administration
Body System	E	Physiological Systems and Anatomical Regions
Root Operation	0	Introduction
Body System	1	Subcutaneous Tissue
Approach	3	Percutaneous
Substance	V	Hormone
Qualifier	G	Insulin

INDEX: Introduction of substance in or on subcutaneous tissue, hormone (insulin)

8. **Principal Diagnosis:**   **E66.2** Obesity with alveolar hypoventilation

   Secondary Diagnoses: **Z68.42** Body mass index (BMI), adult, 45.0–49.9;
   I10 Hypertension, (essential);
   E78.5, Hyperlipidemia;
   G47.33 Apnea, sleep, obstructive (adult);
   E88.81 Resistance, insulin;
   M16.0 Osteoarthritis, primary, hip, bilateral;
   M17.0 Osteoarthritis, primary, knee, bilateral

Principal Procedure:

Character	Code	Explanation
Section	0	Medical and Surgical
Body System	D	Gastrointestinal System
Root Operation	1	Bypass
Body Part	6	Stomach
Approach	4	Percutaneous Endoscopic
Device	Z	No Device
Qualifier	A	Jejunum

INDEX: Bypass, Stomach (Bypass was from stomach to jejunum; see guidelines for bypass procedures B3.6a.)

Secondary Procedure(s): None indicated by the documentation provided

9. **Principal Diagnosis:** **E66.1** Obesity, morbid, due to excess calories

   Secondary Diagnoses: **I10** Hypertension, (essential);
   E11.44 Diabetes, type 2 with diabetic amyotrophy;
   E78.5 Hyperlipidemia;
   Z96.653. See the Index main term Presence, knee-joint implant. The seventh character, 3 for bilateral, is found in the Tabular;
   Z68.43, Body, mass index, adult, 50.0–59.9

Principal Procedure:

Character	Code	Explanation
Section	0	Medical and Surgical
Body System	D	Gastrointestinal System
Root Operation	V	Restriction
Body Part	6	Stomach
Approach	4	Percutaneous Endoscopic
Device	C	Extraluminal Device
Qualifier	Z	No Qualifier

INDEX: Banding, see Restriction, Stomach; insertion of port is part of procedure

Secondary Procedure(s): None indicated by the documentation provided

10. **First-Listed Diagnosis:** **Z71.3** Counseling, Dietary. For this outpatient encounter, assign this code first as it was the reason for the office visit. See the instruction note in the Tabular to use an additional code for any associated underlying medical condition, as below.

    Secondary Diagnoses: **E78.0** Hypercholesterolemia, familial;
    Z87.891 History, Personal, nicotine dependence

11. **Principal Diagnosis:** **E89.1** Postprocedural hypoinsulinemia. The guidelines concerning secondary diabetes mellitus due to pancreatectomy advise that this code is sequenced first, followed by the additional codes listed below (Guideline I.C.4.6(b)i).

    Secondary Diagnoses: **E13.9** Diabetes, secondary or Diabetes, postpancreatectomy, see Diabetes, specified type NEC;.
    Z90.411 Absence, pancreas, acquired, partial;
    Z79.4, Long term drug therapy, Insulin

    Principal Procedure: None indicated by the documentation provided

    Secondary Procedure(s): None indicated by the documentation provided

12. **Principal Diagnosis:** **E87.5** Hyperkalemia

    Secondary Diagnoses: **N28.9** Insufficiency, renal, (acute);
    I12.9 Hypertension, kidney, with stage 1 through stage 4 chronic kidney disease;
    N18.1 Disease, kidney, chronic, stage 1;
    I25.10 Disease, artery, coronary;

Z95.0 Presence of cardiac pacemaker;
I48.0 Fibrillation, atrial;
Z91.14 Noncompliance, with medication;
Z91.11 Noncompliance with dietary regimen

Principal Procedure: None indicated by the documentation provided

Secondary Procedure(s): None indicated by the documentation provided

13. **Principal Diagnosis:** **E10.11** Diabetes, type 1 with ketoacidosis with coma

    Secondary Diagnoses: **E10.21** Diabetes, type 1 with nephropathy;
    E10.341 Diabetes, type 1 with retinopathy, nonproliferative, severe with macular edema;
    N39.0 Infection, Urinary (tract);
    B96.20 Infection, Escherichia coli [E. Coli];
    F10.229 Dependence, Alcohol with intoxication;
    Z91.19 Noncompliance with medical treatment

    Principal Procedure: None indicated by the documentation provided

    Secondary Procedure(s): None indicated by the documentation provided

14. **Principal Diagnosis:** **E86.0** Dehydration

    Secondary Diagnoses: **E87.6** Hypokalemia;
    K52.9 Gastroenteritis;
    J18.9 Pneumonia;
    L22 Diaper rash

    Principal Procedure: None indicated by the documentation provided

    Secondary Procedure(s): None indicated by the documentation provided

15. **Principal Diagnosis:** **E76.1** Mucopolysaccharidosis, type II or Hunter syndrome. See the Index main term Hunter's, syndrome, or Index main term Mucopolysaccharidosis, type, II.

    Secondary Diagnoses: None indicated by the documentation provided

    Principal Procedure: None indicated by the documentation provided

    Secondary Procedure(s): None indicated by the documentation provided

16. **Principal Diagnosis:** **E86.0** Dehydration. Code E86.0 is assigned as the principal diagnosis because the provider documented it as the reason for admission.

    Secondary Diagnoses: **K52.9** Noninfective gastroenteritis and colitis, unspecified.
    Code K52.9 is assigned as the secondary diagnosis. Although it was not the reason for admission or warranted admission if it were the only diagnosis, gastroenteritis was treated.

    Principal Procedure: None indicated by the documentation provided

    Secondary Procedure(s): None indicated by the documentation provided

Chapter 5

Mental, Behavioral, and Neurodevelopmental Disorders

1. **Principal Diagnosis:**   **F10.231** Dependence, Alcohol with withdrawal delirium

   Secondary Diagnoses: **F10.251** Dependence, Alcohol with alcohol-induced psychotic disorder with hallucinations;
   F17.210 Dependence, Nicotine , cigarettes, (uncomplicated)

   Principal Procedure: None indicated by the documentation provided

   Secondary Procedure(s):   None indicated by the documentation provided

2. **Principal Diagnosis:**   **F41.8** Anxiety depression

   Secondary Diagnoses: **F40.01** Agoraphobia with panic disorder

   Principal Procedure: None indicated by the documentation provided

   Secondary Procedure(s):   None indicated by the documentation provided

3. **Principal Diagnosis:**   **F14.20** Dependence, drug, Cocaine, (uncomplicated)

   Secondary Diagnoses: None indicated by the documentation provided

   Principal Procedure:

Character	Code	Explanation
Section	H	Substance Abuse Treatment
Body System	Z	None
Root Type	2	Detoxification Services
Type Qualifier	Z	None
Qualifier	Z	None
Qualifier	Z	None
Qualifier	Z	None

INDEX: Detoxification Services, for substance abuse

Secondary Procedure(s):

Character	Code	Explanation
Section	G	Mental Health
Body System	Z	None
Root Type	G	Narcosynthesis
Type Qualifier	Z	None
Qualifier	Z	None
Qualifier	Z	None
Qualifier	Z	None

INDEX: Narcosynthesis

4. **Principal Diagnosis:** **G47.10** Hypersomnia, (organic)

Note: A code from category F19 Other psychoactive substance related disorders is not assigned because the lithium carbonate was not associated with a mental or behavioral disorder—the lithium carbonate was being taken to treat the patient's bipolar disorder. Reference ICD-10-CM official coding guidelines I.C.5.b.3.

Secondary Diagnoses: **T43.595A** Table of Drugs and Chemicals, Lithium carbonate, Adverse effect, initial encounter;

F31.31 Disorder, Bipolar, current episode depressed, mild

Principal Procedure:

Character	Code	Explanation
Section	G	Mental Health
Body System	Z	None
Root Type	3	Medication Management
Type Qualifier	Z	None
Qualifier	Z	None
Qualifier	Z	None
Qualifier	Z	None

INDEX: Medication Management (Not for substance abuse, this is a prescribed medication for mental health disorder.)

Secondary Procedure(s): None indicated by the documentation provided

5. **Principal Diagnosis:** **F41.0** Disorder, Panic

Secondary Diagnoses: **R07.89** Pain, chest, non-cardiac

Principal Procedure: None indicated by the documentation provided

Secondary Procedure(s): None indicated by the documentation provided

6. **Principal Diagnosis:** **F45.41** Disorder, Pain, exclusively related to psychological factors

Secondary Diagnoses: **F42** Obsessive-compulsive neurosis

Principal Procedure: None indicated by the documentation provided

Secondary Procedure(s): None indicated by the documentation provided

7. **Principal Diagnosis:** **F11.23** Dependence, drug, Opioid with withdrawal

Secondary Diagnoses: **F11.281** Dependence, drug, Opioid with opioid-induced sexual dysfunction

Principal Procedure:

Character	Code	Explanation
Section	H	Substance Abuse Treatment
Body System	Z	None
Root Type	2	Detoxification Services
Type Qualifier	Z	None
Qualifier	Z	None
Qualifier	Z	None
Qualifier	Z	None

INDEX: Detoxification Services, for substance abuse

Secondary Procedure(s):

Character	Code	Explanation
Section	H	Substance Abuse Treatment
Body System	Z	None
Root Type	3	Individual Counseling
Type Qualifier	7	Motivational Enhancement
Qualifier	Z	None
Qualifier	Z	None
Qualifier	Z	None

INDEX: Substance Abuse Treatment, Individual, motivational

8. **Principal Diagnosis:** **F60.3** Disorder, personality, borderline
    Secondary Diagnoses: **F12.21** Dependence, drug, Cannabis, in remission
    Principal Procedure: None indicated by the documentation provided
    Secondary Procedure(s): None indicated by the documentation provided

9. **First-Listed Diagnosis:** **F20.0** Schizophrenia, Paranoid schizophrenia
    Secondary Diagnoses: **Z91.120** Patient's intentional underdosing of medication regimen due to financial hardship, see the Index main term Underdosing, subterm intentional

10. **Principal Diagnosis:** **F50.01** Anorexia nervosa, restricting type
    Secondary Diagnoses: **E87.8** Disorder, electrolyte;
    Z68.1 Body mass index (BMI) 19 or less, adult
    Principal Procedure: None indicated by the documentation provided
    Secondary Procedure(s): None indicated by the documentation provided

11. **Principal Diagnosis:** **F33.2** Disorder, depressive, recurrent, current episode, severe
    Secondary Diagnoses: **S13.4xxA** Sprain, cervical, Initial encounter;
    X83.8xxA Suicide, hanging;
    Y92.015 External Cause Index, Place of occurrence, residence, house, garage;
    G89.4 Syndrome, Chronic pain;
    F11.20 Dependence, drug, methadone, see Opioid (uncomplicated). The patient is taking methadone, so he is still dependent on opioids.

Principal Procedure: None indicated by the documentation provided

Secondary Procedure(s): None indicated by the documentation provided

12. **First-Listed Diagnosis:** **F10.220** Dependence, Alcohol with intoxication, (uncomplicated)

   Secondary Diagnoses: **Y90.7** Blood alcohol level of 220-239 mg/100 ml (External cause)

13. **First-Listed Diagnosis:** **F20.81** Disorder, Schizophreniform disorder

   Secondary Diagnoses: **F91.2** Disorder, Conduct, adolescent-onset type;
   F90.1 Disorder, Attention-deficit hyperactivity, predominantly hyperactive type;
   F81.9 Disability, learning;
   F63.1, Pyromania;
   Z81.8 History, Family mental disorders

14. **Principal Diagnosis:** **F14.23** Dependence, drug, Cocaine with withdrawal

   Secondary Diagnoses: **F12.20** Dependence, drug, Cannabis, uncomplicated;
   F14.282 Dependence, Cocaine with cocaine-induced sleep disorder

Principal Procedure:

Character	Code	Explanation
Section	H	Substance Abuse Treatment
Body System	Z	None
Root Type	2	Detoxification Services
Type Qualifier	Z	None
Qualifier	Z	None
Qualifier	Z	None
Qualifier	Z	None

INDEX: Detoxification Services, for substance abuse

Secondary Procedure(s): None indicated by the documentation provided

15. **Principal Diagnosis:** **F43.12** Disorder, Post-traumatic stress, chronic

   Secondary Diagnoses: **R45.851** Ideation, Suicidal

Principal Procedure:

Character	Code	Explanation
Section	G	Mental Health Services
Body System	Z	None
Root Type	5	Individual Psychotherapy
Type Qualifier	6	Supportive
Qualifier	Z	None
Qualifier	Z	None
Qualifier	Z	None

INDEX: Psychotherapy, Individual, Mental Health Services, Supportive

Secondary Procedure(s):

Character	Code	Explanation
Section	G	Mental Health Services
Body System	Z	None
Root Type	5	Individual Psychotherapy
Type Qualifier	2	Cognitive
Qualifier	Z	None
Qualifier	Z	None
Qualifier	Z	None

INDEX: Psychotherapy, Individual, Mental Health Services, Cognitive

Chapter 6

Diseases of the Nervous System

1. **First-Listed Diagnosis:** **G30.1** Disease, Alzheimer's, late onset, with behavioral disturbance

   Secondary Diagnoses: **F02.81** Disease, Alzheimer's, late onset, with behavioral disturbances. Requires second code for behavioral disturbance

2. **First-Listed Diagnosis:** **G80.0** Palsy, cerebral, spastic, quadriplegic

   Secondary Diagnoses: **G40.909** Seizure, recurrent;
   J45.909 Asthma;
   Z93.1 Status, gastrostomy

3. **Principal Diagnosis:** **G20** Parkinson's disease, see Parkinsonism

   Secondary Diagnoses: **L02.212** Abscess, cutaneous, see Abscess by site—back

   Principal Procedure:

Character	Code	Explanation
Section	0	Medical and Surgical
Body System	J	Subcutaneous Tissue and Fascia
Root Operation	9	Drainage
Body Part	7	Subcutaneous Tissue and Fascia, Back
Approach	0	Open
Device	Z	No Device
Qualifier	Z	No Qualifier

INDEX: Incision, abscess, see Drainage, subcutaneous, back

Secondary Procedure(s): None indicated by the documentation provided

4. **First-Listed Diagnosis:**   **G40.A09** Epilepsy, childhood absence

   Secondary Diagnoses: None indicated by the documentation provided

5. **Principal Diagnosis:**   **A41.9** Sepsis

   Secondary Diagnoses: **R65.21** Sepsis, severe, with septic shock;
   N17.9 Failure, renal, acute;
   K72.00 Failure, hepatic, acute;
   G31.83 Lewy body dementia;
   F02.90 Dementia without behavioral disturbance. See the note to use additional code for the dementia;
   J69.0 Pneumonia, aspiration, due to food;
   R13.10 Difficulty, swallowing, see Dysphagia;
   Z74.01 Status, bed, confinement;
   Z66 DNR
   L89.153 Ulcer, pressure, sacrum, stage III

   Principal Procedure: None indicated by the documentation provided

   Secondary Procedure(s):   None indicated by the documentation provided

6. **Principal Diagnosis:**   **G50.0** Neuralgia, trigeminal

   Secondary Diagnoses: **I10** Hypertension (essential)

   Principal Procedure:

Character	Code	Explanation
Section	0	Medical and Surgical
Body System	0	Central Nervous System
Root Operation	N	Release
Body Part	K	Trigeminal Nerve
Approach	0	Open
Device	Z	No Device
Qualifier	Z	No Qualifier

INDEX: Release, nerve, trigeminal

   Secondary Procedure(s):   None indicated by the documentation provided

7. **First-Listed Diagnosis:**   **G51.0** Palsy, Bell's, or facial nerve

   Secondary Diagnoses: **E11.9** Diabetes, type 2;
   F17.210 Dependence, drug, nicotine, cigarettes

8. **Principal Diagnosis:**   **G00.0** Meningitis, bacterial, H. influenzae

    Secondary Diagnoses: **H66.001** Otitis, media, suppurative, acute

    Principal Procedure:

Character	Code	Explanation
Section	0	Medical and Surgical
Body System	0	Central Nervous System
Root Operation	9	Drainage
Body Part	U	Spinal Canal
Approach	3	Percutaneous
Device	Z	No Device
Qualifier	X	Diagnostic

INDEX: Drainage, spinal canal

    Secondary Procedure(s):   None indicated by the documentation provided

9. **Principal Diagnosis:**   **A37.01** Whooping cough due to Bordetella pertussis with pneumonia

    Secondary Diagnoses: None indicated by the documentation provided

    Principal Procedure: None indicated by the documentation provided

    Secondary Procedure(s):   None indicated by the documentation provided

10. **Principal Diagnosis:**   **G45.9** Attack, transient ischemic

    Secondary Diagnoses: **I69.354** Sequela, infarction, cerebral, hemiplegia, left nondominant;
    I10 Hypertension, (essential);
    E11.22 Diabetes, type 2, with chronic kidney disease;
    N18.2 Disease, kidney, chronic, stage 2

    Principal Procedure: None indicated by the documentation provided

    Secondary Procedure(s):   None indicated by the documentation provided

11. **First-Listed Diagnosis:**   **F07.81** Syndrome, postconcussionial. See the Tabular instruction note to Use additional code to identify associated post-traumatic headache (G44.3-).

    Secondary Diagnoses: **G44.321** Headache, posttraumatic, chronic, intractable. See the Tabular instruction note after code F07.81: Use additional code to identify associated post-traumatic headache if applicable.

12. **Principal Diagnosis:**   **G90.01** Syndrome, carotid, sinus

    Secondary Diagnoses: None indicated by the documentation provided

Principal Procedure:

Character	Code	Explanation
Section	0	Medical and Surgical
Body System	J	Subcutaneous Tissue and Fascia
Root Operation	H	Insertion
Body Part	6	Subcutaneous Tissue and Fascia, Chest
Approach	0	Open
Device	6	Pacemaker Dual Chamber
Qualifier	Z	No Qualifier

INDEX: Pacemaker, Dual Chamber, Chest

Secondary Procedure(s):

Character	Code	Explanation
Section	0	Medical and Surgical
Body System	2	Heart and Great Vessels
Root Operation	H	Insertion
Body Part	6	Atrium, Right
Approach	3	Percutaneous
Device	J	Cardiac Lead, Pacemaker
Qualifier	Z	No Qualifier

INDEX: Insertion of device in Atrium, right

Secondary Procedure(s):

Character	Code	Explanation
Section	0	Medical and Surgical
Body System	2	Heart and Great Vessels
Root Operation	H	Insertion
Body Part	L	Ventricle, Left
Approach	3	Percutaneous
Device	J	Cardiac Lead, Pacemaker
Qualifier	Z	No Qualifier

INDEX: Insertion of device, in Ventricle, left

13. **Principal Diagnosis:** **M48.06** Stenosis, spinal, lumbar region
    Secondary Diagnoses: **G97.41** Tear, dura
    Principal Procedure:

Character	Code	Explanation
Section	0	Medical and Surgical
Body System	S	Lower Joints
Root Operation	B	Excision
Body Part	2	Lumbar Vertebral Disc
Approach	0	Open
Device	Z	No Device
Qualifier	Z	No Qualifier

INDEX: Excision, Disc, Lumbar Vertebral

Secondary Procedure(s):

Character	Code	Explanation
Section	0	Medical and Surgical
Body System	0	Central Nervous System
Root Operation	Q	Repair
Body Part	2	Dura Mater
Approach	0	Open
Device	Z	No Device
Qualifier	Z	No Qualifier

INDEX: Repair, Dura Mater

14. **Principal Diagnosis:** **T60.0x1D** Table of Drugs, Organophosphate, poisoning, accidental. Assign 7th character D for Subsequent encounter, as the patient had been seen for this condition one month prior to this admission.

    Secondary Diagnoses: **G62.2** Polyneuropathy, in organophosphate. See the Tabular instruction to Code first (T51–65) to identify toxic agent.

    Principal Procedure: None indicated by the documentation provided

    Secondary Procedure(s): None indicated by the documentation provided

15. **Principal Diagnosis:** **G89.21** Pain, chronic, due to trauma

    Secondary Diagnoses: **S34.5xxS** Sequela, injury.
    The original injury to the sympathetic lumbosacral nerve is coded with the 7th character "S" for sequela episode.

Principal Procedure:

Character	Code	Explanation
Section	3	Administration
Physiological System	E	Physiological Systems and Anatomic
Root Operation	0	Introduction
Body System or Region	T	Peripheral Nerves and Plexi
Approach	3	Percutaneous
Substance	C	Regional Anesthetic
Qualifier	Z	No Qualifier

INDEX: Introduction of substance in or on, Nerve, Peripheral, Anesthetic, regional

Secondary Procedure(s): None indicated by the documentation provided

16. **Principal Diagnosis:** **G00.1** Meningitis, bacterial, pneumococcal

    Secondary Diagnoses: **J13** Pneumonia, Streptococcus pneumoniae;
    H66.003 Otitis, media, suppurative, acute, bilateral

Principal Procedure:

Character	Code	Explanation
Section	0	Medical and Surgical
Body System	0	Central Nervous System
Root Operation	9	Drainage
Body Part	U	Spinal Canal
Approach	3	Percutaneous
Device	Z	No Device
Qualifier	X	Diagnostic

INDEX: Drainage, spinal canal

Secondary Procedure(s): None indicated by the documentation provided

17. **Principal Diagnosis:** **G93.3** Syndrome, postviral, fatigue

    Secondary Diagnoses: **B94.8** Sequelae, infectious disease, specified

    Principal Procedure: None indicated by the documentation provided

    Secondary Procedure(s): None indicated by the documentation provided

Chapter 7

Diseases of the Eye and Adnexa

1. **First-Listed Diagnosis:** **H40.123** Glaucoma, Low-tension see glaucoma, open angle, primary, low tension, bilateral

   Secondary Diagnoses: None indicated by the documentation provided

2. **Principal Diagnosis:** **H33.011** Detachment, retina, with retinal break, single, right eye

   Secondary Diagnoses: **Z98.42** Status, cataract extraction, left eye;

   Z63.31 Absence, family member, see also Disruption, family, due to absence of family member due to military deployment

   Principal Procedure:

Character	Code	Explanation
Section	0	Medical and Surgical
Body System	8	Eye
Root Operation	Q	Repair
Body Part	E	Retina, Right
Approach	3	Percutaneous
Device	Z	No Device
Qualifier	Z	No Qualifier

   INDEX: Cryoretinopexy—Repair, retina, right

   Secondary Procedure(s): None indicated by the documentation provided

3. **First-Listed Diagnosis:** **H11.052** Pterygium, peripheral, progressive, left eye

   Secondary Diagnoses: None indicated by the documentation provided

4. **Principal Diagnosis:** **H50.012** Esotropia, see Strabismus, convergent concomitant, monocular, left eye

   Secondary Diagnoses: None indicated by the documentation provided

   Principal Procedure:

Character	Code	Explanation
Section	0	Medical and Surgical
Body System	8	Eye
Root Operation	T	Resection
Body Part	M	Extraocular Muscle, Left
Approach	0	Open

Device	Z	No Device
Qualifier	Z	No Qualifier

INDEX: Resection, muscle, extraocular, left

Secondary Procedure(s): None indicated by the documentation provided

5. **First-Listed Diagnosis:** **E11.339** Diabetes, type 2 with retinopathy, nonproliferative, moderate without macular edema

   Secondary Diagnoses: None indicated by the documentation provided

6. **First-Listed Diagnosis:** **H02.001** Entropion, right, lower
   Secondary Diagnoses: **H50.10** Exotropia, see Strabismus, divergent concomitant;
   H10.45 Conjunctivitis, allergic, chronic

7. **Principal Diagnosis:** **H16.072** Ulcer, cornea, perforated, left

   Secondary Diagnoses: **Z94.7** Transplant (status), cornea;
   Q90.9 Syndrome, Down

Principal Procedure:

Character	Code	Explanation
Section	0	Medical and Surgical
Body System	8	Eye
Root Operation	R	Replacement
Body Part	9	Cornea, Left
Approach	3	Percutaneous
Device	K	Nonautologous Tissue Substitute
Qualifier	Z	No Qualifier

INDEX: Transplant see Replacement, cornea, left

Secondary Procedure(s): None indicated by the documentation provided

8. **First-Listed Diagnosis:** **H27.02** Aphakia, acquired

   Secondary Diagnoses: **H21.42** Membrane, pupillary. Cataract extraction status not coded due to Excludes1 note with code H27.02.

9. **First-Listed Diagnosis:** **H25.11** Cataract, nuclear, sclerosis, see Cataract, senile nuclear

   Secondary Diagnoses: **H40.2213** Glaucoma, angle closure, chronic, right, severe stage

10. **First-Listed Diagnosis:** **H02.014** Entropion, cicatricial, left, upper

    Secondary Diagnoses: **H02.114** Ectropion, cicatricial, left upper;
    H16.212 Keratoconjunctivitis, exposure;
    L90.5 Scar/scarring;
    Z85.828 History, personal, malignant, skin

11. **Ophthalmology Diagnosis: H44.011** Panophthalmitis

    Ophthalmology Procedure:

Character	Code	Explanation
Section	0	Medical and Surgical
Body System	8	Eye
Root Operation	9	Drainage
Body Part	4	Vitreous Right
Approach	3	Percutaneous
Device	Z	No Device
Qualifier	Z	No Qualifier

INDEX: Sclerotomy, see Drainage, eye, vitreous

Ophthalmology Procedure:

Character	Code	Explanation
Section	3	Administration
Physiological System	E	Physiological Systems and Anatomical Regions
Root Operation	0	Introduction
Body System/Region	C	Eye
Approach	3	Percutaneous
Substance	2	Anti-infective
Qualifier	9	Other Anti-infectives

INDEX: Introduction of substance into eye anti-infective

12. **First-Listed Diagnosis:**   **H02.834** Dermatochalasis, eyelid, left

    Secondary Diagnoses: **H02.831** Dermatochalasis, eyelid, right;
    H02.432 Ptosis, eyelid, see Blepharoptosis, paralytic, left upper;
    G51.0 Palsy, Bell's, see Palsy, facial

13. **First-Listed Diagnosis:**   **H40.31x2** Glaucoma secondary to trauma, moderate stage

    Secondary Diagnoses: **T26.41xS** Burn, eye, sequela

14. **First-Listed Diagnosis:**   **H18.731** Descemetocele, right

    Secondary Diagnoses: **T85.398D** Complication, graft, cornea, mechanical, specified type;
    Z94.7 Transplant status cornea

15. **First-Listed Diagnosis:**   **H44.511** Glaucoma, absolute

    Secondary Diagnoses: **H57.11** Pain, ocular, right eye

Chapter 8

Diseases of the Ear and Mastoid Process

1. **First-Listed Diagnosis:** **H90.41** Loss, hearing, see also Deafness, sensorineural, unilateral, right ear
   (There is no hearing loss on left side.)

   Secondary Diagnoses: None indicated by the documentation provided

2. **First-Listed Diagnosis:** **H93.11** Tinnitus, see category H93.1, right ear

   Secondary Diagnoses: None indicated by the documentation provided

3. **First-Listed Diagnosis:** **H81.10** Vertigo, benign positional

   Secondary Diagnoses: None indicated by the documentation provided

4. **First-Listed Diagnosis:** **H61.23** Cerumen, bilateral

   Secondary Diagnoses: None indicated by the documentation provided

5. **First-Listed Diagnosis:** **H72.02** Perforation, tympanic (membrane), central, left ear

   Secondary Diagnoses: None indicated by the documentation provided

6. **First-Listed Diagnosis:** **H90.42** Loss, hearing, see also Deafness, sensorineural, unilateral, left

   Secondary Diagnoses: **H65.22** Otitis, media, chronic, serous, see nonsuppurative, chronic, serous.
   The possible perforation of the tympanic membrane is not coded in the
   outpatient setting.

7. **First-Listed Diagnosis:** **H60.42** Cholesteatoma, external ear, left

   Secondary Diagnoses: **H66.92** Otitis, media, chronic, left

8. **First-Listed Diagnosis:** **H92.03** Pain, ear, see category H92.0, bilateral

   Secondary Diagnoses: **J06.9** Infection, respiratory, upper (acute)
   According to ICD-10-CM coding guidelines, the possible conditions are not coded
   as this is an outpatient encounter. See Section IV, H, Uncertain Diagnosis.

9. **First-Listed Diagnosis:** **H66.002** Otitis, media, suppurative, acute, recurrent, left

   Secondary Diagnoses: None indicated by the documentation provided

10. **First-Listed Diagnosis:** **H70.001**, Mastoiditis, acute, right ear

    Secondary Diagnoses: **H66.001** Otitis, media, purulent, acute, see suppurative, right

11. **First-Listed Diagnosis:** **H60.21** Otitis externa, malignant, right

    Secondary Diagnoses: **E11.65** Diabetes, type 2, with, hyperglycemia

12. **First-Listed Diagnosis:** **H60.333** Swimmer's ear, bilateral

    Secondary Diagnoses: None indicated by the documentation provided

13. **First-Listed Diagnosis:**   **H81.09** Meniere disease, unspecified

    Secondary Diagnoses: None indicated by the documentation provided

14. **First-Listed Diagnosis:**   **H65.192** Otitis (acute), with effusion, see also Otitis, media, nonsuppurative, acute, left

    Secondary Diagnoses: None indicated by the documentation provided

15. **First-Listed Diagnosis:**   **H81.23** Neuronitis, vestibular, bilateral

    Secondary Diagnoses: None indicated by the documentation provided

Chapter 9

Diseases of the Circulatory System

1. **Principal Diagnosis:**   **I21.19** Infarction, myocardium, ST elevation, inferior

    Secondary Diagnoses: **I25.10** Arteriosclerosis, coronary;
I25.83 Arteriosclerosis, coronary, due to lipid rich plaque (A code first coronary atherosclerosis note is present at I25.83.);
I48.0 Fibrillation, atrial

Principal Procedure:

Character	Code	Explanation
Section	4	Measurement and Monitoring
Body System	A	Physiological Systems
Root Operation	0	Measurement
Body System	2	Cardiac
Approach	3	Percutaneous
Function Device	N	Sampling and Pressure
Qualifier	8	Bilateral (right and left heart)

INDEX: Catheterization, heart, see Measurement, Cardiac

Secondary Procedure(s):

Character	Code	Explanation
Section	B	Imaging
Body System	2	Heart
Root Type	0	Fluoroscopy
Body Part	6	Heart, Right and Left
Contrast	1	Low Osmolar
Qualifier	Z	None
Qualifier	Z	None

INDEX: Angiocardiography, combined right and left heart

Secondary Procedure(s):

Character	Code	Explanation
Section	B	Imaging
Body System	2	Heart
Root Type	1	Fluoroscopy
Body Part	1	Coronary Arteries, Multiple
Contrast	1	Low Osmolar
Qualifier	Z	None
Qualifier	Z	None

INDEX: Arteriography, see Fluoroscopy, heart

2. **Principal Diagnosis:**   **I25.10** Disease, artery, coronary, see Arteriosclerosis, coronary (artery)

   Secondary Diagnoses: **T81.718A** Complication, surgical procedure, vascular, artery, specified NEC

   Principal Procedure:

Character	Code	Explanation
Section	0	Medical and Surgical
Body System	2	Heart and Great Vessels
Root Operation	1	Bypass
Body Part	3	Coronary Artery, Four or More Sites
Approach	0	Open
Device	9	Autologous Venous Tissue
Qualifier	W	Aorta

INDEX: Bypass, artery, coronary, four or more sites

Secondary Procedure(s):

Character	Code	Explanation
Section	0	Medical and Surgical
Body System	6	Lower Veins
Root Operation	B	Excision
Body Part	Q	Greater Saphenous Veins Left
Approach	0	Open
Device	Z	No Device
Qualifier	Z	No Qualifier

INDEX: Excision, vein, greater saphenous

Secondary Procedure(s):

Character	Code	Explanation
Section	5	Extracorporeal Assistance and Performance
Physiological Systems	A	Physiological systems
Root Operation	1	Performance
Body System	2	Cardiac
Duration	2	Continuous
Function	1	Output
Qualifier	Z	No Qualifier

INDEX: Bypass, cardiopulmonary

3. **First-Listed Diagnosis:** **I69.351** Hemiplegia, following, cerebrovascular disease, cerebral infarction

   Secondary Diagnoses: **I69.321** Dysphasia, following, cerebrovascular disease, cerebral infarction;
   I10 Hypertension;
   I48.0 Fibrillation, atrial

4. **Principal Diagnosis:** **I63.411** Infarction, cerebral, due to embolism, cerebral arteries

   Secondary Diagnoses: **R13.10** Dysphagia;
   G81.94 Hemiplegia (Left nondominant side) (Report any neurological deficits caused by a CVA, even if it has resolved at the time of discharge.);
   I10 Hypertension

Principal Procedure:

Character	Code	Explanation
Section	B	Imaging
Body System	0	Central Nervous System
Root Type	2	Computerized Tomography (CT scan)
Body Part	0	Brain
Contrast	1	Low Osmolar
Qualifier	Z	None
Qualifier	Z	None

INDEX: Computerized tomography, brain

Secondary Procedure(s): None indicated by the documentation provided

5. **First-Listed Diagnosis:** **I46.9** Arrest, cardiac
   This case is an outpatient visit in the emergency room. The physician describes the myocardial infarction as "probable." Probable conditions are not coded for outpatient cases. See Coding Guideline IV.H.

Secondary Diagnoses: **I11.9** Hypertension, heart (Cardiomegaly is not coded because it is not stated as a diagnosis by the physician.);
Y93.H1 External cause code—Activity, shoveling, snow;
Y99.8 External cause status, specified;
Y92.014 Place of occurrence, residence, house, single family, driveway (Additional codes are added to indicate the activity of the patient causing the cardiopulmonary arrest).

6. **First-Listed Diagnosis:**   **I13.0** Hypertension, cardiorenal, with heart failure with stage 1 through stage 4 chronic kidney disease

Secondary Diagnoses: **I50.9** Failure, heart, congestive;
N18.2 Disease, kidney, chronic stage 2;
E11.42 Diabetes, type 2, with polyneuropathy

7. **Principal Diagnosis:**   **I25.10** Atherosclerosis, coronary artery
Secondary Diagnoses: **I24.9** Syndrome, coronary
Principal Procedure:

Character	Code	Explanation
Section	0	Medical and Surgical
Body System	2	Heart and Great Vessels
Root Operation	7	Dilation
Body Part	0	Coronary Artery, One Site
Approach	3	Percutaneous
Device	D	Intraluminal Device
Qualifier	Z	No Qualifier

INDEX: PTCA, see dilation, heart and great vessels

Secondary Procedure(s):

Character	Code	Explanation
Section	4	Measurement and Monitoring
Body System	A	Physiological Systems
Root Operation	0	Measurement
Body Part	2	Cardiac
Approach	3	Percutaneous
Device	N	Sampling and Pressure
Qualifier	7	Left Heart

INDEX: Catheterization, heart, see Measurement, Cardiac

Secondary Procedure(s):

Character	Code	Explanation
Section	B	Imaging
Body System	2	Heart
Root Operation	1	Fluoroscopy
Body Part	1	Coronary Arteries Multiple
Approach	1	Low Osmolar
Device	Z	None
Qualifier	Z	None

INDEX: Arteriography, see Fluoroscopy, Heart

Secondary Procedure(s):

Character	Code	Explanation
Section	3	Administration
Physiological System	E	Physiological Systems and Anatomical Regions
Root Operation	0	Introduction
Body System	3	Peripheral vein
Approach	3	Percutaneous
Substance	P	Platelet Inhibitor
Qualifier	Z	No Qualifier c

INDEX: Administration, other substance, see Introduction of substance in or on

8. **Principal Diagnosis:**   **I71.4** Aneurysm, abdominal

   Secondary Diagnoses: **I10** Hypertension;

   M1A.0510 Arthritis, gouty—see Gout, idiopathic, Gout, chronic, idiopathic, hip

Principal Procedure:

Character	Code	Explanation
Section	0	Medical and Surgical
Body System	4	Lower arteries
Root Operation	U	Supplement
Body Part	0	Abdominal aorta
Approach	3	Percutaneous
Device	J	Synthetic substitute
Qualifier	Z	No Qualifier

INDEX: Graft, see Supplement, aorta, abdominal

Secondary Procedure(s):

Character	Code	Explanation
Section	B	Imaging
Body System	4	Lower Arteries
Root Type	4	Ultrasonography
Body Part	0	Abdominal Aorta
Contrast	Z	None
Qualifier	Z	None
Qualifier	3	Intravascular

INDEX: Ultrasonography, Aorta, Abdominal intravascular

9. **Principal Diagnosis:**   **I82.431** Thrombosis, vein, popliteal

   Secondary Diagnoses: **I50.9** Failure, heart, congestive

   Principal Procedure:

Character	Code	Explanation
Section	B	Imaging
Body System	5	Veins
Root Type	4	Ultrasonography
Body Part	B	Lower Extremity Veins, Right
Contrast	Z	None
Qualifier	Z	None
Qualifier	3	Intravascular

INDEX: Ultrasonography, vein, lower extremity, right, intravascular

Secondary Procedure(s): None indicated by the documentation provided

10. **Principal Diagnosis:**   **I50.9** Failure, heart, congestive

    Secondary Diagnoses: **Z86.718** History, personal, thrombosis;
    Z79.01 Long-term drug therapy, anticoagulants

   Principal Procedure:

Character	Code	Explanation
Section	B	Imaging
Body System	5	Veins
Root Type	4	Ultrasonography
Body Part	B	Lower Extremity Veins, Right
Contrast	Z	None
Qualifier	Z	None
Qualifier	3	Intravascular

INDEX: Ultrasonography, vein, lower extremity, right, intravascular

Secondary Procedure(s): None indicated by the documentation provided

11. **Principal Diagnosis:**   **I50.42** Failure, heart, systolic combined with diastolic, chronic

    Secondary Diagnoses: **J96.10** Failure, respiratory, chronic;
    I10 Hypertension;
    Z99.81 Dependence, oxygen;
    S52.502A Fracture, traumatic, radius, lower end;
    W18.11xA External cause, fall, from toilet;
    Y92.013 External cause, place of occurrence, residence, house, single family, bedroom;
    N39.0 Infection, urinary;
    Y99.8 External cause status, specified;
    Z87.440 History, personal, urinary (tract) infection

Principal Procedure:

Character	Code	Explanation
Section	2	Placement
Anatomical Regions	W	Anatomical Regions
Root Operation	3	Immobilization
Body Region	D	Lower Arm Left
Approach	X	External
Device	1	Splint
Qualifier	7	No Qualifier

INDEX: Splinting, musculoskeletal, see Immobilization, anatomical regions

Secondary Procedure(s): None indicated by the documentation provided

12. **Principal Diagnosis:**   **I20.9** Angina

    Secondary Diagnoses: **F14.20** Dependence, drug, cocaine;
    F10.10 Abuse, alcohol;
    F17.210 Dependence, drug, nicotine, cigarettes;
    F31.9 Disorder, bipolar;
    J18.9 Pneumonia

    Principal Procedure: None indicated by the documentation provided
    Secondary Procedure(s): None indicated by the documentation provided

13. **Principal (Nursing Home) Diagnosis:**   **I50.32** Failure, heart, diastolic

    Secondary Diagnoses: None indicated by the documentation provided

14. **Principal Diagnosis:**   **I50.33** Failure, heart, diastolic, chronic (congestive) and acute

    Secondary Diagnoses: **I10** Hypertension;
    E11.40 Diabetes, type 2, with neuropathy

    Principal Procedure: None indicated by the documentation provided
    Secondary Procedure(s): None indicated by the documentation provided

15. **Principal Diagnosis:**   **I21.09** Infarct, myocardium, ST elevation, anterior

    Secondary Diagnoses: **I25.10** Disease, artery, coronary

    Principal Procedure:

Character	Code	Explanation
Section	0	Medical and Surgical
Body System	2	Heart and Great Vessels
Root Operation	7	Dilation
Body Part	1	Coronary Artery, Two Sites
Approach	3	Percutaneous
Device	D	Intraluminal device
Qualifier	Z	No qualifier

INDEX: PTCA, see Dilation, heart and great vessels

Secondary Procedure(s):

Character	Code	Explanation
Section	0	Medical and Surgical
Body System	2	Heart and Great Vessels
Root Operation	7	Dilation
Body Part	1	Coronary Artery, Two Sites
Approach	3	Percutaneous
Device	Z	No Device
Qualifier	Z	No qualifier

INDEX: PTCA, see Dilation, heart and great vessels

16. **Principal Diagnosis:**   **I25.119** Disease, artery, coronary, with angina pectoris—see Arteriosclerosis, coronary. Arteriosclerosis, coronary, native vessel, with, angina pectoris. This combination code, which incorporates the diagnoses coronary artery disease and angina pectoris, eliminates the question of sequencing either diagnosis as the principal diagnosis.

    Secondary Diagnoses: **I10** Hypertension

Principal Procedure:

Character	Code	Explanation
Section	4	Measurement and Monitoring
Body System	A	Physiological Systems
Root Operation	0	Measurement
Body System	2	Cardiac
Approach	3	Percutaneous
Function Device	N	Sampling and Pressure
Qualifier	7	Left Heart

INDEX: Catheterization, heart, see Measurement, Cardiac

Secondary Procedure(s):

Character	Code	Explanation
Section	B	Imaging
Body System	2	Heart
Root Type	1	Fluoroscopy
Body Part	5	Heart, left
Contrast	0	High Osmolar
Qualifier	Z	None
Qualifier	Z	None

INDEX: Ventriculogram, left, see Fluoroscopy, heart left

Secondary Procedure(s):

Character	Code	Explanation
Section	B	Imaging
Body System	2	Heart
Root Type	1	Fluoroscopy
Body Part	1	Coronary arteries multiple
Contrast	0	High Osmolar
Qualifier	Z	None
Qualifier	Z	None

INDEX: Arteriography, see Fluoroscopy, heart

17. **Principal Diagnosis:** **I08.3** Insufficiency, mitral, with, aortic valve disease.
Multiple heart valve disease specified as rheumatic or unspecified are assigned as rheumatic disorders.

Secondary Diagnoses: **I50.32** Failure, heart, diastolic, chronic (congestive);
I12.0 Hypertensive kidney with stage 5 chronic kidney disease or end-stage renal disease;
N18.6 Disease, renal, End stage;
Z99.2 Dependence on renal dialysis;
D63.1 Anemia in chronic kidney disease (note that this is a manifestation code and must be sequenced after the code for the underlying disease.);
E78.5 Hyperlipidemia, unspecified;
Z86.19 History, Personal, hepatitis C

Principal Procedure:

Character	Code	Explanation
Section	0	Medical and Surgical
Body System	2	Heart and Great Vessels
Root Operation	R	Replacement
Body Part	F	Aortic Valve
Approach	0	Open
Device	8	Zooplastic Tissue (porcine)
Qualifier	Z	No qualifier

INDEX: Replacement, valve, aortic

Secondary Procedure(s):

Character	Code	Explanation
Section	0	Medical and Surgical
Body System	2	Heart and Great Vessels
Root Operation	U	Supplement
Body Part	G	Mitral Valve
Approach	0	Open
Device	J	Synthetic Substitute
Qualifier	Z	No qualifier

INDEX: Annuloplasty ring is supplementing the function of the mitral valve. Annuloplasty, see Supplement, Heart and Great Vessels.

Secondary Procedure(s):

Character	Code	Explanation
Section	5	Extracorporeal Assistance and Performance
Physiological Systems	A	Physiological systems
Root Operation	1	Performance
Body System	2	Cardiac
Duration	2	Continuous
Function	1	Output
Qualifier	Z	No Qualifier

INDEX: Bypass, cardiopulmonary

18. **Principal Diagnosis:** I50.23 Failure, heart, systolic, acute and chronic (congestive)

    Secondary Diagnoses: E11.9 Diabetes, type 2;
    I10 Hypertension.
    Do not assign Z79.4 Long term (current) use of insulin because the insulin was given during the hospitalization only.

    Principal Procedure: None indicated by the documentation provided

    Secondary Procedure(s): None indicated by the documentation provided

19. **Principal Diagnosis:** I25.110 Disease, artery, coronary, with angina pectoris—see Arteriosclerosis, coronary. Arteriosclerosis, coronary, native vessel, with angina pectoris, unstable

    Secondary Diagnoses: F17.210 Dependence, nicotine, cigarettes

    Principal Procedure:

Character	Code	Explanation
Section	0	Medical and Surgical
Body System	2	Heart and Great Vessels
Root Operation	1	Bypass
Body Part	2	Coronary Artery, Three Sites
Approach	0	Open
Device	9	Autologous venous tissue
Qualifier	W	Aorta

INDEX: Bypass, artery, coronary, three sites

Secondary Procedure(s):

Character	Code	Explanation
Section	0	Medical and Surgical
Body System	6	Lower Veins
Root Operation	B	Excision
Body Part	Q	Greater Saphenous Veins Left
Approach	0	Open
Device	Z	No Device
Qualifier	Z	No Qualifier

INDEX: Excision, vein, greater saphenous, left

Secondary Procedure(s):

Character	Code	Explanation
Section	5	Extracorporeal Assistance and Performance
Physiological Systems	A	Physiological systems
Root Operation	1	Performance
Body System	2	Cardiac
Duration	2	Continuous
Function	1	Output
Qualifier	Z	No Qualifier

INDEX: Bypass, cardiopulmonary

20. **Principal Diagnosis:**   **I65.23** Occlusion, artery, carotid

    Secondary Diagnoses: **G45.3** Amaurosis fugax

    Principal Procedure:

Character	Code	Explanation
Section	0	Medical and Surgical
Body System	3	Upper Arteries
Root Operation	C	Extirpation
Body Part	K	Internal carotid artery right
Approach	4	Percutaneous endoscopic
Device	Z	No device
Qualifier	Z	No Qualifier

INDEX: Endarterectomy, see Extirpation, upper arteries

Secondary Procedure(s):

Character	Code	Explanation
Section	B	Imaging
Body System	3	Upper arteries
Root Type	0	Plain radiography
Body Part	8	Internal carotid artery bilateral
Contrast	Z	None
Qualifier	Z	None
Qualifier	Z	None

INDEX: Arteriography, see Plain radiology, upper arteries

21. **First-Listed Diagnosis:**   **I69.320** Sequelae, stroke NOS, aphasia

    Secondary Diagnoses: **I69.392** Sequelae, stroke NOS, facial weakness

22. **Principal (Nursing Home) Diagnosis:**   **I69.365** Sequelae, stroke, paralytic syndrome
    Assign sixth character "5" to designate bilateral

    Secondary Diagnoses: **G82.50** Quadriplegia
    Use additional code at I69.36 directs users to assign the quadriplegia if present

    Principal Procedure: None indicated by the documentation provided

    Secondary Procedure(s):   None indicated by the documentation provided

23. **Principal (Nursing Home) Diagnosis:**   **I69.398** Sequelae, stroke, specified effect
    Use additional code to identify sequelae present

    Secondary Diagnoses: **G40.909** Disorder, seizure

    Principal Procedure: None indicated by the documentation provided

    Secondary Procedure(s):   None indicated by the documentation provided

24. **Principal Diagnosis:**   **I69.398** Sequelae, stroke, specified effect
    Use additional code to identify sequelae present

    Secondary Diagnoses: **M62.442** Contracture, tendon, hand;
    I10 Hypertension, (essential);
    J41.0 Bronchitis, chronic, simple

Principal Procedure:

Character	Code	Explanation
Section	0	Medical and Surgical
Body System	L	Tendons
Root Operation	X	Transfer
Body Part	8	Hand Tendon Left

Approach	O	Open
Device	Z	No Device
Qualifier	Z	No Qualifier

INDEX: Transfer, tendon, hand, left

Secondary Procedure(s): None indicated by the documentation provided

Chapter 10

Diseases of the Respiratory System

1. **Principal Diagnosis:** **J44.1** Disease, lung, obstructive

   Secondary Diagnoses: **Z87.891** History, personal, nicotine dependence (smoking)
   The respiratory insufficiency is integral to COPD and not coded.

   Principal Procedure: None indicated by the documentation provided

   Secondary Procedure(s): None indicated by the documentation provided

2. **Principal Diagnosis:** **J69.0** Pneumonia, aspiration

   Secondary Diagnoses: **J15.9** Pneumonia, bacterial

   Principal Procedure: None indicated by the documentation provided

   Secondary Procedure(s): None indicated by the documentation provided

3. **First-Listed Diagnosis:** **J45.909** Asthma
   Note: Allergic rhinitis is not coded separately; see the Tabular List includes note under category J45—asthma.

   Secondary Diagnoses: None indicated by the documentation provided

4. **Principal Diagnosis:** **J35.3** Hypertrophy, tonsils, with adenoids

   Secondary Diagnoses: None indicated by the documentation provided

   Principal Procedure:

Character	Code	Explanation
Section	0	Medical and Surgical
Body System	C	Mouth and Throat
Root Operation	T	Resection
Body Part	P	Tonsils
Approach	0	Open
Device	Z	No Device
Qualifier	Z	No Qualifier

INDEX: Tonsillectomy, see resection, mouth and throat

Secondary Procedure(s):

Character	Code	Explanation
Section	0	Medical and Surgical
Body System	C	Mouth and Throat
Root Operation	T	Resection
Body Part	Q	Adenoids
Approach	0	Open
Device	Z	No Device
Qualifier	Z	No Qualifier

INDEX: Adenoidectomy, see resection, adenoids

5. **Principal Diagnosis:**   **J18.9** Pneumonia

   Secondary Diagnoses: **D61.810** Pancytopenia, antineoplastic, chemotherapy induced (Note: Pancytopenia is a type of aplastic anemia that represents a deficiency of all 3 elements of the blood only the code for pancytopenia should be assigned);
   C90.00 Myeloma;
   F32.9 Depression

   Principal Procedure:

Character	Code	Explanation
Section	3	Administration
Physiological System	0	Circulatory
Root Operation	2	Transfusion
Body System/Region	3	Peripheral vein
Approach	3	Percutaneous
Substance	N	Red Blood Cells
Qualifier	1	Nonautologous

INDEX: Transfusion, vein, peripheral, blood, red cells

Secondary Procedure(s): None indicated by the documentation provided

6. **First-Listed Diagnosis:**   **J45.909** Asthma

   Secondary Diagnoses: **Z79.52** Long-term (current) use of systemic steroids

7. **First-Listed Diagnosis:**   **J02.0** Pharyngitis, streptococcal

   Secondary Diagnoses: **H66.003** Otitis, media, suppurative, acute
   "Possible" early tonsillar abscess is not coded because this is an outpatient record.

8. **Principal Diagnosis:** **J44.0** Disease, lung, obstructive, with acute bronchitis

   Secondary Diagnoses: **I10** Hypertension;
   I25.10 Disease, heart, ischemic, atherosclerotic;
   Z95.1 Presence of, aortocoronary graft;
   I50.9 Failure, heart, congestive;
   I69.354 Hemiplegia, following, cerebrovascular infarction

   Principal Procedure: None indicated by the documentation provided

   Secondary Procedure(s): None indicated by the documentation provided

9. **First-Listed Diagnosis:** **J01.10** Sinusitis, frontal, acute

   Secondary Diagnoses: **J01.00** Sinusitis, maxillary, acute

10. **Principal Diagnosis:** **J93.12** Pneumothorax, spontaneous, secondary

    Secondary Diagnoses: **J90** Effusion, pleura;
    J44.9 Obstructive, lung, chronic;
    Z99.81 Dependence, oxygen

Principal Procedure:

Character	Code	Explanation
Section	0	Medical and Surgical
Body System	W	Anatomical Regions, General
Root Operation	9	Drainage
Body Part	B	Pleural cavity, right
Approach	3	Percutaneous
Device	0	Drainage Device
Qualifier	Z	No Qualifier

INDEX: Drainage, chest wall

Secondary Procedure(s): None indicated by the documentation provided

11. **Principal Diagnosis:** **R09.1** Pleurisy

    Secondary Diagnoses: **M32.14** Lupus, systemic, with organ involvement;
    E86.0 Dehydration;
    R19.7 Diarrhea;
    E87.1 Hyponatremia;
    E87.6 Hypokalemia;
    R79.89 Azotemia

    Principal Procedure: None indicated by the documentation provided

    Secondary Procedure(s): None indicated by the documentation provided

12. **Principal Diagnosis:**   **J44.0** Disease, lung, obstructive, with acute bronchitis

   Secondary Diagnoses: **I27.81** Cor, pulmonale;
                              Z99.81 Dependence, oxygen;
                              Z51.5 Palliative care

   Principal Procedure: None indicated by the documentation provided

   Secondary Procedure(s): None indicated by the documentation provided

13. **Principal Diagnosis:**   **J12.9** Pneumonia, viral

   Secondary Diagnoses: **E86.0** Dehydration

   Principal Procedure: None indicated by the documentation provided

   Secondary Procedure(s): None indicated by the documentation provided

14. **Principal Diagnosis:**   **J15.1** Pneumonia, pseudomonas

   Secondary Diagnoses: **J44.1** Asthma, with chronic obstructive pulmonary disease, exacerbation;
                              R91.8 Mass, lung;
                              E09.9 Diabetes, steroid-induced;
                              I50.9 Failure, heart, congestive;
                              J96.00 Failure, respiratory;
                              F17.218 Dependence, drug, nicotine, with disorder, specified disorder NEC;
                              Z51.5 Palliative care;
                              Z79.52 Long-term drug therapy, steroids, systemic

   Principal Procedure: None indicated by the documentation provided

   Secondary Procedure(s): None indicated by the documentation provided

15. **Principal Diagnosis:**   **C34.12** Neoplasm table, lung, upper lobe

   Secondary Diagnoses: **J91.0** Effusion, pleura, malignant

   Principal Procedure:

Character	Code	Explanation
Section	0	Medical and Surgical
Body System	W	Anatomical Regions, General
Root Operation	9	Drainage
Body Part	B	Pleural cavity left
Approach	3	Percutaneous
Device	Z	No device
Qualifier	Z	No qualifier

INDEX: Thoracentesis, see Drainage, Anatomical Regions, General

Secondary Procedure(s): None indicated by the documentation provided

16. **Principal Diagnosis:**   **J90** Pleural effusion, not elsewhere classified

    Secondary Diagnoses: **J96.21** Acute respiratory failure with hypoxia (This diagnosis is sequenced second as it was not present on admission.);
    C16.0 Malignant neoplasm of cardia (Includes gastroesophageal junction.)

Principal Procedure:

Character	Code	Explanation
Section	0	Medical and Surgical
Body System	W	Anatomical Regions, General
Root Operation	9	Drainage
Body Part	B	Pleural Cavity Left
Approach	3	Percutaneous
Device	0	Drainage Device
Qualifier	Z	No Qualifier

INDEX: Drainage, pleural cavity, left, chest tube left in place

Secondary Procedure(s):

Character	Code	Explanation
Section	5	Extracorporeal Assistance & Performance
Physiological System	A	Physiological Systems
Root Operation	1	Performance
Body Part	9	Respiratory
Duration	4	24-96 Consecutive hours
Function	5	Ventilation
Qualifier	Z	No Qualifier

INDEX: Mechanical ventilation, see Performance, Respiratory

Note: Mechanical ventilation is coded to the extracorporeal assistance and performance section. Insertion of the endotracheal tube as part of a mechanical ventilation procedure is not coded as a separate device insertion procedure, because it is merely the interface between the patient and the equipment used to perform the procedure, rather than an end in itself. On the other hand, insertion of an endotracheal tube in order to maintain an airway in patients who are unconscious or unable to breathe on their own is the central objective of the procedure. Therefore, insertion of an endotracheal tube as an end in itself is coded to the root operation INSERTION and the device ENDOTRACHEAL AIRWAY. Refer to Appendix C in the *ICD-10-PCS Reference Manual*—page C.8–9

17. **Principal Diagnosis:**   **J69.0** Pneumonitis due to inhalation of food and vomit

      Secondary Diagnoses: **J96.00** Failure, respiratory, acute

Note: 2012 draft ICD-10-CM is missing J96.00 in Alpha Index but it is included in Tabular List.

Principal Procedure:

Character	Code	Explanation
Section	5	Extracorporeal Assistance & Performance
Physiological System	A	Physiological Systems
Root Operation	0	Performance
Body Part	9	Respiratory
Duration	4	24-96 consecutive hours
Function	5	Ventilation
Qualifier	8	Intermittent positive airway pressure

INDEX: Intermittent positive airway pressure, 24–96 consecutive hours, ventilation

Secondary Procedure(s): None indicated by the documentation provided

18. **Principal Diagnosis:**   **J96.10** Failure, respiratory, chronic

      Secondary Diagnoses: **T50.901S** Poisoning, Drug NEC, sequelae;

                                F19.20 Dependency, drug/polysubstance;

                                Z99.11 Dependency, on respirator;

                                Z93.0 Tracheostomy status

Principal Procedure:

Character	Code	Explanation
Section	5	Extracorporeal Assistance & Performance
Physiological System	A	Physiological Systems
Root Operation	1	Performance
Body Part	9	Respiratory
Duration	5	Greater than 96 consecutive hours
Function	5	Ventilation
Qualifier	Z	No qualifier

INDEX: Mechanical ventilation, see Performance, respiratory

Secondary Procedure(s): None indicated by the documentation provided

Chapter 11

Diseases of the Digestive System

1. **Principal Diagnosis:**   **K80.10** Calculus, gallbladder, with cholecystitis, chronic

   Secondary Diagnoses: None indicated by the documentation provided

   Principal Procedure:

Character	Code	Explanation
Section	0	Medical and Surgical
Body System	F	Hepatobiliary System and Pancreas
Root Operation	T	Resection
Body Part	4	Gallbladder
Approach	0	Open
Device	Z	No Device
Qualifier	Z	No Qualifier

INDEX: Cholecystectomy, see Resection, gallbladder

Note: ICD-10-PCS guidelines B3.3. If the intended procedure was discontinued, code the procedure to the root operation performed.

Secondary Procedure(s):

Character	Code	Explanation
Section	0	Medical and Surgical
Body System	F	Hepatobiliary System and Pancreas
Root Operation	J	Inspection
Body Part	4	Gallbladder
Approach	4	Percutaneous endoscopic
Device	Z	No Device
Qualifier	Z	No Qualifier

INDEX: Laparoscopy, see Inspection.

Note: ICD-10-PCS guideline B3.2.d. During the same operative episode, multiple procedures are coded if the intended root operation is attempted using one approach but is converted to a different approach. Example, Laparoscopic cholecystectomy converted to open cholecystectomy as percutaneous endoscopic inspection and open resection.

2. **Principal Diagnosis:** **K50.012** Disease, Crohn's—see Enteritis, regional, small intestine, with intestinal obstruction

   Secondary Diagnoses: **L52** Erythema, nodosum

   Principal Procedure:

Character	Code	Explanation
Section	0	Medical and Surgical
Body System	D	Gastrointestinal System
Root Operation	B	Excision
Body Part	B	Ileum
Approach	0	Open
Device	Z	No Device
Qualifier	Z	No Qualifier

INDEX: Excision, ileum.

Note: A partial resection meets the definition of the root operation for excision rather than resection because only part of the ileum was excised during this encounter. Also end-to-end anastomosis part of the procedure.

Secondary Procedure(s): None indicated by the documentation provided

3. **Principal Diagnosis:** **K40.90** Hernia, inguinal

   Secondary Diagnoses: **R07.2** Pain, chest, precordial;
   I10 Hypertension;
   J44.9 Disease, lung, obstructive;
   Z53.09 Canceled procedure, because of contraindication

   Principal Procedure: None indicated by the documentation provided

   Secondary Procedure(s): None indicated by the documentation provided

4. **Principal Diagnosis:** **K29.01** Gastritis, acute, with bleeding

   Secondary Diagnoses: **K25.4** Ulcer, stomach, chronic, with hemorrhage;
   K44.9 Hernia, hiatal;
   B96.81 Infection, Helicobacter pylori, as cause of disease classified elsewhere;
   K31.7 Polyp, stomach;
   D12.0, Polyp, colon, cecum;
   K57.30 Diverticulosis, large intestine;
   I50.9 Failure, heart, congestive;
   I48.0 Fibrillation, atrial

   Principal Procedure:

Character	Code	Explanation
Section	0	Medical and Surgical
Body System	D	Gastrointestinal System

	Code	
Root Operation	B	Excision
Body Part	7	Stomach, Pylorus
Approach	8	Via Natural or Artificial Opening Endoscopic
Device	Z	No Device
Qualifier	X	Diagnostic

INDEX: Biopsy, see Excision by site with qualifier diagnostic, stomach, pylorus

Secondary Procedure(s):

Character	Code	Explanation
Section	0	Medical and Surgical
Body System	D	Gastrointestinal System
Root Operation	5	Destruction
Body Part	6	Stomach
Approach	8	Via Natural or Artificial Opening Endoscopic
Device	Z	No Device
Qualifier	Z	No Qualifier

INDEX: Cauterization, see Destruction, stomach

Secondary Procedure(s):

Character	Code	Explanation
Section	0	Medical and Surgical
Body System	D	Gastrointestinal System
Root Operation	B	Excision
Body Part	H	Cecum
Approach	8	Via Natural or Artificial Opening Endoscopic
Device	Z	No Device
Qualifier	Z	No Qualifier

INDEX: Excision, cecum

5. **Principal Diagnosis:** **K52.9** Gastroenteritis

   Secondary Diagnoses: **E86.0** Dehydration;
   J18.9 Pneumonia;
   K44.9 Hernia, hiatal;
   K21.0 Esophagitis, reflux

   Principal Procedure: None indicated by the documentation provided

   Secondary Procedure(s): None Indicated by the documentation provided

6. **Principal Diagnosis:**   **K28.4** Ulcer, gastrojejunal, with hemorrhage

   Secondary Diagnoses: **K44.9** Hernia, hiatal;

                                         K21.0 Esophagitis, reflux;

                                         Z95.1 Presence of, aortocoronary graft;

                                         I25.2 Infarct, myocardium, healed or old,

                                         Z79.82 Long-term drug therapy aspirin;

                                         Z86.718 History, personal, venous thrombosis or embolism;

                                         Z86.711, History, personal, venous thrombosis or embolism, pulmonary;

                                         Z79.01 Long-term drug therapy, anticoagulants;

                                         I50.9 Failure, heart, congestive;

                                         M19.90 Arthritis;

                                         E78.5 Hyperlipidemia

Principal Procedure:

Character	Code	Explanation
Section	0	Medical and Surgical
Body System	D	Gastrointestinal System
Root Operation	J	Inspection
Body Part	0	Upper Intestinal Tract
Approach	8	Via Natural or Artificial Opening Endoscopic
Device	Z	No Device
Qualifier	Z	No Qualifier

INDEX: EGD (esophagogastroduodenoscopy)

Secondary Procedure(s):

Character	Code	Explanation
Section	3	Administration
Physiological System	0	Circulatory
Root Operation	2	Transfusion
Body System	3	Peripheral vein
Approach	3	Percutaneous
Substance	L	Fresh Plasma
Qualifier	1	Nonautologous

INDEX: Transfusion, Vein, peripheral, plasma, fresh

7. **Principal Diagnosis:**   **I86.4** Varix, gastric

   Secondary Diagnoses: **K92.0** Hematemesis;

                                           F10.20 Alcoholism;

                                           K70.30 Cirrhosis, alcoholic;

                                           K70.10 Hepatitis, alcoholic;

                                           I85.00 Varix, esophageal

Principal Procedure:

Character	Code	Explanation
Section	0	Medical and Surgical
Body System	6	Lower Veins
Root Operation	1	Bypass
Body Part	8	Portal Vein
Approach	3	Percutaneous
Device	D	Intraluminal Device
Qualifier	Y	Lower Vein

INDEX: Shunt creation, see Bypass, vein, portal

Secondary Procedure(s): None indicated by the documentation provided

8. **Principal Diagnosis:** **K80.65** Calculus, gallbladder and bile duct, with cholecystitis, chronic with obstruction

Secondary Diagnoses: **K85.9** Pancreatitis, acute

Principal Procedure:

Character	Code	Explanation
Section	0	Medical and Surgical
Body System	F	Hepatobiliary System and Pancreas
Root Operation	T	Resection
Body Part	4	Gallbladder
Approach	0	Open
Device	Z	No Device
Qualifier	Z	No Qualifier

INDEX: Cholecystectomy, see Resection, gallbladder

Secondary Procedure(s):

Character	Code	Explanation
Section	0	Medical and Surgical
Body System	F	Hepatobiliary System and Pancreas
Root Operation	J	Inspection
Body Part	B	Hepatobiliary
Approach	0	Open
Device	Z	No Device
Qualifier	Z	No Qualifier

INDEX: Exploration, see Inspection, duct, hepatobiliary (common bile duct)

9. **Principal Diagnosis:**   **K85.9** Pancreatitis, acute

    Secondary Diagnoses: **K86.1** Pancreatitis, chronic;

    F10.229 Alcohol, intoxication, with dependence

    Principal Procedure: None indicated by the documentation provided

    Secondary Procedure(s):   None indicated by the documentation provided

10. **Principal Diagnosis:**   **K02.53** Caries, dental, chewing surface, penetrating into pulp

    Secondary Diagnoses: **K04.5** Periodontitis, apical;

    Z79.01 Long-term drug therapy, anticoagulant;

    Z51.81 Monitoring, therapeutic drug level;

    Z95.2 Presence, heart valve implant;

    F71 Disability, Intellectual, moderate

Principal Procedure:

Character	Code	Explanation
Section	0	Medical and Surgical
Body System	C	Mouth and Tract
Root Operation	D	Extraction
Body Part	W	Upper Tooth
Approach	X	External
Device	Z	No Device
Qualifier	1	Multiple

INDEX: Extraction, tooth, upper

Secondary Procedure(s):

Character	Code	Explanation
Section	0	Medical and Surgical
Body System	C	Mouth and Tract
Root Operation	D	Extraction
Body Part	X	Lower Tooth
Approach	X	External
Device	Z	No Device
Qualifier	1	Multiple

INDEX: Extraction, tooth, lower

11. **Principal Diagnosis:**   **K55.0** Gangrene, intestine

    Secondary Diagnoses: **J96.00** Failure, respiratory, acute;
                               A41.51 Sepsis;
                               R65.20 Sepsis, severe, Escherichia coli;
                               I10 Hypertension;
                               E03.9 Hypothyroidism;
                               Z51.5 Palliative care

Principal Procedure:

Character	Code	Explanation
Section	0	Medical and Surgical
Body System	W	Anatomical Regions, General
Root Operation	J	Inspection
Body Part	G	Peritoneal cavity
Approach	0	Open
Device	Z	No device
Qualifier	Z	No qualifier

INDEX: Laparotomy, exploratory, see Inspection, Peritoneal cavity

Secondary Procedure(s):

Character	Code	Explanation
Section	5	Extracorporeal Assistance & Performance
Physiological System	A	Physiological systems
Root Operation	1	Performance
Body System	9	Respiratory
Duration	4	24-96 consecutive hours
Function	5	Ventilation
Qualifier	Z	No qualifier

INDEX: Mechanical ventilation, see Performance, respiratory

Note: Mechanical ventilation is coded to the extracorporeal assistance and performance section. Insertion of the endotracheal tube as part of a mechanical ventilation procedure is not coded as a separate device insertion procedure, because it is merely the interface between the patient and the equipment used to perform the procedure, rather than an end in itself. On the other hand, insertion of an endotracheal tube in order to maintain an airway in patients who are unconscious or unable to breathe on their own is the central objective of the procedure. Therefore, insertion of an endotracheal tube as an end in itself is coded to the root operation INSERTION and the device ENDOTRACHEAL AIRWAY. Refer to Appendix C in the *ICD-10-PCS Reference Manual*—page C.8–9

12. **Principal Diagnosis:** **K63.1** Perforated, bowel

   Secondary Diagnoses: **K65.1** Abscess, peritoneal;
   J95.03 Complication, tracheostomy, malfunction;
   J96.10 Failure, respiratory, chronic,
   Z99.11 Dependence, on, respirator;
   M33.91 Dermatopolymyositis, with respiratory involvement;
   A41.51 Sepsis, Escherichia coli

Principal Procedure:

Character	Code	Explanation
Section	0	Medical and Surgical
Body System	D	Gastrointestinal System
Root Operation	T	Resection
Body Part	L	Transverse colon
Approach	0	Open
Device	Z	No Device
Qualifier	Z	No Qualifier

INDEX: Colectomy, see Resection, Colon, Transverse

Secondary Procedure(s):

Character	Code	Explanation
Section	0	Medical and Surgical
Body System	D	Gastrointestinal System
Root Operation	1	Bypass
Body Part	B	Ileum
Approach	0	Open
Device	Z	No Device
Qualifier	4	Cutaneous

INDEX: Ileostomy, see Bypass, Ileum

Secondary Procedure(s):

Character	Code	Explanation
Section	0	Medical and Surgical
Body System	D	Gastrointestinal System
Root Operation	9	Drainage
Body Part	V	Mesentery
Approach	0	Open

Character	Code	Explanation
Device	Z	No Device
Qualifier	Z	No Qualifier

INDEX: Drainage, mesentery

Secondary Procedure(s):

Character	Code	Explanation
Section	0	Medical and Surgical
Body System	B	Respiratory System
Root Operation	W	Revision
Body Part	1	Trachea
Approach	0	Open
Device	F	Tracheostomy Device
Qualifier	Z	No Qualifier

INDEX: Revision of device in trachea

Secondary Procedure(s):

Character	Code	Explanation
Section	5	Extracorporeal Assistance & Performance
Physiological System	A	Physiological systems
Root Operation	1	Performance
Body System	9	Respiratory
Duration	5	Greater than 96 consecutive hours
Function	5	Ventilation
Qualifier	Z	No Qualifier

INDEX: Mechanical ventilation, see Performance, respiratory

13. **First-Listed Diagnosis:** **K21.9** Reflux, gastroesophageal

   Secondary Diagnoses: **K44.9** Hernia, hiatal;
   K26.7 Ulcer, duodenum, chronic
   Note: May also code R19.5 for tarry or abnormal stool color, as It was an indication for the visit, but no cause was identified and patient instructed to discontinue use of the over-the-counter medications that could have possibly been causing problem.

14. **Principal Diagnosis:** **K26.4** Ulcer, duodenum, chronic, with hemorrhage

   Secondary Diagnoses: **K80.51** Calculus, bile duct, with obstruction

Principal Procedure:

Character	Code	Explanation
Section	0	Medical and Surgical
Body System	F	Hepatobiliary System and Pancreas
Root Operation	C	Extirpation
Body Part	9	Common Bile Duct
Approach	8	Via Natural or Artificial Opening Endoscopic
Device	Z	No Device
Qualifier	Z	No Qualifier

INDEX: Extirpation, Duct, common bile

Secondary Procedure(s):

Character	Code	Explanation
Section	0	Medical and Surgical
Body System	F	Hepatobiliary System and Pancreas
Root Operation	9	Drainage
Body Part	9	Common bile duct
Approach	8	Via Natural or Artificial Opening Endoscopic
Device	Z	No Device
Qualifier	Z	No Qualifier

INDEX: Drainage, common bile duct

Secondary Procedure(s):

Character	Code	Explanation
Section	B	Imaging
Body System	F	Hepatobiliary System and Pancreas
Root Type	1	Fluoroscopy
Body Part	4	Gallbladder, Bile ducts and Pancreatic Ducts
Contrast	1	Low Osmolar
Qualifier	Z	None
Qualifier	Z	None

INDEX: ERCP, see Fluoroscopy, Hepatobiliary System and Pancreas (gallbladder, bile duct)

15. **Principal Diagnosis:** **K70.30** Disease, liver, alcoholic, cirrhosis

Secondary Diagnoses: **I85.11** Varix, esophageal, in cirrhosis of liver, bleeding;
F10.239 Dependence, alcohol, with withdrawal;
D69.6 Thrombocytopenia

Principal Procedure:

Character	Code	Explanation
Section	0	Medical and Surgical
Body System	D	Gastrointestinal System
Root Operation	J	Inspection
Body Part	0	Upper intestinal tract
Approach	8	Via Natural or Artificial Opening Endoscopic
Device	Z	No Device
Qualifier	Z	No Qualifier

INDEX: EGD (esophagogastroduodenoscopy)

Secondary Procedure(s):

Character	Code	Explanation
Section	H	Substance Abuse Treatment
Body System	Z	None
Root Type	2	Detoxification Services
Type Qualifier	Z	None
Qualifier	Z	None
Qualifier	Z	None
Qualifier	Z	None

INDEX: Detoxification Services for substance abuse

16. **Principal Diagnosis:** **K26.0** Ulcer, duodenum, acute, with hemorrhage

 Secondary Diagnoses: **K57.30** Diverticulosis, large intestine

Principal Procedure:

Character	Code	Explanation
Section	0	Medical Surgical
Body System	D	Gastrointestinal System
Root Operation	B	Excision
Body Part	9	Duodenum
Approach	8	Via Natural or Artificial Opening Endoscopic
Device	Z	No Device
Qualifier	X	Diagnostic

INDEX: Biopsy—see Excision with qualifier Diagnostic, Excision, Duodenum

Secondary Procedure(s):

Character	Code	Explanation
Section	0	Medical Surgical
Body System	D	Gastrointestinal
Root Operation	J	Inspection
Body Part	D	Lower Intestinal Tract
Approach	8	Via Natural or Artificial Opening Endoscopic
Device	Z	No Device
Qualifier	Z	No Qualifier

INDEX: Colonoscopy

17. **Principal Diagnosis:**   **K40.91** Hernia, inguinal, unilateral, recurrent

   Secondary Diagnoses: None indicated by the documentation provided

   Principal Procedure:

Character	Code	Explanation
Section	0	Medical and Surgical
Body System	Y	Anatomical Regions, Lower Extremities
Root Operation	Q	Repair
Body Part	5	Inguinal region right
Approach	0	Open
Device	Z	No device
Qualifier	Z	No qualifier

INDEX: Herniorrhaphy, see Repair, anatomical regions, lower extremities.

Note: includes inguinal area

Secondary Procedure(s): None indicated by the documentation provided

18. **Principal Diagnosis:**   **K80.10** Calculus, gallbladder, with cholecystitis, chronic

   Secondary Diagnoses: **D13.4** Adenoma see Neoplasm, benign, bile duct, intrahepatic

   Principal Procedure:

Character	Code	Explanation
Section	0	Medical and Surgical
Body System	F	Hepatobiliary System and Pancreas
Root Operation	T	Resection
Body Part	4	Gallbladder
Approach	4	Percutaneous Endoscopic

Character	Code	Explanation
Device	Z	No Device
Qualifier	Z	No Qualifier

INDEX: Cholecystectomy, see Resection, gallbladder

Secondary Procedure(s):

Character	Code	Explanation
Section	0	Medical and Surgical
Body System	F	Hepatobiliary System and Pancreas
Root Operation	B	Excision
Body Part	1	Liver, Right Lobe
Approach	4	Percutaneous Endoscopic
Device	Z	No Device
Qualifier	X	Diagnostic

INDEX: Biopsy, see Excision with qualifier diagnostic, liver, right lobe

19. **Principal Diagnosis:**   **K56.5** Obstruction, intestine with adhesions

    Secondary Diagnoses: **E03.9** Hypothyroidism;
    I10 Hypertension;
    E78.5 Hyperlipidemia;
    F43.0 Reaction, stress, acute
Note: Code R03.0 Elevated blood-pressure reading, without diagnosis of hypertension, is not assigned. See the instruction note in the Index and Tabular. This code is not assigned for patients who have a diagnosis of hypertension.

Principal Procedure:

Character	Code	Explanation
Section	0	Medical and Surgical
Body System	D	Gastrointestinal System
Root Operation	N	Release
Body Part	8	Small Intestine
Approach	0	Open
Device	Z	No Device
Qualifier	Z	No Qualifier

INDEX: Lysis, see Release, intestine, small

Secondary Procedure(s):

Character	Code	Explanation
Section	3	Administration
Physiological System	E	Physiological System and Anatomical Regions
Root Operation	0	Introduction
Body System/Region	M	Peritoneal Cavity
Approach	0	Open
Substance	5	Adhesion Barrier
Qualifier	Z	No Qualifier

INDEX: Introduction of substance in or on, peritoneal cavity, adhesions barrier

20. **Principal Diagnosis:**   **K70.40** Encephalopathy, hepatic—see Failure, hepatic, alcoholic

    Secondary Diagnoses: **K70.30** Cirrhosis, liver, alcoholic;
                                        F10.229 Dependence, alcohol, with intoxication with delirium;
                                        Y90.5 External Cause Index, Blood alcohol level of 100-119 mg/100 ml.

    Principal Procedure: None indicated by the documentation provided

    Secondary Procedure(s):   None indicated by the documentation provided

21. **Principal Diagnosis:**   **K26.0** Ulcer, duodenum, acute, with hemorrhage

    Secondary Diagnoses: **K44.9** Hernia, hiatal

    Principal Procedure:

Character	Code	Explanation
Section	0	Medical and Surgical
Body System	D	Gastrointestinal System
Root Operation	5	Destruction
Body Part	9	Duodenum
Approach	8	Via Natural or Artificial Opening Endoscopic
Device	Z	No Device
Qualifier	Z	No Qualifier

INDEX: Cauterization, see Destruction, duodenum

Secondary Procedure(s):   None indicated by the documentation provided

Chapter 12

Diseases of the Skin and Subcutaneous Tissue

1. **Principal Diagnosis:**   **L89.313** Ulcer, pressure, buttock

   Secondary Diagnoses: **L97.411** Ulcer, lower limb, right;

                                     I70.203 Arteriosclerosis, lower limb, leg, bilateral

Principal Procedure:

Character	Code	Explanation
Section	0	Medical and Surgical
Body System	K	Muscle
Root Operation	B	Excision
Body Part	N	Hip muscle, right
Approach	0	Open
Device	Z	No Device
Qualifier	Z	No Qualifier

INDEX: Debridement, excisional, see Excision, Muscle

Secondary Procedure(s):

Character	Code	Explanation
Section	0	Medical and Surgical
Body System	H	Skin and Breast
Root Operation	B	Excision
Body Part	M	Skin, right foot
Approach	X	External
Device	Z	No Device
Qualifier	Z	No Qualifier

INDEX: Debridement, excisional, see Excision, Skin

2. **Principal Diagnosis:**　　**L05.01** Cyst, pilonidal, with abscess
   Secondary Diagnoses:　None indicated by documentation provided
   Principal Procedure:

Character	Code	Explanation
Section	0	Medical and Surgical
Body System	H	Skin and Breast
Root Operation	9	Drainage
Body Part	8	Skin buttock
Approach	X	External
Device	Z	No Device
Qualifier	Z	No Qualifier

INDEX: Drainage, skin, buttock

Secondary Procedure(s):　None indicated by the documentation provided

3. **First-Listed Diagnosis:**　　**L23.2** Dermatitis, contact, allergic, due to cosmetics
   Secondary Diagnoses:　　**T49.8x5A** Drugs table, cosmetics, poisoning, adverse effect;
   L70.0 Acne, cystic

4. **First-Listed Diagnosis:**　　**S81.832A** Puncture, leg, left
   Secondary Diagnoses:　　**L03.116** Cellulitis, lower limb

5. **Dermatology Diagnosis:**　**L56.5** DSAP

   Secondary Dermatology Diagnoses:　**X32.xxxA** External cause table, exposure, sunlight
   　　Note: See additional code note under category L56 for inclusion of this code.

   Dermatology Procedure:

Character	Code	Explanation
Section	0	Medical and Surgical
Body System	H	Skin and Breast
Root Operation	B	Excision
Body Part	D	Skin, right lower arm
Approach	X	External
Device	Z	No Device
Qualifier	X	Diagnostic

INDEX: Biopsy, see Excision with qualifier diagnostic

Secondary Dermatology Procedure:　None indicated by the documentation provided

6. **First-Listed Diagnosis:** **L74.510** Hyperhidrosis, focal, axilla

   Secondary Diagnoses: **L74.513** Hyperhidrosis, focal, soles;

   L74.512 Hyperhidrosis, focal, palms

7. **First-Listed Diagnosis:** **L23.81** Dermatitis, contact, allergic, dander

   Secondary Diagnoses: None indicated by the documentation provided

8. **First-Listed Diagnosis:** **K51.50** Colitis, left sided

   Secondary Diagnoses: **L52** Erythema, nodosum

9. **First-Listed Diagnosis:** **E10.621** Diabetes, type I, with foot ulcer

   Secondary Diagnoses: **L97.411** Ulcer, lower limb, heel, right, with skin breakdown only

10. **First-Listed Diagnosis:** **L42** Pityriasis, rosea

    Secondary Diagnoses: None indicated by documentation provided

11. **Dermatology Diagnosis:** **C44.41** Neoplasm, scalp, basal cell carcinoma

    Secondary Dermatology Diagnoses: **L57.0** Keratosis, actinic

    Dermatology Procedure:

Character	Code	Explanation
Section	0	Medical and Surgical
Body System	H	Skin and Breast
Root Operation	B	Excision
Body Part	0	Skin, scalp
Approach	X	External
Device	Z	No Device
Qualifier	X	Diagnostic

INDEX: Punch biopsy, see Excision with qualifier Diagnostic

Dermatology Procedure:

Character	Code	Explanation
Section	0	Medical and Surgical
Body System	H	Skin and Breast
Root Operation	B	Excision
Body Part	0	Skin, scalp
Approach	X	External
Device	Z	No Device
Qualifier	Z	No Qualifier

INDEX: Excision, Skin, Scalp

12. **Principal Diagnosis:**   **L02.212** Abscess, back

    Secondary Diagnoses: **B95.62** Infection, bacterial, staphylococcus, methicillin resistant (MRSA);
    Z16.29 Resistance, organism to drug, antibiotic, specified;
    E11.65 Diabetes, with hyperglycemia;
    I10 Hypertension

    Principal Procedure:

Character	Code	Explanation
Section	0	Medical and Surgical
Body System	H	Skin and Breast
Root Operation	9	Drainage
Body Part	6	Skin, back
Approach	X	External
Device	0	Drainage device
Qualifier	Z	No Qualifier

INDEX: Incision, abscess, see Drainage

    Secondary Procedure(s):   None indicated by the documentation provided

13. **Principal Diagnosis:**   **L03.311** Cellulitis, abdominal wall

    Secondary Diagnoses: **R78.81** Bacteremia;
    A49.8 Infection, pseudomonas;
    I87.2 Dermatitis, stasis;
    L03.115 Cellulitis, lower limb;
    L03.116 Cellulitis, lower limb;
    K70.30 Cirrhosis, alcoholic;
    E88.09 Hypoalbuminemia;
    E66.01 Obesity, morbid

    Principal Procedure: None indicated by the documentation provided
    Secondary Procedure(s):   None indicated by the documentation provided

14. **Principal Diagnosis:**   **L51.3** Stevens-Johnson syndrome

    Secondary Diagnoses: **T36.0x5A** Table of drugs, penicillin, adverse effect;
    L49.2 Exfoliation, 20–29 percent of body surface;
    H02.841; H02.8422; H02.844; H02.845 Edema, eyelid

    Principal Procedure: None indicated by the documentation provided
    Secondary Procedure(s):   None indicated by the documentation provided

15. **Principal Diagnosis:**   **L89.154** Ulcer, pressure, sacral region

    Secondary Diagnoses: **I50.32** Failure, heart, diastolic, chronic;
    I25.10 Arteriosclerosis, coronary;
    I25.82 Occlusion, coronary, chronic total

Principal Procedure:

Character	Code	Explanation
Section	0	Medical and Surgical
Body System	Q	Lower Bones
Root Operation	B	Excision
Body Part	S	Coccyx
Approach	0	Open
Device	Z	No Device
Qualifier	Z	No Qualifier

INDEX: Debridement, excisional was done down to the bone, body system is lower bones—See Excision, coccyx

Secondary Procedure(s): None indicated by the documentation provided

16. **First-Listed Diagnosis:** **L90.5**, Scar see cicatrix, skin

    Secondary Diagnoses: **T24.301S** Burn, leg see lower limb, right, third degree, sequela; **X02.0xxS** Exposure, fire, controlled, building

Chapter 13

Diseases of the Musculoskeletal System and Connective Tissue

1. **Principal Diagnosis:** **M51.26** Displacement, intervertebral disc, lumbar

   Secondary Diagnoses: **M47.20** Osteoarthritis, spine—See Spondylosis, Spondylosis, with radiculopathy

Principal Procedure:

Character	Code	Explanation
Section	0	Medical and Surgical
Body System	S	Lower Joints
Root Operation	B	Excision
Body Part	2	Lumbar vertebral disc
Approach	0	Open
Device	Z	No Device
Qualifier	Z	No Qualifier

INDEX: Excision, disc, lumbar vertebral

Note: the laminotomy is the approach for this procedure and not coded separately.

Secondary Procedure(s): None indicated by the documentation provided

2. **Principal Diagnosis:** **M80.08xA** Osteoporosis, age-related, with current pathological fracture, vertebra

   Secondary Diagnoses: None indicated by documentation provided

   Principal Procedure:

Character	Code	Explanation
Section	3	Administration
Physiological Systems	E	Physiological Systems and Anatomical Regions
Root Operation	0	Introduction
Body System	R	Spinal Canal
Approach	3	Percutaneous
Substance	3	Anti-inflammatory
Qualifier	Z	No Qualifier

INDEX: Injection, see Introduction of substance in or on, Spinal canal, anti-inflammatory

Note: The substance value anti-inflammatory is used because the anesthetic is only added to lessen the pain of the injection.

   Secondary Procedure(s): None indicated by the documentation provided

3. **First Listed Diagnosis:** **M15.9** Arthritis, degenerative—See Osteoarthritis, Osteoarthritis, generalized

   Secondary Diagnoses: **M47.817** Spondylosis, without myelopathy, lumbosacral spine;
   I10 Hypertension;
   I25.719 Disease, artery, coronary, with angina pectoris—See Arteriosclerosis, coronary, artery, bypass graft, autologous vein, with angina pectoris
   Note: There is an Excludes2 note under section M15–M19 for osteoarthritis of spine M47 so an additional code can be used to describe the osteoarthritis of spine for this patient.

   Principal Procedure: None indicated by the documentation provided

   Secondary Procedure(s): None indicated by the documentation provided

4. **Principal Diagnosis:** **M32.14** Lupus, systemic, with organ or system involvement, renal

   Secondary Diagnoses: **M32.19** Lupus, systemic, with organ or system involvement, specified organ or system NEC;
   G72.49 Myopathy, inflammatory;
   D63.8 Anemia, due to, chronic disease, classified elsewhere;
   M20.039 Deformity, finger, swan-neck

Principal Procedure:

Character	Code	Explanation
Section	3	Administration
Physiological System	E	Physiological Systems and Anatomical Regions
Root Operation	0	Introduction
Body System	4	Central vein
Approach	3	Percutaneous
Substance	0	Antineoplastic
Qualifier	5	Other Antineoplastic

INDEX: Infusion, see Introduction of substance in or on, vein, central

Secondary Procedure(s): None indicated by the documentation provided

5. **First Listed Diagnosis:** **M84.361A** Fracture, traumatic, stress, tibia, right

   Secondary Diagnoses: **M84.362A** Fracture, traumatic, stress, tibia, left;
   M84.374A Fracture, traumatic, stress, metatarsus, right foot;
   S39.012A, Strain, low back;
   Y93.01 Index to external cause, Activity, walking and running;
   Y99.8 Index to external cause, recreation or sport not for income or while a student

6. **Principal Diagnosis:** **M86.161** Osteomyelitis, acute, fibula

   Secondary Diagnoses: **B95.8** Infection, bacterial, as cause of disease classified elsewhere, staphylococcus

Principal Procedure:

Character	Code	Explanation
Section	0	Medical and Surgical
Body System	Q	Lower bones
Root Operation	B	Excision
Body Part	J	Fibula right
Approach	0	Open
Device	Z	No device
Qualifier	Z	No qualifier

INDEX: Debridement, excisional, see Excision, fibula, right

Secondary Procedure(s): None indicated by the documentation provided

7. **Principal Diagnosis:** **T84.032A** Complication, joint, mechanical, loosening, knee

   Secondary Diagnoses: **M10.061** Gout, idiopathic, knee, right;
   M10.062 Gout, idiopathic, knee, left

Principal Procedure:

Character	Code	Explanation
Section	0	Medical and Surgical
Body System	S	Lower joints
Root Operation	R	Replacement
Body Part	C	Knee joint, right
Approach	0	Open
Device	J	Synthetic substitute
Qualifier	9	Cemented

INDEX: Replacement, joint, knee, right

Secondary Procedure(s):

Character	Code	Explanation
Section	0	Medical and Surgical
Body System	S	Lower joints
Root Operation	P	Removal
Body Part	C	Knee joint, right
Approach	0	Open
Device	J	Synthetic substitute
Qualifier	Z	No qualifier

INDEX: Removal of device from, joint, knee, right

8. **First-Listed Diagnosis:** All of the symptoms in this case could be coded as secondary since a rule out diagnosis cannot be coded in the physician office. There is no guideline on the sequencing of codes. Because there are so many sites that could be coded in this case, the coder should ask the physician to identify the significant pain sites and then coding could be limited to fewer sites.

   Secondary Diagnoses: **M79.641; M79.642; M79.644; M79.645; M25.531; M25.532; M25.561; M25.562; M79.671; M79.672** Pain, joint or limb as specified—hand, fingers, wrists, knees and feet;
   M25.642; M25.642; M25.631; M25.632; M25.661; M25.662; M25.674; M25.675 Stiffness of sites;
   M25.431; M25.432; M25.441; M25.442; M25.461; M25.462; M25.474; M25.475 Swelling, joint—see Effusion, joint (specified site);

R53.83 Fatigue;
R63.0 Anorexia;
R63.4 Weight loss;
Z82.61 History, family, arthritis

9. **First Listed Diagnosis:**   **M24.411** Dislocation, recurrent, shoulder

    Secondary Diagnoses: **M12.511** Arthritis, traumatic—see Arthropathy, traumatic, shoulder

10. **Principal Diagnosis:**   **M75.121** Tear, rotator cuff, complete

    Secondary Diagnoses: **M65.811** Tenosynovitis, shoulder region;
    I10 Hypertension

Principal Procedure:

Character	Code	Explanation
Section	0	Medical and Surgical
Body System	R	Upper joints
Root Operation	B	Excision
Body Part	J	Shoulder Joint Right
Approach	4	Percutaneous Endoscopic
Device	Z	No Device
Qualifier	Z	No Qualifier

INDEX: Synovectomy upper joint, see Excision, upper joint

Secondary Procedure(s):

Character	Code	Explanation
Section	0	Medical and Surgical
Body System	L	Tendons
Root Operation	M	Reattachment
Body Part	1	Shoulder tendon, right
Approach	4	Percutaneous endoscopic
Device	Z	No device
Qualifier	Z	No qualifier

INDEX: Reattachment, tendon, shoulder, right

11. **Principal Diagnosis:**   **M23.221** Tear, meniscus old—see Derangement, knee, meniscus, due to old tear, medial posterior horn

    Secondary Diagnoses: **I11.9** Hypertension, heart (disease)

    Principal Procedure:

Character	Code	Explanation
Section	0	Medical and Surgical
Body System	S	Lower joints
Root Operation	B	Excision
Body Part	C	Knee joint, right
Approach	4	Percutaneous endoscopic
Device	Z	No device
Qualifier	Z	No qualifier

INDEX: Meniscectomy, see excision, lower joints

Secondary Procedure(s):   None indicated by the documentation provided

12. **First-Listed Diagnosis:**   **M20.12** Hallux, valgus, left foot

    Secondary Diagnoses: **M20.11** Hallux valgus, right foot;
    J44.9 Bronchitis, asthmatic, chronic;
    Q21.0 Defect, ventricular septal

13. **Principal Diagnosis:**   **M54.5** Pain, low back

    Secondary Diagnoses: **C50.911** Neoplasm breast, malignant, primary;
    D75.81 Myelofibrosis, secondary;
    D46.9 Myelodysplastic syndrome;
    T45.1x5S, Table of drugs, antineoplastic, adverse effect. This instance would use the 7th character of "S" since this patient had developed the myelodysplastic syndrome previously and not during this current episode of care.

    Principal Procedure: None indicated by the documentation provided

    Secondary Procedure(s):   None indicated by the documentation provided

14 **Principal Diagnosis:**   **S83.511A** Tear, ligament, see Sprain, knee, cruciate ligament, anterior

    Secondary Diagnoses: **S83.411A** Tear, ligament see Sprain, knee, collateral ligament, medial;
    M23.221 Tear meniscus, see Derangement, knee, meniscus, due to old tear or injury, medial, posterior horn

    Principal Procedure:

Character	Code	Explanation
Section	0	Medical and Surgical
Body System	M	Bursae and Ligaments
Root Operation	Q	Repair

Body Part	N	Knee Bursa and Ligament , Right
Approach	4	Percutaneous Endoscopic
Device	Z	No Device
Qualifier	Z	No Qualifier

INDEX: Repair, bursa and ligament, knee right (ACL repair)

Secondary Procedure(s):

Character	Code	Explanation
Section	0	Medical and Surgical
Body System	M	Bursae and Ligaments
Root Operation	Q	Repair
Body Part	N	Knee Bursa and Ligament Right
Approach	4	Percutaneous Endoscopic
Device	Z	No Device
Qualifier	Z	No Qualifier

INDEX: Repair, bursa and ligament knee right (MCL repair)

Note: This procedure is coded twice due to the multiple procedure guideline B3.2—Duplicate procedure codes are assigned because the same root operation is repeated at the different body sites that are included in the same body part value.

Secondary Procedure(s):

Character	Code	Explanation
Section	0	Medical and Surgical
Body System	M	Bursae and Ligaments
Root Operation	U	Supplement
Body Part	N	Knee Bursa and Ligament Right
Approach	4	Percutaneous endoscopic
Device	K	Nonautologous tissue substitute
Qualifier	Z	No Qualifier

INDEX: Graft, see Supplement, bursa and ligament, knee

Note: A supplement procedure is coded to account for the patellar tendon graft for the ACL repair.

Secondary Procedure(s):

Character	Code	Explanation
Section	0	Medical and Surgical
Body System	S	Lower joints
Root Operation	B	Excision
Body Part	C	Knee joint, right
Approach	4	Percutaneous Endoscopic
Device	Z	No Device
Qualifier	Z	No Qualifier

INDEX: Menisectomy, see Excision, lower joints

15. **Principal Diagnosis:**   **M22.42** Chondromalacia patella

      Secondary Diagnoses: **M70.42** Bursitis, prepatellar;
                                       K26.9 Ulcer, duodenum;
                                       K21.9 GERD (gastroesophageal reflux disease);
                                       N40.1 Enlarged prostate with lower urinary tract symptoms [LUTS];
                                       R33.8 Retention, urine, specified NEC

Principal Procedure:

Character	Code	Explanation
Section	0	Medical and Surgical
Body System	S	Lower Joints
Root Operation	B	Excision
Body Part	D	Knee Joint Left
Approach	4	Percutaneous Endoscopic
Device	Z	No Device
Qualifier	Z	No Qualifier

INDEX: Debridement, excisional, see Excision, joint, knee, left

Secondary Procedure(s): None indicated by the documentation provided

16. **Principal Diagnosis:**   **M51.17** Disorder, disc, (intervertebral) with radiculopathy, lumbosacral region

      Secondary Diagnoses: **G56.01** Syndrome, carpal tunnel

Principal Procedure:

Character	Code	Explanation
Section	0	Medical and Surgical
Body System	S	Lower Joints
Root Operation	T	Resection
Body Part	4	Lumbosacral Disc
Approach	0	Open
Device	Z	No Device
Qualifier	Z	No Qualifier

INDEX: Discectomy, see Resection, lower joints

Secondary Procedure(s): None indicated by the documentation provided

17. **Principal Diagnosis:** **M16.4** Osteoarthritis post-traumatic hip bilateral

Secondary Diagnoses: None indicated by the documentation provided

Principal Procedure:

Character	Code	Explanation
Section	0	Medical and Surgical
Body System	S	Lower Joints
Root Operation	R	Replacement
Body Part	B	Hip joint left
Approach	0	Open
Device	3	Synthetic substitute, ceramic
Qualifier	9	Cemented

INDEX: Replacement, joint, hip, left

Secondary Procedure(s): None indicated by the documentation provided

18. **Principal Diagnosis:** **M81.0** Osteoporosis, senile see Osteoporosis age-related

Secondary Diagnoses: **S52.532D** Fracture, Colles' see Colles' fracture (Subsequent encounter for closed fracture with routine healing);
W09.2xxD External cause, Fall from playground equipment, jungle gym;
Y92.211 External cause, place of occurrence, school, elementary;
Y93.39 External cause, Activity, climbing NEC.
Note: These external cause codes are assigned as secondary diagnoses because the fracture was treated and still in the process of healing. Assign "D" as the 7th character extension to indicate that this is a subsequent encounter for closed fracture with routine healing.

Principal Procedure:

Character	Code	Explanation
Section	0	Medical and Surgical
Body System	P	Upper bones
Root Operation	P	Removal
Body Part	J	Radius Left
Approach	X	External
Device	5	External Fixation Device
Qualifier	Z	No Qualifier

INDEX: Removal of device from radius, left (external fixator)

Secondary Procedure(s):

Character	Code	Explanation
Section	0	Medical and Surgical
Body System	P	Upper Bones
Root Operation	S	Reposition
Body Part	J	Radius Left
Approach	0	Open
Device	Z	No Device
Qualifier	Z	No Qualifier

INDEX: Reduction fracture see Reposition radius, left (open, no fixation)

Secondary Procedure(s):

Character	Code	Explanation
Section	0	Medical and Surgical
Body System	P	Upper bones
Root Operation	U	Supplement
Body Part	J	Radius left
Approach	0	Open
Device	K	Nonautologous tissue substitute
Qualifier	Z	No qualifier

INDEX: Graft, see Supplement, radius (Bone graft) left

19. **First-Listed Diagnosis:**   **M53.1** Syndrome, cervicobrachial

     Secondary Diagnoses: **S13.4xxS** Whiplash injury sequela;
     V43.52xS Accident, transport, car occupant, driver, collision with car

20. **First-Listed Diagnosis:**   **M62.561** Atrophy, muscle, lower leg, right

     Secondary Diagnoses: **M62.562** Atrophy, muscle, lower leg, left;
     G14, Syndrome, postpolio (Note: Code G14, a more specific neurological condition, has an Excludes1 note for code B91 for sequela of polio.)

21. **Principal Diagnosis:**   **M12.552** Arthritis, traumatic, see arthropathy traumatic hip

     Secondary Diagnoses: **S72.002S** Fracture, traumatic, femur, neck, see upper end neck;
     V43.63xS External cause, Accident, transport, car occupant, passenger, collision, pick up truck (with selection of "S" as the 7th character for sequela)

Principal Procedure:

Character	Code	Explanation
Section	0	Medical and Surgical
Body System	S	Lower joints
Root Operation	R	Replacement
Body Part	B	Hip joint left
Approach	0	Open
Device	3	Synthetic substitute ceramic
Qualifier	A	Uncemented

INDEX: Replacement, joint, hip, left

Secondary Procedure(s): None indicated by the documentation provided

Chapter 14

Diseases of the Genitourinary System

1. **Principal Diagnosis:**   **N39.0** Infection, urinary (tract)

     Secondary Diagnoses: **B96.4** Infection, bacteria, as cause of disease classified elsewhere, proteus;
     I10 Hypertension;
     I25.10 Arteriosclerosis, coronary (artery);
     Z98.61 Status (post), angioplasty, coronary artery;
     J44.9 Disease, lung, obstructive;
     Z87.440 History, personal, urinary infection(s)

     Principal Procedure: None indicated by the documentation provided

     Secondary Procedure(s):   None indicated by the documentation provided

2. **Principal Diagnosis:** **N40.1** Hyperplasia, prostate, with lower urinary tract symptoms

   Secondary Diagnoses: **R33.8** Retention, urinary, C61 Neoplasm table, prostate

   Principal Procedure:

Character	Code	Explanation
Section	0	Medical and Surgical
Body System	V	Male Reproductive System
Root Operation	B	Excision
Body Part	0	Prostate
Approach	7	Via Natural or Artificial Opening
Device	Z	No Device
Qualifier	Z	No Qualifier

INDEX: TURP (transurethral resection of prostate)

Secondary Procedure(s): None indicated by the documentation provided

3. **Principal Diagnosis:** **N81.12** Cystocele, female, paravaginal

   Secondary Diagnoses: **N39.3** Incontinence, stress;
   E11.9 Diabetes, type 2

   Principal Procedure:

Character	Code	Explanation
Section	0	Medical and Surgical
Body System	U	Female Reproductive System
Root Operation	Q	Repair
Body Part	G	Vagina
Approach	0	Open
Device	Z	No Device
Qualifier	Z	No Qualifier

INDEX: Colporrhaphy, see Repair, vagina

Secondary Procedure(s): None indicated by the documentation provided

4. **Principal Diagnosis:** **N17.9** Failure, renal, acute

   Secondary Diagnoses: **N40.1** Hyperplasia, prostate, with lower urinary tract symptoms;
   N13.8 Obstruction, urinary
   Note: It is important to follow all instructional notes with both codes for proper sequencing.

Principal Procedure:

Character	Code	Explanation
Section	0	Medical and Surgical
Body System	T	Urinary System
Root Operation	9	Drainage
Body Part	B	Bladder
Approach	7	Via Natural or Artificial Opening
Device	0	Drainage Device
Qualifier	Z	No Qualifier

INDEX: Catheterization, see Drainage, bladder

Secondary Procedure(s):

Character	Code	Explanation
Section	B	Imaging
Body System	T	Urinary System
Root Type	1	Fluoroscopy
Body Part	4	Kidneys, Ureters, Bladder
Contrast	1	Low Osmolar
Qualifier	Z	None
Qualifier	Z	None

INDEX: Pyelography, see Fluoroscopy, urinary system

5. **Principal Diagnosis:**   **N10** Pyelonephritis, acute

   Secondary Diagnoses: **N17.9** Failure, renal, acute;
   I10 Hypertension;
   Z87.442 History, personal, calculi, renal

Principal Procedure:

Character	Code	Explanation
Section	0	Medical and Surgical
Body System	T	Urinary System
Root Operation	9	Drainage
Body Part	B	Bladder
Approach	7	Via Natural or Artificial Opening
Device	0	Drainage Device
Qualifier	Z	No Qualifier

INDEX: Catheterization, see Drainage, bladder

Secondary Procedure(s): None indicated by the documentation provided

6. **Principal Diagnosis:** **N18.3** Disease, kidney, chronic, stage 3

   Secondary Diagnoses: **I15.1** Hypertension, secondary, due to renal disorders NEC;
   Q61.3 Polycystic kidney

   Principal Procedure: None indicated by the documentation provided

   Secondary Procedure(s): None indicated by the documentation provided

7. **Principal Diagnosis:** **N80.0** Endometriosis, uterus

   Secondary Diagnoses: **N80.1** Endometriosis, ovary;
   N80.2 Endometriosis, fallopian tube;
   N80.3 Endometriosis, peritoneal;
   D06.9 Neoplasm, cervix, carcinoma in situ

Principal Procedure:

Character	Code	Explanation
Section	0	Medical and Surgical
Body System	U	Female Reproductive System
Root Operation	T	Resection
Body Part	9	Uterus
Approach	7	Via Natural or Artificial Opening
Device	Z	No Device
Qualifier	Z	No Qualifier

INDEX: Hysterectomy, see Resection, Uterus

Secondary Procedure(s):

Character	Code	Explanation
Section	0	Medical and Surgical
Body System	U	Female Reproductive System
Root Operation	T	Resection
Body Part	7	Fallopian Tubes, Bilateral
Approach	7	Via Natural or Artificial Opening
Device	Z	No Device
Qualifier	Z	No Qualifier

INDEX: Salpingectomy, see Resection, Female Reproductive System

Secondary Procedure(s):

Character	Code	Explanation
Section	0	Medical and Surgical
Body System	U	Female Reproductive System
Root Operation	T	Resection

Body Part	2	Ovaries, Bilateral
Approach	7	Via Natural or Artificial Opening
Device	Z	No Device
Qualifier	Z	No Qualifier

INDEX: Oophorectomy, see Resection, Female Reproductive System

8. **First-Listed Diagnosis:** **N30.00** Cystitis, acute

   Secondary Diagnoses: **B96.20** Infection, bacterial, as cause of disease classified elsewhere E. coli; **Z87.440** History, personal, urinary (tract) infection

9. **First-Listed Diagnosis:** **N20.0** Calculus, kidney
   Note: Renal colic is not coded as it is a symptom of the calculus.

   Secondary Diagnoses: None indicated by the documentation provided

10. **Principal Diagnosis:** **N20.1** Calculus, ureter

    Secondary Diagnoses: None indicated by the documentation provided

    Principal Procedure:

Character	Code	Explanation
Section	0	Medical and Surgical
Body System	T	Urinary System
Root Operation	F	Fragmentation
Body Part	6	Ureter Right
Approach	X	External
Device	Z	No Device
Qualifier	Z	No Qualifier

INDEX: Lithotripsy, see Fragmentation, ureter right and ureter left

Secondary Procedure(s):

Character	Code	Explanation
Section	0	Medical and Surgical
Body System	T	Urinary System
Root Operation	F	Fragmentation
Body Part	7	Ureter Left
Approach	X	External
Device	Z	No Device
Qualifier	Z	No Qualifier

INDEX: Lithotripsy, see Fragmentation, ureter right and ureter left

11. **Principal Diagnosis:**   **N39.0** Infection, urinary (tract)

    Secondary Diagnoses: **E86.0** Dehydration;
    C67.5 Neoplasm, bladder, neck, malignant, primary;
    I25.10 Disease, artery, coronary, see Arteriosclerosis, coronary;
    Z95.1 Status, aortocoronary bypass;
    Z93.6 Status, nephrostomy;
    E11.9 Diabetes, type 2;
    E78.0 Hypercholesterolemia

    Principal Procedure: None indicated by the documentation provided

    Secondary Procedure(s):   None indicated by the documentation provided

12. **Principal Diagnosis:**   **N92.1** Menometrorrhagia

    Secondary Diagnoses: **N94.6** Dysmenorrhea;
    D25.9 Fibroid, uterus;
    D62 Anemia, blood loss, acute;
    D68.9 Defect, coagulation;
    T39.315A Table of Drugs, ibuprofen, adverse effect;
    K66.0 Adhesions, peritoneum;
    N99.71 Complication, intraoperative, puncture or laceration, genitourinary organ or structure;
    R50.82 Fever, postoperative;
    J98.11 Atelectasis;
    J95.89 Complication, respiratory system, postoperative;
    N13.30 Hydronephrosis;
    R09.02 Hypoxemia,
    F17.210 Dependence, drug, nicotine cigarettes

    Principal Procedure:

Character	Code	Explanation
Section	0	Medical and Surgical
Body System	U	Female Reproductive System
Root Operation	T	Resection
Body Part	9	Uterus
Approach	0	Open
Device	Z	No Device
Qualifier	Z	No Qualifier

INDEX: Hysterectomy, see Resection Uterus

Secondary Procedure(s):

Character	Code	Explanation
Section	0	Medical and Surgical
Body System	U	Female Reproductive System
Root Operation	T	Resection
Body Part	C	Cervix
Approach	0	Open
Device	Z	No Device
Qualifier	Z	No Qualifier

INDEX: Resection, cervix

Secondary Procedure(s):

Character	Code	Explanation
Section	0	Medical and Surgical
Body System	U	Female Reproductive System
Root Operation	T	Resection
Body Part	7	Fallopian Tubes, Bilateral
Approach	0	Open
Device	Z	No Device
Qualifier	Z	No Qualifier

INDEX: Salpingectomy, see Resection, Female Reproductive System

Secondary Procedure(s):

Character	Code	Explanation
Section	0	Medical and Surgical
Body System	U	Female Reproductive System
Root Operation	T	Resection
Body Part	2	Ovaries, Bilateral
Approach	0	Open
Device	Z	No Device
Qualifier	Z	No Qualifier

INDEX: Oophorectomy, see Resection, Female Reproductive System

Secondary Procedure(s):

Character	Code	Explanation
Section	0	Medical and Surgical
Body System	D	Gastrointestinal System
Root Operation	N	Release
Body Part	W	Peritoneum
Approach	0	Open
Device	Z	No Device
Qualifier	Z	No Qualifier

INDEX: Lysis, see Release, peritoneum

Secondary Procedure(s):

Character	Code	Explanation
Section	0	Medical and Surgical
Body System	D	Gastrointestinal System
Root Operation	Q	Repair
Body Part	8	Small Intestine
Approach	0	Open
Device	Z	No Device
Qualifier	Z	No Qualifier

INDEX: Suture, laceration, see Repair, small bowel

Secondary Procedure(s):

Character	Code	Explanation
Section	0	Medical and Surgical
Body System	T	Urinary system
Root Operation	9	Drainage
Body Part	6	Ureter, Right
Approach	8	Via Natural or Artificial Opening Endoscopic
Device	0	Drainage Device
Qualifier	Z	No Qualifier

INDEX: Drainage, ureter, right

Secondary Procedure(s):

Character	Code	Explanation
Section	B	Imaging
Body System	T	Urinary System
Root Type	1	Fluoroscopy
Body Part	4	Kidneys, Ureter, Bladder (pyelogram)
Contrast	1	Low Osmolar
Qualifier	Z	None
Qualifier	Z	None

INDEX: Pyelogram, see Fluoroscopy, urinary system: retrograde pyelogram examines kidney, ureter, bladder

13. **Principal Diagnosis:** **N17.9** Failure, renal, acute

   Secondary Diagnoses: **E86.0** Dehydration

   Principal Procedure: None indicated by the documentation provided

   Secondary Procedure(s): None indicated by the documentation provided

14. **Principal Diagnosis:** **N39.3** Incontinence, urine, stress

   Secondary Diagnoses: **J44.9** Disease, lung, obstructive;
   Z99.81 Dependence, oxygen

   Principal Procedure:

Character	Code	Explanation
Section	0	Medical and Surgical
Body System	T	Urinary System
Root Operation	S	Reposition
Body Part	C	Bladder Neck
Approach	0	Open
Device	Z	No Device
Qualifier	Z	No Qualifier

INDEX: Sling, levator muscle for urethral suspension, see Reposition, bladder neck

   Secondary Procedure(s): None indicated by the documentation provided

15. **First-Listed Diagnosis:**   **N93.8** Bleeding, uterus, dysfunctional

    Secondary Diagnoses: **Z30.2** Encounter (for), sterilization

16. **Principal Diagnosis:**   **N13.6** Hydronephrosis, with obstruction, ureteral or renal calculus with infection

    Secondary Diagnoses: None indicated by the documentation provided

    Principal Procedure:

Character	Code	Explanation
Section	0	Medical Surgical
Body System	T	Urinary System
Root Operation	7	Dilation
Body Part	4	Kidney Pelvis Left
Approach	8	Via Natural or Artificial Opening Endoscopic
Device	D	Intraluminal Device
Qualifier	Z	No Qualifier

INDEX: Dilation of left kidney pelvic with insertion of intraluminal device (stent)

Secondary Procedure(s):

Character	Code	Explanation
Section	B	Imaging
Body System	T	Urinary System
Root Type	1	Fluoroscopy
Body Part	4	Kidneys Ureter Bladder (Pyelogram)
Contrast	Z	None
Qualifier	Z	None
Qualifier	Z	None

INDEX: Pyelogram, see Fluoroscopy, urinary system: retrograde pyelogram examines kidney, ureter, bladder no contrast

17. **Principal Diagnosis:**   **N39.0** Infection, urinary (tract)

    Secondary Diagnoses: **N41.00** Prostatitis acute;

    N41.10 Prostatitis chronic;

    N40.0 Enlarged prostate without lower urinary tract symptoms [LUTS];

    I48.91 Fibrillation, Atrial;

    Z79.01 Long term drug therapy (current) anticoagulants

    Principal Procedure: None indicated by the documentation provided

    Secondary Procedure(s):   None indicated by the documentation provided

Chapter 15

Pregnancy, Childbirth, and the Puerperium

1. **First-Listed Diagnosis:** **O99.810** Pregnancy, complicated by, abnormal glucose tolerance

   Secondary Diagnoses: **Z3A.22** Pregnancy weeks of gestation 22 weeks

2. **Principal Diagnosis:** **O03.4** Abortion, incomplete

   Secondary Diagnoses: **Z3A.10** Pregnancy weeks of gestation 10 weeks;
   O16.1 Hypertension, complicating pregnancy

   Principal Procedure:

Character	Code	Explanation
Section	1	Obstetrics
Body System	0	Pregnancy
Root Operation	D	Extraction
Body Part	1	Products of Conception Retained
Approach	7	Via Natural or Artificial Opening
Device	Z	No Device
Qualifier	Z	No Qualifier

   INDEX: Extraction, products of conception, retained (Refer to PCS coding guideline C.2 for procedures following delivery or abortion.)

   Secondary Procedure(s): None indicated by the documentation provided

3. **Principal Diagnosis:** **O33.9** Delivery, cesarean, cephalopelvic disproportion

   Secondary Diagnoses: **O34.21** Delivery, cesarean, previous cesarean delivery;
   Z3A.39 Pregnancy, weeks of gestation, 39 weeks;
   Z37.0 Outcome of delivery, single, liveborn

   Principal Procedure:

Character	Code	Explanation
Section	1	Obstetrics
Body System	0	Pregnancy
Root Operation	D	Extraction
Body Part	0	Products of conception
Approach	0	Open
Device	Z	No Device
Qualifier	1	Low Cervical

   INDEX: Cesarean section, see Extraction, products of conception

   Secondary Procedure(s): None indicated by the documentation provided

4. **Principal Diagnosis:** **009.513** Pregnancy, complicated by, elderly, primigravida

   Secondary Diagnoses: **Z3A.38** Pregnancy, weeks of gestation, 38 weeks;

   Z37.0 Outcome of delivery, single, liveborn

   Principal Procedure:

Character	Code	Explanation
Section	1	Obstetrics
Body System	0	Pregnancy
Root Operation	E	Delivery
Body Part	0	Products of Conception
Approach	X	External
Device	Z	No Device
Qualifier	Z	No Qualifier

INDEX: Delivery, manually assisted

Secondary Procedure(s): None indicated by the documentation provided

5. **Principal Diagnosis:** **O80** Delivery, normal

   Secondary Diagnoses: **Z3A.40** Pregnancy, weeks of gestation, 40 weeks;

   Z37.0 Outcome of delivery, single, liveborn

   Principal Procedure:

Character	Code	Explanation
Section	1	Obstetrics
Body System	0	Pregnancy
Root Operation	E	Delivery
Body Part	0	Products of Conception
Approach	X	External
Device	Z	No Device
Qualifier	Z	No Qualifier

INDEX: Delivery, manually assisted

Secondary Procedure(s):

Character	Code	Explanation
Section	1	Obstetrics
Body System	0	Pregnancy
Root Operation	9	Drainage
Body Part	0	Products of Conception
Approach	7	Via Natural or Artificial Opening
Device	Z	No Device
Qualifier	D	Fluid Other

INDEX: Induction of labor, artificial rupture of membranes, see Drainage, pregnancy, products of conception, fluid

6. **First-Listed Diagnosis:** **O99.322** Pregnancy, complicated by, drug use, second trimester

   Secondary Diagnoses: **F14.20** Dependence, drug, cocaine;
   O23.42 Pregnancy, complicated by, infection, urinary (tract), second trimester;
   Z34.15, Pregnancy, weeks of gestation, 15 weeks

7. **First-Listed Diagnosis:** **O91.12** Abscess, breast, puerperal—see Mastitis, obstetric, purulent associated with puerperium

   Secondary Diagnoses: None indicated by the documentation provided

8. **Principal Diagnosis:** **O99.63** Puerperal, gastrointestinal disease NEC

   Secondary Diagnoses: **K80.00** Calculus, gallbladder, with cholecystitis, acute

   Principal Procedure:

Character	Code	Explanation
Section	0	Medical and Surgical
Body System	F	Hepatobiliary System and Pancreas
Root Operation	T	Resection
Body Part	4	Gallbladder
Approach	4	Percutaneous Endoscopic
Device	Z	No Device
Qualifier	Z	No Qualifier

INDEX: Resection, gallbladder

Secondary Procedure(s): None indicated by the documentation provided

9. **Principal Diagnosis:** **O07.1** Abortion, attempted, complicated by, hemorrhage

   Secondary Diagnoses: **O99.019** Pregnancy, complicated by anemia,
   D62 Anemia, blood loss, acute

   Principal Procedure:

Character	Code	Explanation
Section	1	Obstetrics
Body System	0	Pregnancy
Root Operation	D	Extraction
Body Part	1	Products of Conception Retained
Approach	7	Via Natural or Artificial Opening
Device	Z	No Device
Qualifier	Z	No Qualifier

INDEX: Extraction, products of conception, retained (Refer to PCS coding guideline C.2 for procedures following delivery or abortion.)

Secondary Procedure(s): None indicated by the documentation provided

10. **Principal Diagnosis:** **O02.1** Abortion, missed
    Secondary Diagnoses: **Z3A.12** Pregnancy, weeks of gestation, 12 weeks
    Principal Procedure:

Character	Code	Explanation
Section	1	Obstetrics
Body System	0	Pregnancy
Root Operation	D	Extraction
Body Part	1	Products of Conception Retained
Approach	7	Via Natural or Artificial Opening
Device	Z	No Device
Qualifier	Z	No Qualifier

INDEX: Extraction, products of conception, retained (Refer to PCS coding guideline C.2 for procedures following delivery or abortion.)

Secondary Procedure(s): None indicated by the documentation provided

11. **Principal Diagnosis:** **O44.13** Pregnancy, complicated by, placenta previa, third trimester
    Secondary Diagnoses: **O30.043** Pregnancy, twin, dichorionic/diamniotic, third trimester;
    O60.14x1 Pregnancy, complicated by, preterm labor, third trimester;
    O61.14x2 Pregnancy, complicated by, preterm labor, third trimester;
    O99.013 Pregnancy, complicated by, anemia, third trimester;
    D62 Anemia, blood loss, acute;
    Z3A.35 Pregnancy, weeks of gestation 35 weeks;
    Z37.2 Outcome of delivery, twins, both liveborn

    Principal Procedure:

Character	Code	Explanation
Section	1	Obstetrics
Body System	0	Pregnancy
Root Operation	D	Extraction
Body Part	0	Products of Conception
Approach	0	Open
Device	Z	No Device
Qualifier	1	Low Cervical

INDEX: Cesarean section, see Extraction, Products of Conception

Secondary Procedure(s): None indicated by the documentation provided

12. **Principal Diagnosis:**   **O36.8130** Pregnancy, complicated by, decreased fetal movement

    Secondary Diagnoses: **O34.21** Delivery, cesarean delivery, previous cesarean delivery;
    O09.43 Pregnancy, complicated, grand multiparity;
    O99.013 Pregnancy, complicated by, anemia;
    D50.9 Anemia, iron deficiency;
    O13.3 Hypertension, gestational;
    Z30.2 Encounter for sterilization;
    Z3A.38 Pregnancy, weeks of gestation, 38 weeks;
    Z37.0 Outcome of delivery, single, liveborn

Principal Procedure:

Character	Code	Explanation
Section	1	Obstetrics
Body System	0	Pregnancy
Root Operation	D	Extraction
Body Part	0	Products of Conception
Approach	0	Open
Device	Z	No Device
Qualifier	1	Low Cervical

INDEX: Cesarean section, see Extraction, Products of Conception

Secondary Procedure(s):

Character	Code	Explanation
Section	0	Medical and Surgical
Body System	U	Female Reproductive System
Root Operation	L	Occlusion
Body Part	7	Fallopian Tubes Bilateral
Approach	0	Open
Device	Z	No Device
Qualifier	Z	No Qualifier

INDEX: Ligation, see Occlusion, Fallopian tubes, bilateral

13. **Principal Diagnosis:**   **O76** Pregnancy, fetal, heart rate irregularity

    Secondary Diagnoses: **O99.013** Pregnancy, complicated by, anemia;
    D50.9 Anemia, iron deficiency;
    Z3A.38, Pregnancy, weeks of gestation, 38 weeks;
    Z37.0 Outcome of delivery, single, liveborn

Principal Procedure:

Character	Code	Explanation
Section	1	Obstetrics
Body System	0	Pregnancy
Root Operation	D	Extraction
Body Part	0	Products of Conception
Approach	0	Open
Device	Z	No Device
Qualifier	1	Low Cervical

INDEX: Cesarean section, see Extraction, Products of Conception

Secondary Procedure(s):

Character	Code	Explanation
Section	1	Obstetrics
Body System	0	Pregnancy
Root Operation	9	Drainage
Body Part	0	Products of Conception
Approach	7	Via Natural or Artificial Opening
Device	Z	No Device
Qualifier	C	Fluid Other

INDEX: Induction of labor, artificial rupture of membranes, see Drainage, pregnancy, products of conception, fluid other

Secondary Procedure(s):

Character	Code	Explanation
Section	4	Measurement and Monitoring
Physiologic System	A	Physiological system
Root Operation	1	Monitoring
Body System	H	Products of Conception Cardiac
Approach	X	External
Function/Device	C	Rate
Qualifier	Z	No Qualifier

INDEX: Monitoring, Products of conception, cardiac, rate

14. **Principal Diagnosis:** **060.14x0** Pregnancy, complicated by, preterm labor, third trimester

    Secondary Diagnoses: **034.83** Pregnancy, complicated by, cystocele;

    009.523 Pregnancy, complicated by elderly multigravida;

    Z30.2 Encounter, sterilization;

    Z3A.36 Pregnancy, weeks of gestation, 36 weeks;

    Z37.0 Outcome of delivery, single, liveborn

Principal Procedure:

Character	Code	Explanation
Section	1	Obstetrics
Body System	0	Pregnancy
Root Operation	E	Delivery
Body Part	0	Products of Conception
Approach	X	External
Device	Z	No Device
Qualifier	Z	No Qualifier

INDEX: Delivery, manually assisted

Secondary Procedure(s):

Character	Code	Explanation
Section	4	Measurement and Monitoring
Physiologic System	A	Physiological Systems
Root Operation	1	Monitoring
Body System	H	Products of Conception Cardiac
Approach	X	External
Function/Device	C	Rate
Qualifier	Z	No Qualifier

INDEX: Monitoring, products of conception, cardiac, rate

Secondary Procedure(s):

Character	Code	Explanation
Section	0	Medical and Surgical
Body System	U	Female Reproductive System
Root Operation	L	Occlusion
Body Part	7	Fallopian Tubes Bilateral
Approach	8	Via Natural or Artificial Opening Endoscopic
Device	Z	No Device
Qualifier	Z	No Qualifier

INDEX: Ligation, see Occlusion, fallopian tubes, bilateral

15. **Principal Diagnosis:**   **O44.13** Delivery, cesarean for, placenta previa, third trimester

     Secondary Diagnoses: **O32.8xx0** Delivery, cesarean for, breech presentation, incomplete;
         O13.3 Hypertension, gestational;
         O41.1230 Pregnancy, complicated by, Chorioamnionitis;
         Z3A.32 Pregnancy, weeks of gestation, 32 weeks;
         Z37.0 Outcome of delivery, single, liveborn

Principal Procedure:

Character	Code	Explanation
Section	1	Obstetrics
Body System	0	Pregnancy
Root Operation	D	Extraction
Body Part	0	Products of Conception
Approach	0	Open
Device	Z	No Device
Qualifier	1	Low Cervical

INDEX: Cesarean section, see Extraction, products of conception

Secondary Procedure(s): None indicated by the documentation provided

Chapter 16

Certain Conditions Originating in the Perinatal Period

1. **Principal Diagnosis:**   **P07.03** Low, birthweight, extreme, with weight of 750–999 grams

     Secondary Diagnoses: **P07.32** Premature, newborn, less than 37 completed weeks, see Preterm infant, newborn, gestational age, 29 completed weeks;
         P22.0 Syndrome, respiratory, distress, newborn
         (See the note located under Category P07 Disorders of newborn related to short gestation and low birth weight, not elsewhere classified: When both birth weight and gestational age of the newborn are available, both should be coded with birth weight sequenced before gestational age.)

     Principal Procedure: None indicated by the documentation provided

     Secondary Procedure(s): None indicated by the documentation provided

2. **Principal Diagnosis:**   **P36.0** Sepsis, newborn, due to Streptococcus, group B

     Secondary Diagnoses: None indicated by the documentation provided

     Principal Procedure: None indicated by the documentation provided

     Secondary Procedure(s): None indicated by the documentation provided

3. **First-Listed Diagnosis:**   **Z00.111** Newborn, examination, 8 to 28 days old

       Note: The purpose of the visit was for the well baby exam. Use additional code for any identified abnormal findings appears under code Z00.11.

    Secondary Diagnoses: **P38.9** Omphalitis without hemorrhage

4. **Principal Diagnosis:**   **P70.1** Syndrome, infant, of diabetic mother

    Secondary Diagnoses: **P00.2** Newborn, affected by, maternal, infectious disease

    Principal Procedure: None indicated by the documentation provided

    Secondary Procedure(s):   None indicated by the documentation provided

5. **Principal Diagnosis:**   **P29.3** Hypertension, pulmonary, of newborn

    Secondary Diagnoses: **P84** Hypoxemia, newborn

    Principal Procedure:

Character	Code	Explanation
Section	5	Extracorporeal Assistance and Performance
Physiological System	A	Physiological Systems
Root Operation	1	Performance
Body System	5	Circulatory
Duration	2	Continuous
Function	2	Oxygenation
Qualifier	3	Membrane

INDEX: ECMO, see Performance Circulatory

Secondary Procedure(s):

Character	Code	Explanation
Section	B	Imaging
Body System	2	Heart
Root Type	4	Ultrasonography
Body Part	D	Pediatric Heart
Contrast	Y	Other Contrast
Qualifier	Z	None
Qualifier	Z	None

INDEX: Echocardiogram, see Ultrasonography, Heart pediatric

6. **Principal Diagnosis:** **P24.01** Pneumonia, aspiration, meconium

    Secondary Diagnoses: **P05.18** Small-for-dates with weight of 2200 grams

    Principal Procedure: None indicated by the documentation provided

    Secondary Procedure(s): None indicated by the documentation provided

7. **Principal Diagnosis:** **P96.1** Withdrawal state, newborn infant of dependent mother

    Secondary Diagnoses: **P05.18** Small-for-dates with weight of 2400 grams

    Principal Procedure: None indicated by the documentation provided

    Secondary Procedure(s): None indicated by the documentation provided

8. **First-Listed Diagnosis:** **Z00.1** Newborn, examination, 8 to 28 days old
    Note: The purpose of the visit was for the well baby exam. Use additional code for any identified abnormal findings appears under code Z00.11.

    Secondary Diagnoses: **P05.9** Newborn, affected by, fetal, growth retardation;
    P07.16 Low, birth weight, with weight of 1500–1749 grams;
    P07.39 Preterm infant, newborn, gestational age, 36 completed weeks

9. **First-Listed Diagnosis:** **P04.41** Crack baby

    Secondary Diagnoses: **P22.1** Tachypnea, transitory, of newborn

10. **First-Listed Diagnosis:** **P92.8** Feeding, problem, newborn, specified, NEC

    Secondary Diagnoses: **P02.5** Newborn, affected by, umbilical cord around neck

11. **Principal Diagnosis:** **Z38.01** Newborn, delivered by cesarean

    Secondary Diagnoses: **P05.07** Light-for-dates with weight of 1920 grams;
    P07.35 Preterm infant, newborn gestational age, 32 completed weeks;
    P00.2 Newborn, affected by (suspected), maternal condition, infectious disease

    Principal Procedure: None indicated by the documentation provided

    Secondary Procedure(s): None indicated by the documentation provided

12. **Principal Diagnosis:** **Z38.00** Newborn, born in hospital

    Secondary Diagnoses: **P05.18** Small-for-dates, weight 2035 grams;

    P00.2 Newborn, affected by (suspected), maternal condition, infectious disease;

    P22.8 Distress, respiratory, newborn; P84 Acidosis, newborn;

    P59.0 Newborn, jaundice, of prematurity; P71.8 Hypermagnesemia, neonatal

    Principal Procedure: None indicated by the documentation provided

    Secondary Procedure(s): None indicated by the documentation provided

13. **First-Listed Diagnosis:** **Z00.110** Newborn, examination, under 8 days old.

    Secondary Diagnoses: **P39.1** Conjunctivitis, chlamydial, neonatal

14. **Principal Diagnosis:** **P35.2** Herpes, simplex, congenital

   Secondary Diagnoses: **P05.18** Small-for-dates, weight 2040 grams

   Principal Procedure: None indicated by the documentation provided

   Secondary Procedure(s): None indicated by the documentation provided

15. **Principal Diagnosis:** **P07.16** Low, birth weight, with weight of 1600 grams

   Secondary Diagnoses: **P07.36** Preterm infant, newborn, gestational age 33 completed weeks; **Q76.0** Spina Bifida occulta

   Principal Procedure: None indicated by the documentation provided

   Secondary Procedure(s): None indicated by the documentation provided

Chapter 17

Congenital Malformations, Deformations, and Chromosomal Abnormalities

1. **Principal Diagnosis:** **H90.6** Loss, hearing, see also Deafness, mixed, bilateral

   Secondary Diagnoses: **Q16.5** anomaly, ear, inner

   Principal Procedure:

Character	Code	Explanation
Section	0	Medical and Surgical
Body System	9	Ear, Nose, Sinus
Root Operation	H	Insertion
Body Part	D	Inner Ear, Right
Approach	0	Open
Device	5	Hearing Device, Single Channel Cochlear Prosthesis
Qualifier	Z	No Qualifier

INDEX: Cochlear Implant, single channel, use Hearing Device, Single Channel Cochlear Prosthesis, Right

Secondary Procedure(s):

Character	Code	Explanation
Section	0	Medical and Surgical
Body System	9	Ear, Nose, Sinus
Root Operation	H	Insertion
Body Part	E	Inner Ear, Left
Approach	0	Open
Device	5	Hearing Device, Single Channel Cochlear Prosthesis
Qualifier	Z	No Qualifier

INDEX: Cochlear Implant, single channel, use Hearing Device, Single Channel Cochlear Prosthesis, Left

2. **Principal Diagnosis:** **Q44.2** Atresia, bile duct

   Secondary Diagnoses: **Q44.3** Obstruction, bile duct, congenital

   Principal Procedure:

Character	Code	Explanation
Section	0	Medical and Surgical
Body System	F	Hepatobiliary System and Pancreas
Root Operation	1	Bypass
Body Part	4	Gallbladder
Approach	0	Open
Device	Z	No Device
Qualifier	B	Small Intestine

INDEX: Roux-en-Y Hepatobiliary System and Pancreas

Note: ICD-10-PCS coding guidelines B3.6a: Bypass procedures are coded by identifying the body part bypassed "from" and the body part bypassed "to." The fourth character body part specifies the body part bypassed from, and the qualifier specifies the body part bypassed to.

Secondary Procedure(s):

Character	Code	Explanation
Section	B	Imaging
Body System	F	Hepatobiliary System and Pancreas
Root Type	1	Fluoroscopy
Body Part	3	Gallbladder and Bile Ducts
Contrast	1	Low Osmolar
Qualifier	Z	None
Qualifier	Z	None

INDEX: Cholangiogram, see Fluoroscopy, Hepatobiliary System and Pancreas

3. **Principal Diagnosis:** **Q25.1** Coarctation, aorta

   Secondary Diagnoses: None indicated by the documentation provided

   Principal Procedure:

Character	Code	Explanation
Section	0	Medical and Surgical
Body System	2	Heart and Great Vessels
Root Operation	B	Excision
Body Part	W	Thoracic, Aorta

Approach	0	Open
Device	Z	No Device
Qualifier	Z	No Qualifier

INDEX: Excision, Aorta, Thoracic

Secondary Procedure(s):

Character	Code	Explanation
Section	5	Extracorporeal Assistance and Performance
Physiological System	A	Physiological Systems
Root Operation	1	Performance
Body System	2	Cardiac
Duration	2	Continuous
Function	1	Output
Qualifier	Z	No Qualifier

INDEX: Bypass, Cardiopulmonary

4. **First-Listed Diagnosis:** **Z00.111** Newborn, examination, 8 to 28 days old

   Secondary Diagnoses: **Q65.6** Dislocatable hip, congenital provided

5. **Principal Diagnosis:** **Q22.1** Stenosis, pulmonary valve, congenital

   Secondary Diagnoses: **Q25.6** Stenosis, pulmonary artery;
   Z98.89 History, personal, surgery;
   Z87.74 History, personal, congenital malformation, circulatory system

Principal Procedure:

Character	Code	Explanation
Section	0	Medical and Surgical
Body System	2	Heart and Great Vessels
Root Operation	R	Replacement
Body Part	H	Pulmonary Valve
Approach	0	Open
Device	K	Nonautologous Tissue Substitute
Qualifier	Z	No Qualifier

INDEX: Replacement, valve, pulmonary

Secondary Procedure(s):

Character	Code	Explanation
Section	0	Medical and Surgical
Body System	2	Heart and Great Vessels
Root Operation	Q	Repair
Body Part	R	Pulmonary Artery, Left
Approach	0	Open
Device	Z	No Device
Qualifier	Z	No Qualifier

INDEX: Arterioplasty, see Repair, Heart and Great Vessels

Secondary Procedure(s):

Character	Code	Explanation
Section	0	Medical and Surgical
Body System	2	Heart and Great Vessels
Root Operation	Q	Repair
Body Part	Q	Pulmonary Artery, Right
Approach	0	Open
Device	Z	No Device
Qualifier	Z	No Qualifier

INDEX: Arterioplasty, see Repair, Heart and Great Vessels

Secondary Procedure(s):

Character	Code	Explanation
Section	5	Extracorporeal Assistance and Performance
Physiological System	A	Physiological Systems
Root Operation	1	Performance
Body System	2	Cardiac
Duration	2	Continuous
Function	1	Output
Qualifier	Z	No Qualifier

INDEX: Bypass, Cardiopulmonary

Secondary Procedure(s):

Character	Code	Explanation
Section	B	Imaging
Body System	2	Heart
Root Type	4	Ultrasonography
Body Part	D	Pediatric Heart
Contrast	Z	None
Qualifier	Z	None
Qualifier	4	Transesophageal

INDEX: Echocardiogram, see Ultrasonography Heart Pediatric

6. **First-Listed Diagnosis:**   **Q40.0** Hypertrophic, pylorus, congenital

   Secondary Diagnoses: None indicated by the documentation provided

7. **First-Listed Diagnosis:**   **Q37.8** Cleft, lip, bilateral, with cleft palate

   Secondary Diagnoses: **R63.3** Difficult, feeding

8. **Principal Diagnosis:**   **Q43.1** Hirschsprung's Disease

   Secondary Diagnoses: None indicated by the documentation provided

   Principal Procedure:

Character	Code	Explanation
Section	0	Medical and Surgical
Body System	D	Gastrointestinal System
Root Operation	1	Bypass
Body Part	N	Sigmoid Colon
Approach	0	Open
Device	Z	No Device
Qualifier	4	Cutaneous

INDEX: Colostomy, see Bypass, Gastrointestinal System

Secondary Procedure(s):

Character	Code	Explanation
Section	0	Medical and Surgical
Body System	D	Gastrointestinal System
Root Operation	B	Excision
Body Part	N	Sigmoid Colon
Approach	0	Open
Device	Z	No Device
Qualifier	X	Diagnostic

INDEX: Biopsy, see Excision with qualifier Diagnostic

9. **First-Listed Diagnosis:** **Q13.4**, Embryotoxon (congenital corneal malformation)

   Secondary Diagnoses: **Q91.7** Trisomy 13

10. **Principal Diagnosis:** **Q23.4** Hypoplastic, left heart syndrome

    Secondary Diagnoses: **Q21.0** Defect, ventricular septal;
    P36.4 Newborn, sepsis, due to Escherichia coli

11. **First-Listed Diagnosis:** **Q30.0** Atresia, choanal

    Secondary Diagnoses: None indicated by the documentation provided

12. **First-Listed Diagnosis:** **Z00.121** Examination, child, with abnormal findings

    Secondary Diagnoses: **Q53.10** Undescended, testicle—see Cryptorchid, unilateral

13. **First-Listed Diagnosis:** **Q51.3** Bicornate uterus

    Secondary Diagnoses: None indicated by the documentation provided

14. **Principal Diagnosis:** **Q31.5** Laryngomalacia

    Secondary Diagnoses: None indicated by the documentation provided

    Principal Procedure: None indicated by the documentation provided

    Secondary Procedure(s): None indicated by the documentation provided

15. **First-Listed Diagnosis:** **Q54.0** Hypospadias, balanic

    Secondary Diagnoses: None indicated by the documentation provided

Chapter 18

Symptoms, Signs, and Abnormal Clinical and Laboratory Findings, Not Elsewhere Classified

1. **Principal Diagnosis:** **R19.4** Change, bowel habits

   Secondary Diagnoses: **Z80.0** History, family, malignant neoplasm, gastrointestinal tract

Principal Procedure:

Character	Code	Explanation
Section	0	Medical and Surgical
Body System	D	Gastrointestinal System
Root Operation	J	Inspection
Body Part	D	Lower Intestinal Tract
Approach	8	Via Natural or Artificial Opening Endoscopic
Device	Z	No Device
Qualifier	Z	No Qualifier

INDEX: Colonoscopy

Secondary Procedure(s): None indicated by the documentation provided

2. **First-Listed Diagnosis:** **R93.3** Findings, abnormal, inconclusive, without diagnosis, radiologic, gastrointestinal tract

   Secondary Diagnoses: **R10.84** Pain, abdominal, generalized;
   R53.83 Fatigue;
   R11.0 Nausea

3. **Principal Diagnosis:** **R91.8** Lung mass

   Secondary Diagnoses: **R05** Cough;
   R07.89 Chest pressure;
   R00.1 Bradycardia;
   Z53.09 Procedure not done because of contraindication

Principal Procedure:

Character	Code	Explanation
Section	0	Medical and Surgical
Body System	B	Respiratory System
Root Operation	J	Inspection
Body Part	0	Tracheobronchial Tree
Approach	8	Via Natural or Artificial Opening Endoscopic
Device	Z	No Device
Qualifier	Z	No Qualifier

INDEX: Bronchoscopy

Secondary Procedure(s): None indicated by the documentation provided

4. **Principal Diagnosis:**   **R07.89** Chest pain, atypical

   Secondary Diagnoses: **I20.9** Angina pectoris;

                                       K21.9 Gastroesophageal reflux disease

Principal Procedure:

Character	Code	Explanation
Section	0	Medical and Surgical
Body System	D	Gastrointestinal System
Root Operation	J	Inspection
Body Part	0	Upper Intestinal Tract
Approach	8	Via Natural or Artificial Opening Endoscopic
Device	Z	No Device
Qualifier	Z	No Qualifier

INDEX: EGD (Esophagogastroduodenoscopy)

Secondary Procedure(s):

Character	Code	Explanation
Section	4	Measurement and Monitoring
Physiological System	A	Physiological Systems
Root Operation	0	Measurement
Body System	2	Cardiac
Approach	X	External
Function/Device	M	Total Activity
Qualifier	4	Stress

INDEX: Stress Test

Note: The Alphabetic Index in the *2012 Draft ICD-10-PCS* published by Ingenix/OptumInsight code book lists the code 4A12XM4, which is "monitoring". But a stress test seems to meet the definition of "measurement," which is determining the level of a physiological or physical function at a point in time. Exercises in the *2012 ICD-10-PCS Reference Manual* available on the CMS website gives an example of cardiac stress test, single measurement with the answer of 4A02XMA. The CMS website's PDF file of the 2012 Draft ICD-10-PCS code set lists both codes, 4A02XMA and 4A12XMA.

Secondary Procedure(s):

Character	Code	Explanation
Section	C	Nuclear Medicine
Body System	2	Heart
Root Type	1	Planar Nuclear Medicine Imaging

Body Part	G	Myocardium
Radionuclide	S	Thallium 201
Qualifier	Z	None
Qualifier	Z	None

INDEX: Nuclear Medicine—See Planar Nuclear Medicine Imaging, Myocardium C21G

5. **First-Listed Diagnosis:**   **R20.0** Numbness

    Secondary Diagnoses: **R26.2** Difficulty in walking;
                                                R27.9 Lack of coordination;
                                                R25.1 Tremor

6. **First-Listed Diagnosis:**   **R92.0** Microcalcifications, breast

    Secondary Diagnoses: **N60.11** Fibrocystic disease, breast, see mastopathy, cystic, right breast

7. **First-Listed Diagnosis:**   **R87.810** Human papillomavirus (HPV), DNA test positive, high risk, cervix

    Secondary Diagnoses: None indicated by documentation provided

8. **First-Listed Diagnosis:**   **R19.7** Diarrhea

    Secondary Diagnoses: **R62.51** Failure to thrive

9. **First-Listed Diagnosis:**   **R51** Headache

    Secondary Diagnoses: **R50.9** Fever;
                                                R11.2 Nausea with vomiting;
                                                R29.1 Meningismus

10. **Principal Diagnosis:**   **R10.11** Abdominal pain, right upper quadrant

    Secondary Diagnoses: **R11.2** Nausea and vomiting;
                                                R93.5 Findings, abnormal, radiologic, abdomen;
                                                R03.0 Elevated blood pressure readings

Principal Procedure:

Character	Code	Explanation
Section	B	Imaging
Body System	W	Anatomical Regions
Root Type	4	Ultrasonography
Body Part	0	Abdomen
Contrast	Z	None
Qualifier	Z	None
Qualifier	Z	None

INDEX: Ultrasonography, abdomen

Secondary Procedure(s): None indicated by the documentation provided

11. **Principal Diagnosis:** **R13.10** Dysphagia

    Secondary Diagnoses: **F41.9** Anxiety disorder;
    E86.0 Dehydration

    Principal Procedure:

Character	Code	Explanation
Section	0	Medical and Surgical
Body System	D	Gastrointestinal System
Root Operation	J	Inspection
Body Part	0	Upper Intestinal Tract
Approach	8	Via Natural or Artificial Opening Endoscopic
Device	Z	No Device
Qualifier	Z	No Qualifier

    INDEX: EGD (Esophagogastroduodenoscopy)

    Secondary Procedure(s): None indicated by the documentation provided

12. **First-Listed Diagnosis:** **R50.9** Fever with chills,

    Secondary Diagnoses: **R52** Body aches—see Pain, generalized;
    R53.1 Weakness;
    F53.83 Fatigue

13. **First-Listed Diagnosis:** **R94.39**, Findings, abnormal, stress test

    Secondary Diagnoses: **R03.0** Elevation, blood pressure reading

14. **First-Listed Diagnosis:** **R68.84** Pain, jaw

    Secondary Diagnoses: **M25.519** Pain, shoulder, unspecified;
    R94.31 Abnormal, EKG

15. **First-Listed Diagnosis:** **R10.83** Colic

    Secondary Diagnoses: None indicated by documentation provided

16. **First-Listed Diagnosis:** **R45.4** Irritability (either symptom could be listed first)

    Secondary Diagnoses: **R45.87** Impulsiveness;
    S06.2x0S Sequela, injury, brain (traumatic) diffuse;
    Y36.230S War operations, explosion, IED

Chapter 19A

Injuries, Effects of Foreign Body, Burns and Corrosions, and Frostbite

1. **First-Listed Diagnosis:**   **T21.31xA** Burn, chest wall, third degree, chest, initial encounter

   Secondary Diagnoses: **T22.232A** Burn, above elbow, left, second degree, initial encounter;

          T22.231A Burn, above elbow, right, second degree initial encounter,

          T31.20 Burn, extent, 20–29% with 0–9% third degree burns, initial encounter

2. **Principal Diagnosis:**   **S03.0xxA** Dislocation, mandible, initial encounter

   Secondary Diagnoses: **S61.401A** Laceration, hand, right, initial encounter

   Principal Procedure:

Character	Code	Explanation
Section	0	Medical and Surgical
Body System	N	Head and Facial Bones
Root Operation	S	Reposition
Body Part	V	Mandible, Left
Approach	X	External
Device	Z	No Device
Qualifier	Z	No Qualifier

INDEX: Reduction, dislocation, see Reposition

Secondary Procedure(s):

Character	Code	Explanation
Section	0	Medical and Surgical
Body System	X	Head and Facial Bones
Root Operation	Q	Reposition
Body Part	J	Mandible, Left
Approach	X	External
Device	Z	No Device
Qualifier	Z	No Qualifier

INDEX: Repair, hand, right

3. **Principal Diagnosis:**   **S72.402A** Fracture, traumatic, femur, lower end, initial encounter

   Secondary Diagnoses: **S92.112A** Fracture, traumatic, talus, neck, initial encounter

   Principal Procedure:

Character	Code	Explanation
Section	0	Medical and Surgical
Body System	Q	Lower Bones
Root Operation	S	Reposition
Body Part	C	Lower Femur, Left
Approach	0	Open
Device	4	Internal Fixation Device
Qualifier	Z	No Qualifier

INDEX: Reduction, Fracture, see Reposition, Femur

Secondary Procedure(s):

Character	Code	Explanation
Section	0	Medical and Surgical
Body System	Q	Lower Bones
Root Operation	S	Reposition
Body Part	M	Tarsal, Left
Approach	0	Open
Device	4	Internal Fixation Device
Qualifier	Z	No Qualifier

INDEX: Reduction, Fracture, see Reposition, Talus

4. **Principal Diagnosis:**   **S43.431A** Lesion, SLAP, initial encounter

   Secondary Diagnoses: None indicated by the documentation provided

   Principal Procedure:

Character	Code	Explanation
Section	0	Medical and Surgical
Body System	M	Bursae and Ligaments
Root Operation	Q	Repair
Body Part	1	Shoulder Bursa and Ligament, Right
Approach	0	Open

| Device | Z | No Device |
| Qualifier | Z | No Qualifier |

INDEX: Repair, Bursa and Ligament, see Body Part Key, Glenoid Ligament (Labrum) refers one to Shoulder Bursa and Ligament

Secondary Procedure(s): None indicated by the documentation provided

5. **Principal Diagnosis:** **S06.9x2A** Injury, head, with loss of consciousness initial encounter

Secondary Diagnoses: **S01.419A** Laceration, cheek, initial encounter;
S01.81xA Laceration, forehead and jaw, initial encounter;
S01.511A Laceration, lip, initial encounter;
S60.511A Abrasion, hand, right, initial encounter;
S60.512A Abrasion, hand, left, initial encounter;
S30.1xxA Contusion, abdominal wall, initial encounter;
S80.01xA Contusion, knee, right, initial encounter,
S80.02xA Contusion, knee, left, initial encounter;
S80.11xA, Contusion, lower leg, right, initial encounter;
S80.12xA Contusion, lower leg, left, initial encounter

Principal Procedure:

Character	Code	Explanation
Section	0	Medical and Surgical
Body System	H	Skin and Breast
Root Operation	Q	Repair
Body Part	1	Skin, Face (Cheek)
Approach	X	External
Device	Z	No Device
Qualifier	Z	No Qualifier

INDEX: Suture, Laceration Repair, see Repair

Secondary Procedure(s):

Character	Code	Explanation
Section	0	Medical and Surgical
Body System	H	Skin and Breast
Root Operation	Q	Repair
Body Part	1	Skin, Face (Forehead)
Approach	X	External
Device	Z	No Device
Qualifier	Z	No Qualifier

INDEX: Suture, Laceration Repair, see Repair

Secondary Procedure(s):

Character	Code	Explanation
Section	0	Medical and Surgical
Body System	C	Mouth and Throat
Root Operation	Q	Repair
Body Part	0	Upper Lip
Approach	X	External
Device	Z	No Device
Qualifier	Z	No Qualifier

INDEX: Suture, Laceration Repair, see Repair, lip

Secondary Procedure(s):

Character	Code	Explanation
Section	0	Medical and Surgical
Body System	H	Skin and Breast
Root Operation	Q	Repair
Body Part	1	Skin, Face (Jaw)
Approach	X	External
Device	Z	No Device
Qualifier	Z	No Qualifier

INDEX: Suture, Laceration Repair, see Repair

6. **First-Listed Diagnosis:** **S35.02xA** Injury to aorta, abdominal, laceration major, initial encounter
   Note: Instructional note at S35 to code any associated open wound **S31.-**.

   Secondary Diagnoses: **S31.622A** Laceration, abdominal wall, epigastric region with penetration into peritoneal cavity with foreign body, initial encounter

7. **Principal Diagnosis:** **S97.82xA** Crush, foot, initial encounter
   Note: Instructional note at S97 to code all associate injuries.

   Secondary Diagnoses: **S92.312B** Fracture, traumatic, metatarsal, first, initial encounter

   Principal Procedure:

Character	Code	Explanation
Section	0	Medical and Surgical
Body System	Q	Lower Bones
Root Operation	S	Reposition

Body Part	P	Metatarsal, Left
Approach	0	Open
Device	4	Internal Fixation Device
Qualifier	Z	No Qualifier

INDEX: Reduction, Fracture, see Reposition, Metatarsal

Secondary Procedure(s):

Character	Code	Explanation
Section	0	Medical and Surgical
Body System	J	Skin and Breast
Root Operation	8	Division
Body Part	R	Subcutaneous Tissue and Fascia, Left Foot
Approach	0	Open
Device	Z	No Device
Qualifier	Z	No Qualifier

INDEX: Fasciotomy, see Division, Subcutaneous Tissue and Fascia

8. **Principal Diagnosis:**   **T18.128A** Foreign body, esophagus, causing injury, food, initial encounter

   Secondary Diagnoses: **K21.0** Esophagitis, reflux

   Principal Procedure:

Character	Code	Explanation
Section	0	Medical and Surgical
Body System	D	Gastrointestinal System
Root Operation	C	Extirpation
Body Part	4	Esophagogastric Junction
Approach	8	Via Natural or Artificial Opening Endoscopic
Device	Z	No Device
Qualifier	Z	No Qualifier

INDEX: Extirpation, Esophagus, Lower

Secondary Procedure(s): None indicated with the documentation provided

9. **Principal Diagnosis:**   **S32.022A** Fracture, traumatic, vertebra, lumbar, second, burst, unstable, initial encounter

   Secondary Diagnoses: **S32.032A** Fracture, traumatic, vertebra, lumbar, third, burst, unstable, initial encounter

Principal Procedure:

Character	Code	Explanation
Section	0	Medical and Surgical
Body System	Q	Lower Bones
Root Operation	S	Reposition
Body Part	0	Lumbar Vertebra
Approach	0	Open
Device	Z	No Device
Qualifier	1	No Qualifier

INDEX: Reduction, Fracture, see Reposition, Vertebra, Lumbar

Secondary Procedure(s):

Character	Code	Explanation
Section	0	Medical and Surgical
Body System	S	Lower Joints
Root Operation	G	Fusion
Body Part	0	Lumbar Vertebral Joint
Approach	0	Open
Device	A	Interbody Fusion Device
Qualifier	1	Posterior Approach, Posterior Column

INDEX: Fusion, Lumbar Vertebral 1 Joint

Note: Refer to ICD-10-PCS coding guideline B3.10c: When an interbody fusion device is used to render the joint immobile [alone or containing other material like bone graft], the procedure is coded with the device value Interbody Fusion Device.

Secondary Procedure(s):

Character	Code	Explanation
Section	0	Medical and Surgical
Body System	Q	Lower Bones
Root Operation	B	Excision
Body Part	2	Pelvic Bones, Right
Approach	0	Open
Device	Z	No Device
Qualifier	Z	No Qualifier

INDEX: Excision, Bone, Pelvic, Right

10. **First-Listed Diagnosis:** **S64.02xA** Injury, ulnar nerve, hand, initial encounter
Note: Coding guideline I.C.19.b.2 primary injury with damage to nerves/blood vessels is the reason for the injury of the nerve listed first.

Secondary Diagnoses: **S61.512A** Laceration, wrist, left, initial encounter;
S66.902A Laceration, tendon see Injury, muscle, hand, initial encounter

11. **Principal Diagnosis:** **S36.116A** Laceration, liver, major, initial encounter
Note: Instructional note at S36 directs users to code also any associated open wound.

Secondary Diagnoses: **S36.438A** Laceration, jejunum, initial encounter;
S37.011A Hematoma, kidney, see contusion, initial encounter;
S31.129A Laceration, abdominal wall with foreign body, initial encounter;
S41.001A Laceration, shoulder, right, initial encounter;
S81.801A Laceration, leg (lower), right, initial encounter;
T51.0x1A (Table of Drugs and Chemicals) Poisoning, alcohol, beverage, initial encounter

Principal Procedure:

Character	Code	Explanation
Section	0	Medical and Surgical
Body System	F	Hepatobiliary System and Pancreas
Root Operation	Q	Repair
Body Part	0	Liver
Approach	0	Open
Device	Z	No Device
Qualifier	Z	No Qualifier

INDEX: Repair, Liver

Secondary Procedure(s):

Character	Code	Explanation
Section	0	Medical and Surgical
Body System	D	Gastrointestinal System
Root Operation	Q	Repair
Body Part	A	Jejunum
Approach	0	Open
Device	Z	No Device
Qualifier	Z	No Qualifier

INDEX: Repair, Jejunum

Secondary Procedure(s):

Character	Code	Explanation
Section	0	Medical and Surgical
Body System	T	Urinary System
Root Operation	J	Inspection
Body Part	5	Kidney
Approach	0	Open
Device	Z	No Device
Qualifier	Z	No Qualifier

INDEX: Examination, see Inspection, Kidney

Secondary Procedure(s):

Character	Code	Explanation
Section	0	Medical and Surgical
Body System	D	Gastrointestinal
Root Operation	J	Inspection
Body Part	D	Lower Intestinal Tract
Approach	0	Open
Device	Z	No Device
Qualifier	Z	No Qualifier

INDEX: Examination, see Inspection, Colon – Lower Intestinal Tract

Secondary Procedure(s):

Character	Code	Explanation
Section	0	Medical and Surgical
Body System	J	Subcutaneous Tissue and Fascia
Root Operation	C	Extirpation
Body Part	8	Subcutaneous Tissue and Fascia, Abdomen
Approach	0	Open
Device	Z	No Device
Qualifier	Z	No Qualifier

INDEX: Extirpation, Subcutaneous Tissue and Fascia, Abdomen (Glass)

12. **Principal Diagnosis:**   **S02.0xxB** Fracture, traumatic skull parietal bone, initial encounter for open fracture

    Secondary Diagnoses: **S06.5x7A** Hemorrhage, intracranial, subdural, traumatic;

      S06.1x7A Edema, cerebral, see Injury, intracranial, cerebral, edema, diffuse;

      G93.5 Herniation, brainstem

Note: Cerebral contusion is not coded separately due to Excludes1 note at S06.3 for cerebral contusion.

Principal Procedure:

Character	Code	Explanation
Section	0	Medical and Surgical
Body System	N	Head and Facial Bones
Root Operation	9	Drainage
Body Part	3	Parietal Bone, Right
Approach	0	Open
Device	Z	No Device
Qualifier	Z	No Qualifier

INDEX: Drainage, Bone, Parietal, Right

Secondary Procedure(s):

Character	Code	Explanation
Section	0	Medical and Surgical
Body System	0	Central Nervous System
Root Operation	Q	Repair
Body Part	2	Dura Mater
Approach	0	Open
Device	Z	No Device
Qualifier	Z	No Qualifier

INDEX: Repair, Dura Mater

Secondary Procedure(s):

Character	Code	Explanation
Section	0	Medical and Surgical
Body System	0	Central Nervous System
Root Operation	H	Insertion
Body Part	0	Brain
Approach	0	Open
Device	2	Monitoring Device
Qualifier	Z	No Qualifier

INDEX: Insertion of device, Brain

Secondary Procedure(s):

Character	Code	Explanation
Section	5	Extracorporeal Assistance and Performance
Physiological System	A	Physiological Systems
Root Operation	1	Performance
Body System	9	Respiratory
Duration	4	24-96 Consecutive Hours
Function	5	Ventilation
Qualifier	Z	No Qualifier

INDEX: Mechanical Ventilation, see Performance, Respiratory

Secondary Procedure(s):

Character	Code	Explanation
Section	0	Medical and Surgical
Body System	B	Respiratory System
Root Operation	J	Inspection
Body Part	0	Tracheobronchial Tree
Approach	8	Via Natural or Artificial Opening Endoscopic
Device	Z	No Device
Qualifier	Z	No Qualifier

INDEX: Bronchoscopy

13. **Principal Diagnosis:** **S02.65xA** Fracture, traumatic, mandible, angle, initial encounter

    Secondary Diagnoses: **S02.5xxA** Fracture, traumatic tooth, initial encounter;
    S01.81xA Laceration, jaw—See Laceration, head, specified site NEC, initial encounter;
    N39.0 Infection, urinary tract;
    S60.511A Abrasion, hand, right hand, initial encounter

Principal Procedure:

Character	Code	Explanation
Section	0	Medical and Surgical
Body System	N	Head and Facial Bones
Root Operation	S	Reposition
Body Part	V	Mandible, Left
Approach	0	Open

Device	4	Internal Fixation Device
Qualifier	Z	No Qualifier

INDEX: Reposition Mandible Left

Secondary Procedure(s):

Character	Code	Explanation
Section	0	Medical and Surgical
Body System	N	Head and Facial Bones
Root Operation	S	Reposition
Body Part	T	Mandible, Right
Approach	0	Open
Device	4	Internal Fixation Device
Qualifier	Z	No Qualifier

INDEX: Reposition Mandible Right

Secondary Procedure(s):

Character	Code	Explanation
Section	0	Medical and Surgical
Body System	H	Skin and Breast
Root Operation	Q	Repair
Body Part	1	Skin Face
Approach	X	External
Device	Z	No Device
Qualifier	Z	No Qualifier

INDEX: Repair Skin Face

Secondary Procedure(s):

Character	Code	Explanation
Section	0	Medical and Surgical
Body System	C	Mouth and Throat
Root Operation	D	Extraction
Body Part	X	Lower Tooth
Approach	X	External
Device	Z	No Device
Qualifier	0	Single

INDEX: Extraction Tooth Lower

14. **Principal Diagnosis:**   **S82.101A** Fracture, traumatic, tibia, upper

   Secondary Diagnoses: **D66** Hemophilia, A;
   Z21 HIV positive;
   Z96.651 Status, organ replacement, joint, see presence, knee, joint, implant
   Note: Code Z21 for asymptomatic HIV status; there is no documentation to indicate the patient has AIDS (code B20).

Principal Procedure:

Character	Code	Explanation
Section	0	Medical and Surgical
Body System	Q	Lower Bones
Root Operation	S	Reposition
Body Part	G	Tibia, Right
Approach	X	External
Device	Z	No Device
Qualifier	Z	No Qualifier

INDEX: Reposition, Tibia, Right

Secondary Procedure(s):

Character	Code	Explanation
Section	3	Administration
Physiological System	0	Circulatory
Root Operation	2	Transfusion
Body System/Region	3	Peripheral Vein
Approach	3	Percutaneous
Substance	V	Antihemophilic Factors
Qualifier	1	Nonautologous

INDEX: Transfusion, Antihemophilic Factor, Vein, Peripheral

15. **Principal Diagnosis:**   **S82.852A** Fracture, traumatic, ankle, trimalleolar, initial encounter for closed fracture

   Secondary Diagnoses: **I69.354** Sequela, infarction, cerebral, hemiplegia;
   E11.9 Diabetes, type 2;
   I25.9 Ischemia, heart;
   N39.0 Infection, urinary

Principal Procedure:

Character	Code	Explanation
Section	0	Medical and Surgical
Body System	Q	Lower Bones

Root Operation	S	Reposition
Body Part	H	Tibia Left
Approach	X	External
Device	Z	No Device
Qualifier	Z	No Qualifier

INDEX: Reposition, Tibia, Left

Secondary Procedure(s): None indicated by the documentation provided

16. **Principal Diagnosis:** **S59.211A** Fracture, traumatic, radius, lower end, physeal, Salter-Harris, Type I, right, initial encounter for closed fracture

Secondary Diagnoses: **S59.011A** Fracture, traumatic, ulna, lower end, physeal, Salter-Harris, Type I, right, initial encounter for closed fracture
Note: Either fracture, radius or ulna, code could be sequenced as the principal diagnosis.

Principal Procedure:

Character	Code	Explanation
Section	0	Medical and Surgical
Body System	P	Upper Bones
Root Operation	S	Reposition
Body Part	H	Radius Right
Approach	3	Percutaneous
Device	4	Internal Fixation Device
Qualifier	Z	No Qualifier

INDEX: Reposition, Radius, Right

Secondary Procedure(s):

Character	Code	Explanation
Section	0	Medical and Surgical
Body System	P	Upper Bones
Root Operation	S	Reposition
Body Part	K	Ulna Right
Approach	X	External
Device	Z	No Device
Qualifier	Z	No Qualifier

INDEX: Reposition, Ulna, Right

17. **Principal Diagnosis:** **S72.011A** Fracture, traumatic, femur, subcapital, right, initial encounter for closed fracture

Note: A fracture not indicated as open or closed should be coded to closed.

Secondary Diagnoses: **I10,** Hypertension, (essential);

W10.10xA External cause: Fall, off, stairs/steps, curb, initial encounter (Note: Use one placeholder x character for 6th character in order to apply the 7th character, A);

Y93.01 External cause: Activity, walking, marching and hiking;

Y92.481 External cause, place of occurrence, parking lot;

Y99.8 External cause, Status of external cause, leisure activity or specified NEC (for retired)

Principal Procedure:

Character	Code	Explanation
Section	0	Medical and Surgical
Body System	Q	Lower Bones
Root Operation	H	Insertion
Body Part	6	Upper Femur Right
Approach	0	Open
Device	4	Internal Fixation Device
Qualifier	Z	No Qualifier

INDEX: Fixation, bone, internal, without fracture reduction, see Insertion. Insertion Femur Upper Right

Note: Operative report includes "This showed the fracture to be well reduced on its own" so a reposition procedure was not performed.

Secondary Procedure(s): None indicated by the documentation provided

18. **Principal Diagnosis:** **S82.51xK** Nonunion, fracture, see Fracture, by site: Fracture, tibia, malleolus, see Fracture, ankle medial malleolus, 7th character K for subsequent encounter for fracture with nonunion

Secondary Diagnoses: **W10.9xxD** External cause: Fall, down stairs, subsequent encounter

Principal Procedure:

Character	Code	Explanation
Section	0	Medical and Surgical
Body System	Q	Lower Bones
Root Operation	S	Reposition
Body Part	G	Tibia Right
Approach	0	Open

Device	4	Internal Fixation Device
Qualifier	Z	No Qualifier

INDEX: Reposition, Tibia, Right

Secondary Procedure(s):

Character	Code	Explanation
Section	0	Medical and Surgical
Body System	Q	Lower Bones
Root Operation	R	Replacement
Body Part	G	Tibia Right
Approach	0	Open
Device	7	Autologous Tissue Substitute
Qualifier	Z	No Qualifier

INDEX: Graft, see Replacement, Tibia, Right (Bone graft replaced missing bone from the nonunion fracture.)

Secondary Procedure(s):

Character	Code	Explanation
Section	0	Medical and Surgical
Body System	Q	Lower Bones
Root Operation	B	Excision
Body Part	3	Pelvic Bone Left
Approach	0	Open
Device	Z	No Device
Qualifier	Z	No Qualifier

INDEX: (Harvest) Excision, Bone, Pelvic Bone, Left (Body Part Key: Iliac crest = pelvic bone)

19. **Principal Diagnosis:** **S42.211P** Malunion, fracture—See Fracture, by site, Fracture traumatic, humerus, upper end, surgical neck, with 7th character of P for subsequent encounter for fracture with malunion

    Secondary Diagnoses: **W07.xxxS** External cause: Fall, out of chair;

    I25.10 Disease, arteriosclerotic, heart—See Disease, heart, ischemic, atherosclerotic;
    N18.9 Insufficiency, renal, chronic;
    E11.9 Diabetes, type 2

Principal Procedure:

Character	Code	Explanation
Section	0	Medical and Surgical
Body System	P	Upper Bones
Root Operation	S	Reposition
Body Part	C	Humeral Head Right
Approach	0	Open
Device	4	Internal Fixation Device
Qualifier	Z	No Qualifier

INDEX: Reposition Humeral Head, Right (Body Part Key: Neck of Humerus = Humeral Head)

Secondary Procedure(s):

Character	Code	Explanation
Section	0	Medical and Surgical
Body System	P	Upper Bones
Root Operation	R	Replacement
Body Part	C	Humeral Head Right
Approach	0	Open
Device	7	Autologous Tissue Substitute
Qualifier	Z	No Qualifier

INDEX: Graft, see Replacement Humeral Head, Right

Note: Bone graft replaced missing bone from the malunion of the fracture.

Secondary Procedure(s):

Character	Code	Explanation
Section	0	Medical and Surgical
Body System	Q	Lower Bones
Root Operation	B	Excision
Body Part	3	Pelvic Bone Left
Approach	0	Open
Device	Z	No Device
Qualifier	Z	No Qualifier

INDEX: (Harvest) Excision, Bone, Pelvic Bone, Left (Body Part Key: Iliac crest = pelvic bone)

Chapter 19B

Poisoning by Adverse Effect, Underdosing, Toxic Effects of Substances, Other Effects of External Causes, Certain Early Complications of Trauma, and Complications of Surgical and Medical Care

1. **First-Listed Diagnosis:** **T43.202A** Table of Drugs and Chemicals: Antidepressants, Poisoning, intentional, antidepressants, initial encounter

   Secondary Diagnoses: **T42.4x2A** Table of Drugs and Chemicals: Lorazepam, Poisoning, intentional initial encounter;
   T51.0x2A Table of Drugs and Chemicals, alcohol, beverage, poisoning, intentional, initial encounter;
   F32.9 Depression
   Note: Any of the poisoning codes may be listed first. (Coding Guideline I.C.19.e: "Codes in categories T36–T65 are combination codes that include the substance that was taken as well as the intent. No additional external cause code is required for poisonings, toxic effects, adverse effects and underdosing codes.")

2. **Principal Diagnosis:** **R11.2** Nausea and vomiting

   Secondary Diagnoses: **R53.83** Fatigue;
   T46.0x5A Table of Drugs and Chemicals, digoxin, Adverse effect, initial encounter;
   I50.9 Congestive heart failure;
   I25.2 Myocardial infarction, old

   Principal Procedure: None indicated by the documentation provided

   Secondary Procedure(s): None indicated by the documentation provided

3. **Principal Diagnosis:** **T81.4xxA** Infection, due to surgery

   Secondary Diagnoses: **L03.311** Cellulitis, abdominal wall;
   B95.62 Infection, methicillin resistant staphylococcus aureus;
   E11.9 Diabetes, type 2
   Note: When there is documentation of a current infection (e.g., wound infection, stitch abscess, urinary tract infection) due to MRSA, and that infection does not have a combination code that includes the causal organism, assign the appropriate code to identify the condition along with code B95.62, Methicillin resistant Staphylococcus aureus infection as the cause of diseases classified elsewhere for the MRSA infection. Do not assign a code from subcategory Z16.11, Resistance to penicillins. (*ICD-10-CM Official Guidelines for Coding and Reporting* 2012).

   Principal Procedure: None indicated by the documentation provided

   Secondary Procedure(s): None indicated by the documentation provided

4. **Principal Diagnosis:**   **R04.0** Epistaxis

   Secondary Diagnoses: **T45.515A** Adverse effect, coumadin;
                                        Z79.01 Long-term use, anticoagulant;
                                        I48.91 Fibrillation, atrial;
                                        I50.9 Congestive heart failure;
                                        D50.0 Anemia, chronic blood loss

Principal Procedure:

Character	Code	Explanation
Section	2	Placement
Anatomical Region	Y	Anatomical Orifices
Root Operation	4	Packing
Body Region/Orifice	1	Nasal
Approach	X	External
Device	5	Packing Material
Qualifier	Z	No Qualifier

INDEX: Packing, Nasal

Secondary Procedure(s): None indicated by the documentation provided

5. **First-Listed Diagnosis:**   **L29.9** Pruritis

   Secondary Diagnoses: **T36.3x5A** Table of Drugs and Chemicals, azithromycin, Adverse effect, initial encounter;
                                         H66.90 Otitis media, acute

6. **Principal Diagnosis:**   **T40.5x1A** Table of Drugs and Chemicals, cocaine, Poisoning accidental, initial encounter

   Secondary Diagnoses: **R07.9** Pain, chest;
                                         F14.20 Cocaine dependence;
                                         I10 Hypertension

Principal Procedure:

Character	Code	Explanation
Section	4	Measurement and Monitoring
Physiologic System	A	Physiological Systems
Root Operation	1	Monitoring
Body System	2	Cardiac
Approach	X	External
Function/Device	4	Electrical Activity
Qualifier	Z	No Qualifier

INDEX: Telemetry

Secondary Procedure(s): None indicated by the documentation provided

7. **First-Listed Diagnosis:**   **T82.7xxA** Infection, due to device, implant or graft, electronic, cardiac—or— Complication, cardiovascular device, electronic, pulse generator, infection

    Secondary Diagnoses: **L03.313** Cellulitis, chest wall;

    Z86.14 History, personal, infection, methicillin resistant Staphylococcus aureus

8. **First-Listed Diagnosis:**   **R42** Dizziness

    Secondary Diagnoses: **T44.5x5A** Table of Drugs and Chemicals, angiotensin (Avapro is an angiotensis II receptor antagonist), Adverse effect, initial encounter;

    T44.7x5A Table of Drugs and Chemicals, metoprolol, adverse effect, initial encounter;

    I10 Hypertension

9. **First-Listed Diagnosis:**   **T36.8x1A** Table of Drugs and Chemicals, ciprofloxacin, poisoning, accidental, initial encounter

    Secondary Diagnoses: **R19.7** Diarrhea;

    N39.0 Urinary tract infection;

    B96.20 Infection, Escherichia (E. coli), as cause of disease classified elsewhere

10. **Principal Diagnosis:**   **T80.21xA** Infection due to central venous catheter

    Secondary Diagnoses: **A41.01** Sepsis due to Methicillin susceptible Staphylococcus aureus;

    C18.9 Neoplasm, colon, malignant, primary

    Principal Procedure:

Character	Code	Explanation
Section	0	Medical and Surgical
Body System	5	Upper Veins
Root Operation	P	Removal
Body Part	Y	Upper Vein
Approach	0	Open
Device	3	Infusion Device
Qualifier	Z	No Qualifier

INDEX: Removal of device from, Vein Upper

Secondary Procedure(s): None indicated by the documentation provided

11. **Principal Diagnosis:**   **T84.032A** Complication, joint prosthesis, Internal, mechanical, loosening, knee

    Secondary Diagnoses: **G20** Parkinsonism;

    H54.11 Blindness, one eye, right, low vision on left;

    H40.9 Glaucoma;

    I25.2 Infarction, myocardial, healed or old;

    R94.39 Findings, Abnormal, stress test;

    M15.0 Osteoarthrosis, generalized, primary

Principal Procedure:

Character	Code	Explanation
Section	0	Medical and Surgical
Body System	S	Lower Joints
Root Operation	W	Revision
Body Part	C	Knee Joint Right
Approach	0	Open
Device	J	Synthetic Substitute
Qualifier	Z	No Qualifier

INDEX: Revision of device in Knee, Right

Secondary Procedure(s): None indicated by the documentation provided

12. **Principal Diagnosis:** **T86.19** Complication, transplant, kidney, specified type

   Secondary Diagnoses: **C80.2** Complication, transplant, malignant neoplasm;
   C85.99 Lymphoma, non-Hodgkins;
   N18.6 Disease, ESRD;
   Z99.2 Status, dialysis

Principal Procedure:

Character	Code	Explanation
Section	0	Medical and Surgical
Body System	T	Urinary System
Root Operation	T	Resection
Body Part	1	Kidney Left
Approach	0	Open
Device	Z	No Device
Qualifier	Z	No Qualifier

INDEX: Nephrectomy, see Resection, Urinary System

Secondary Procedure(s):

Character	Code	Explanation
Section	5	Extracorporeal Assistance and Performance
Physiological Systems	A	Physiological Systems
Root Operation	1	Performance
Body System	D	Urinary
Duration	0	Single
Function	0	Filtration
Qualifier	Z	No Qualifier

INDEX: Dialysis, Hemodialysis

13. **Principal Diagnosis:** **T86.49** Complication, transplant, liver, specified type NEC

    Secondary Diagnoses: **D89.810** Disease, graft-versus-host, acute;
    R21 Rash;
    R19.7 Diarrhea;
    R18.8 Ascites

Principal Procedure:

Character	Code	Explanation
Section	O	Medical and Surgical
Body System	H	Skin and Breast
Root Operation	B	Excision
Body Part	5	Skin, Chest
Approach	X	External
Device	Z	No Device
Qualifier	X	Diagnostic

INDEX: Biopsy, see Excision with Qualifier Diagnostic, Skin, Chest

Secondary Procedure(s): None indicated by the documentation provided

14. **First-Listed Diagnosis:** **T78.01xA** Shock, anaphylactic, due to food, peanuts

    Secondary Diagnoses: **Z91.010** Allergy, food, status, peanuts

15. **Principal Diagnosis:** **T40.5x1A** Table of Drugs and Chemicals, cocaine, poisoning, accidental (unintentional), initial encounter

    Secondary Diagnoses: **J96.00** Failure, respiratory, acute;
    N17.9 Failure, kidney, acute;
    F14.221 Dependence, drug, with intoxication delirium

Principal Procedure:

Character	Code	Explanation
Section	5	Extracorporeal Assistance and Performance
Physiological System	A	Physiological Systems
Root Operation	1	Performance
Body System	9	Respiratory
Duration	4	24-96 Consecutive Hours
Function	5	Ventilation
Qualifier	Z	No Qualifier

INDEX: Mechanical Ventilation see Performance, Respiratory

Note: The endotracheal tube associated with the mechanical ventilation procedure is considered a component of the equipment used in performing the procedure and is not coded separately. Reference 3.18 *ICD-10-PCS Reference Manual*.

Secondary Procedure(s): None indicated by the documentation provided

16. **Principal Diagnosis:**   **T78.3xxA** Angioneurotic edema, initial encounter

      Secondary Diagnoses: **L03.211** Cellulitis face;
      E86.0 Dehydration;
      R19.7 Diarrhea;
      C64.1 Neoplasm, kidney, malignant, primary;
      C77.2 Neoplasm, lymph gland intra-abdominal, malignant, secondary;
      C34.12 Neoplasm, lung, upper lobe, malignant, primary;
      C78.1C38.1 Neoplasm, mediastinum, anterior, malignant, secondary,
      E05.90 Thyrotoxicosis;
      A41.01 Sepsis, Staphylococcus aureus;
      Z85.048 History, Personal malignant neoplasm rectum or rectosigmoid junction

      Principal Procedure: None indicated by the documentation provided

      Secondary Procedure(s):   None indicated by the documentation provided

17. **Principal Diagnosis:**   **T82.868A** Complication, graft, vascular, thrombosis, initial encounter

      Secondary Diagnoses: **I12.0** Hypertensive kidney disease with stage 5 chronic kidney disease or end-stage renal disease;
      N18.6 Disease, End stage renal;
      N03.9 Glomerulonephritis, chronic;
      Z99.2 Dependence on renal dialysis

Principal Procedure:

Character	Code	Explanation
Section	0	Medical and Surgical
Body System	5	Upper Vein
Root Operation	C	Extirpation
Body Part	D	Cephalic Vein Right
Approach	0	Open
Device	Z	No Device
Qualifier	Z	No Qualifier

INDEX: Thrombectomy, see Extirpation, Vein, Cephalic, Right

Secondary Procedure(s):

Character	Code	Explanation
Section	0	Medical and Surgical
Body System	5	Upper Vein
Root Operation	H	Insertion
Body Part	N	Internal Jugular Vein Left
Approach	3	Percutaneous

Character	Code	Explanation
Device	3	Infusion Device
Qualifier	Z	No Qualifier

INDEX: Insertion of Device in Internal Jugular Vein, Left

Secondary Procedure(s):

Character	Code	Explanation
Section	5	Extracorporeal Assistance and Performance
Physiological Systems	A	Physiological Systems
Root Operation	1	Performance
Body System	D	Urinary
Duration	0	Single
Function	0	Filtration
Qualifier	Z	No Qualifier

INDEX: Dialysis, Hemodialysis

Chapter 20

External Causes of Morbidity

1. **External cause codes:** **Y04.0XXA** Fight, see Assault, fight, unarmed brawl or fight, initial encounter
   Y92.39 Place of occurrence, stadium
   Y93.82 Activity, spectator at an event
   Y99.8 External cause status, student

2. **External cause codes:** **X72.XXXA** Self inflicted, see Suicide, firearm, handgun, initial encounter
   Y92.015 Place of occurrence, residence, house, single family, garage
   Y99.8 External cause status, unemployed (specified)

3. **External cause codes:** **V43.52XA** Accident, transport, car, driver, collision, care, initial encounter
   Y92.411 Place of occurrence, highway
   Y99.0 External cause status, civilian activity done for income or pay

4. **External cause codes:** **W12.XXXA** Fall, from scaffolding, initial encounter
   Y92.61 Place of occurrence, industrial and construction area, building under construction, initial encounter
   Y99.0 External cause status, civilian activity done for income or pay

5. **External cause codes:** **W11.XXXA** Fall from ladder, initial encounter
   Y92.017 Place of occurrence, residence, house, single family, yard
   Y93.H9 Activity, maintenance, exterior building
   Y99.8 External cause status, unemployed

6. **External cause codes:** **V47.52XA** Accident, transport, car occupant, driver, stationary object, initial encounter
   Y92.411 Place of occurrence, highway
   Y93.C2 Activity, interactive electronic device (cell phone)
   Y99.8 External cause status, student

7. **External cause codes:** **V95.32XA** Accident, transport, aircraft, occupant, powered craft accident, fixed wing, commercial, forced landing, initial encounter
   Y92.520 Place of occurrence, airport
   Y99.8 External cause status, leisure

8. **External cause codes:** **W25.XXXA** Contact with glass, sharp, initial encounter
   Y92.832, Place of occurrence, beach
   Y93.01 Activity, walking
   Y99.8 External cause status, leisure

9. **External cause codes:** **W16.032A** Accident, diving, see Fall, into water, in swimming pool, striking wall, initial encounter
   Y92.016 Place of occurrence, swimming pool, private, single family residence
   Y93.12 Activity, diving
   Y99.8 External cause status, student

10. **External cause codes:** **X93.XXXA** Assault, firearm, handgun, initial encounter
    Y92.414 Place of occurrence, local residential street
    Y93.55 Activity, bike riding
    Y99.8 External cause status, student

11. **External cause codes:** **W06.XXXA** Fall from bed, initial encounter
    Y92.230 Place of occurrence, hospital, patient room
    Y99.8 External cause status, patient

12. **External cause codes:** **X99.1XXA** Assault, knife, initial encounter
    Y92.481 Place of occurrence, parking lot
    Y99.8 External cause status, unemployed

13. **External cause codes:** **W20.8XXA** Tree, falling on or hitting initial encounter
    Y92.017 Place of occurrence, residence, house, single family, yard
    Y99.8 External cause status, leisure

14. **External cause codes:** **X98.1XXA** Scalding, inflicted by other person, stated as intentional, see Assault, burning, hot object, tap water, initial encounter
    Y07.59 Perpetrator of assault, maltreatment and neglect by, non family member specified NEC
    Y92.031 Place of occurrence, residence, apartment, bathroom
    Y93.e1 Activity, bathing
    Y99.8 External cause status, student

15. **External cause codes:** **W92.XXXA** Exposure, excessive heat, man-made, initial encounter
    Y92.63 Place of occurrence, factory
    Y99.0 External cause status, civilian activity for income or pay

16. **External cause codes:** **Y93.h2** Straining, excessive, see overexertion, see category Y93, activity involving gardening and landscaping, initial encounter
    Y92.830 Place of occurrence, park (public)
    Y99.0 External cause status, civilian activity for income or pay

17. **External cause codes:** **V00.131A** Accident, skateboard, see Accident, transport, pedestrian, conveyance, skateboard, fall, initial encounter
    Y92.481 Place of occurrence, parking lot
    Y93.51 Activity, skateboarding
    Y99.8 External cause status, student

18. **External cause codes:** **W03.XXXA** Fall, same level, from collision with other person, initial encounter
    Y92.310 Place of occurrence, basketball court
    Y93.67 Activity, basketball
    Y99.8 External cause status, leisure

19. **External cause codes:** **V00.321A** Fall, same level, involving ice or snow, involving skates, skis, see Accident, transport, pedestrian, conveyance, skis, fall, initial encounter
    Y92.828 Place of occurrence, mountain
    Y93.23 Activity, skiing, downhill
    Y99.8 External cause status, leisure

20. **External cause codes:** **V03.00XA** Accident, transport, pedestrian, on foot, collision, with car, initial encounter
    Y92.414 Place of occurrence, street, local residential
    Y93.02 Activity, running
    Y99.8 External cause status, student

Chapter 21

Factors Influencing Health Status and Contact with Health Services

1. **Principal Diagnosis:** **Z38.01** Newborn, born in hospital, by cesarean
   Secondary Diagnoses: **P07.03** Low birthweight, extreme, 945 grams;
   P07.26 Immaturity, extreme, with gestation of 27 weeks;
   P22.0 Syndrome, respiratory, distress, newborn
   Note: Under Category P07 Disorders of newborn related to short gestation and low birth weight, not elsewhere classified is this direction When both birth weight and gestational age of the newborn are available, both should be coded with birth weight sequenced before gestational age."
   Principal Procedure: None indicated by the documentation provided
   Secondary Procedure(s): None indicated by the documentation provided

2. **Principal Diagnosis:**   **I48.91** Fibrillation, atrial

   Secondary Diagnoses: **Z85.51** History, personal, malignant neoplasm, bladder;
   N40.0 Hypertrophy, prostate—See Enlargement, enlarged prostate without lower urinary tract symptoms

   Principal Procedure:

Character	Code	Explanation
Section	0	Medical and Surgical
Body System	T	Urinary System
Root Operation	J	Inspection
Body Part	B	Bladder
Approach	8	Via Natural or Artificial Opening Endoscopic
Device	Z	No Device
Qualifier	Z	No Qualifier

INDEX: Cystoscopy

Secondary Procedure(s):   None indicate by the documentation provided

3. **Principal Diagnosis:**   **I10** Hypertension

   Secondary Diagnoses: **Z30.2** Encounter, sterilization, or Multiparity requiring contraceptive management—See Contraception, sterilization same code

   Principal Procedure:

Character	Code	Explanation
Section	0	Medical and Surgical
Body System	U	Female Reproductive System
Root Operation	L	Occlusion
Body Part	7	Fallopian Tubes, Bilateral
Approach	4	Percutaneous Endoscopic
Device	C	Extraluminal Device (Falope Rings)
Qualifier	Z	No Qualifier

INDEX: Ligation, see Occlusion, fallopian, tubes, bilateral

Note: Fallope rings are placed on the exterior surface of the fallopian tube to accomplish the occlusion.

Secondary Procedure(s):   None indicated by the documentation provided

4. **Principal Diagnosis:**   **Z38.00** Newborn, born in hospital

   Secondary Diagnoses: **Z03.79** Suspected condition, ruled out, maternal and fetal conditions NEC

   Principal Procedure: None indicated by the documentation provided

   Secondary Procedure(s):   None indicated by the documentation provided

5. **First-Listed Diagnosis:**   **R26.2** Gait abnormality, difficulty walking

   Secondary Diagnoses: **Z96.641** Presence, hip joint implant, right;
   Z79.01 Therapy, drug, long term, anticoagulant;
   Z51.81 Encounter, therapeutic drug level monitoring

6. **Principal Diagnosis:**   **Z38.31** Newborn, twin, born in hospital, by cesarean

   Secondary Diagnoses: **P07.17** Low birthweight, with weight of 1800 grams;
   P07.37 Preterm infant, newborn, with gestation of, 34 weeks;
   P59.0 Newborn jaundice, of prematurity
   Note: Under Category P07 Disorders of newborn related to short gestation and low birth weight, not elsewhere classified is this direction "When both birth weight and gestational age of the newborn are available, both should be coded with birth weight sequenced before gestational age."

Principal Procedure:

Character	Code	Explanation
Section	6	Extracorporeal Therapies
Physiological Systems	A	Physiological Systems
Root Operation	6	Phototherapy
Body Part	0	Skin
Duration	1	Multiple
Qualifier	Z	No Qualifier
Qualifier	Z	No Device

INDEX: Phototherapy, skin

Secondary Procedure(s):   None indicated by the documentation provided

7. **Principal Diagnosis:**   **Z04.1** Observation following accident, transport

   Secondary Diagnoses: **V43.62XA** External Cause: Accident, transport, car occupant, passenger, collision with car, initial encounter;
   Z92.411 External Cause: Place of occurrence, street and highway, interstate highway;
   Y93.89 External Cause: Activity, specified (car occupant);
   Y99.8 External Cause: Status of External Cause, specified (infant)

   Principal Procedure: None indicated by the documentation provided

   Secondary Procedure(s):   None indicated by the documentation provided

8. **First-Listed Diagnosis:**   **O09.12** Pregnancy, supervision, high risk, molar pregnancy, second trimester (14 weeks 0 days to less than 28 weeks 0 days)

   Secondary Diagnoses: **O09.02** Pregnancy, supervision, high risk, infertility, second trimester;
   Z3A.24 Pregnancy, weeks of gestation, 24 weeks

9. **First-Listed Diagnosis:**   **Z00.111** Newborn, examination, 8 to 28 days old

   Secondary Diagnoses: None indicated by documentation provided

10. **Principal Diagnosis:**   **Z52.4** Donor, Kidney

    Secondary Diagnoses: **Z91.040** History, allergy, latex

    Principal Procedure:

Character	Code	Explanation
Section	0	Medical and Surgical
Body System	T	Urinary System
Root Operation	T	Resection
Body Part	1	Kidney, Left
Approach	0	Open
Device	Z	No Device
Qualifier	Z	No Qualifier

INDEX: Nephrectomy, see Resection, Urinary System

Secondary Procedure(s):   None indicated by the documentation provided

11. **First-Listed Diagnosis:**   **Z48.00** Change, dressing(nonsurgical)

    Secondary Diagnoses: **S60.511D** Abrasion, right hand, subsequent care;

                                            S60.512D Abrasion, left hand, subsequent care;

                                            W24.0XXD External Cause: Contact with lifting device, subsequent encounter

12. **First-Listed Diagnosis:**   **S32.9XXD** Fracture, pelvis, subsequent encounter for fracture with routine healing

    Secondary Diagnoses: **V03.10XD** External Cause: Accident, transport, pedestrian, on foot, collision with car in traffic

13. **Principal Diagnosis:**   **Z45.09** Admission, adjustment, device, implanted, cardiac

    Secondary Diagnoses: **Z95.2** Presence, implanted, device, heart valve, prosthetic

    Principal Procedure:

Character	Code	Explanation
Section	0	Medical and Surgical
Body System	2	Heart and Great Vessels
Root Operation	R	Replacement
Body Part	G	Mitral Valve
Approach	0	Open
Device	J	Synthetic Substitute
Qualifier	Z	No Qualifier

INDEX: Replacement, valve, mitral

Secondary Procedure(s):   None indicated by the documentation provided

14. **First-Listed Diagnosis:**   **Z77.098** Contact, chemicals, non-medicinal

    Secondary Diagnoses: None indicated by documentation provided

15. **First-Listed Diagnosis:**   **Z23** Admission, prophylactic vaccination

    Secondary Diagnoses: **P07.33** Preterm infant, with gestation of, 30 weeks
    Note: ICD-10-CM coding guideline I.16.e: Codes from category P07, Disorders of newborn related to short gestation and low birth weight, not elsewhere classified, are for use for a child or adult who was premature or had a low birth weight as a newborn and this is affecting the patient's current health status.

16. **Principal Diagnosis:**   **Z40.02** Admission, prophylactic, organ removal, ovary

    Secondary Diagnoses: **Z40.09** Admission, prophylactic, organ removal, specified organ NEC (for the uterus and fallopian tubes);
    C56.1 Neoplasm, ovary, malignant, primary, right;
    Z80.41 History, family, malignant neoplasm, ovary

Principal Procedure:

Character	Code	Explanation
Section	0	Medical and Surgical
Body System	U	Female Reproductive System
Root Operation	T	Resection
Body Part	9	Uterus
Approach	4	Percutaneous Endoscopic
Device	Z	No Device
Qualifier	Z	No Qualifier

INDEX: Hysterectomy, see Resection, Uterus

Secondary Procedure(s):

Character	Code	Explanation
Section	0	Medical and Surgical
Body System	U	Female Reproductive System
Root Operation	T	Resection
Body Part	C	Cervix
Approach	4	Percutaneous Endoscopic
Device	Z	No Device
Qualifier	Z	No Qualifier

INDEX: Resection, Cervix

Note: With a total hysterectomy both the uterus and cervix are removed, and each body part is coded separately.

Secondary Procedure(s):

Character	Code	Explanation
Section	0	Medical and Surgical
Body System	U	Female Reproductive System
Root Operation	T	Resection
Body Part	7	Fallopian Tubes Bilateral
Approach	4	Percutaneous Endoscopic
Device	Z	No Device
Qualifier	Z	No Qualifier

INDEX: Resection, Fallopian Tubes, Bilateral

Secondary Procedure(s):

Character	Code	Explanation
Section	0	Medical and Surgical
Body System	U	Female Reproductive System
Root Operation	T	Resection
Body Part	2	Ovaries, Bilateral
Approach	4	Percutaneous Endoscopic
Device	Z	No Device
Qualifier	Z	No Qualifier

INDEX: Resection, Ovary, Bilateral

Secondary Procedure(s):

Character	Code	Explanation
Section	8	Other Procedures
Body System	E	Physiological Systems and Anatomical Regions
Root Operation	0	Other Procedures
Body Region	W	Trunk Region
Approach	4	Percutaneous Endoscopic
Method	C	Robotic Assisted Procedure
Qualifier	Z	No Qualifier

INDEX: Robotic Assisted Procedure, Trunk Region

Note: As described in the ICD-10-PCS Reference Manual, an additional code is assigned to identify the fact the surgery was a robotic assisted procedure. The code is included in the section of "Other Procedures" defined as methodologies which attempt to remediate or cure a disease or disorder.